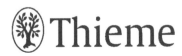

Speech Sound Disorders

Comprehensive Evaluation and Treatment

Kelly Vess, MA, CCC-SLP
Speech-Language Pathologist and Off-Campus Clinical Instructor
Wayne State University
Detroit, Michigan, USA
Eastern Michigan University
Ypsilanti, Michigan, USA

14 illustrations

Thieme
New York • Stuttgart • Delhi • Rio de Janeiro

Library of Congress Cataloging-in-Publication Data
is available from the publisher.

Important note: Medicine is an ever-changing science undergoing continual development. Research and clinical experience are continually expanding our knowledge, in particular our knowledge of proper treatment and drug therapy. Insofar as this book mentions any dosage or application, readers may rest assured that the authors, editors, and publishers have made every effort to ensure that such references are in accordance with **the state of knowledge at the time of production of the book.**

Nevertheless, this does not involve, imply, or express any guarantee or responsibility on the part of the publishers in respect to any dosage instructions and forms of applications stated in the book. **Every user is requested to examine carefully** the manufacturers' leaflets accompanying each drug and to check, if necessary in consultation with a physician or specialist, whether the dosage schedules mentioned therein or the contraindications stated by the manufacturers differ from the statements made in the present book. Such examination is particularly important with drugs that are either rarely used or have been newly released on the market. Every dosage schedule or every form of application used is entirely at the user's own risk and responsibility. The authors and publishers request every user to report to the publishers any discrepancies or inaccuracies noticed. If errors in this work are found after publication, errata will be posted at www.thieme.com on the product description page.

Some of the product names, patents, and registered designs referred to in this book are in fact registered trademarks or proprietary names even though specific reference to this fact is not always made in the text. Therefore, the appearance of a name without designation as proprietary is not to be construed as a representation by the publisher that it is in the public domain.

Thieme Medical Publishers, Inc.
333 Seventh Avenue, 18th Floor
New York, NY 10001, USA
www.thieme.com
+1 800 782 3488, customerservice@thieme.com

5 4 3 2

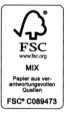

Cover design: Thieme Publishing Group
Typesetting by DiTech Process Solutions, India
Printed in Germany by Beltz Grafische Betriebe

ISBN 978-1-68420-088-7

Also available as an e-book:
eISBN 978-1-68420-089-4

Contents

Videos

Acknowledgment

Thank you to my loving husband, Tyler, who makes me smile even in the hardest of times and to my insightful son, Boden, who inspires me to think from multiple perspectives. I am the most fortunate person in the world for you two.

With deepest gratitude...

To my family, Arline Anderson, John Sr, Dolores, John, and Kathleen, for teaching to love wholeheartedly and abundantly. To my wonderful family who contributed in edits and feedback, especially my playwright father-in-law, James Vess. To Edward Trainor, Christine Felton, and Corey Shipman for your edits and inputs as well. To artists Chris Dean, Katie Murray, and Diane Wright for cover art, photography, and sharing your expertise.

To my wonderful teachers who have instilled a love for intervention and research. I love what I do because of you. To my first mentor, early childhood director, Tina Brown, who provided me with an idealistic idea of what early childhood education could be and then hired me to teach in her preschool classrooms for a couple of years when I was a high school student. Because of her early influence, I knew that developing and providing intervention to preschoolers was my life calling.

To Joan Kaderavek, for teaching me how to practically apply research into practice during my undergraduate years at Eastern Michigan University. To the Institute for the Study of Children, Families, and Communities for giving me the unique opportunity to work as a statistical data analysis researcher as an undergraduate student. This experience paved the way for more advanced research opportunities as a graduate student at Michigan State University.

To Mildred Omar at Michigan State, for providing me with an amazing opportunity of a high-level doctoral position as the project manager on a national level Head Start intervention grant. That hands-on experience in developing assessments, intervention, training staff, and overseeing intervention fidelity across 23 Head Start sites is consistently drawn upon in my current research. To Michael Casby, for his amazing course on research methods. His teachings on evaluating research design memorably ring in my ears 19 years later. To John Eulenberg, for inspiring with his benevolent mindset in giving a voice to all.

To my brilliant colleagues at Barnes Early Childhood Center. The progress our students make is most often jaw dropping due to the amazing teachers and therapists who seamlessly work as one: Marinel Gaitan, Dorothy Heitjan, Dianne Stall, Joseph Evens, Sally Abdella, Sharon Palazzola, Jean Limback, Michele Stopinski, Gina Bordato, and Julie Huellmantel. Thank you also to volunteer extraordinaire, Dana Dykstra. I learn so much from all of you every day and value our close collaboration.

To our Student Services Director Stephanie Hayes and Educational Superintendent Jon Dean, who strongly supported the research and the development of this book. Ms. Hayes and Dr. Dean have generously provided advisement and legal consultation to ensure students' protection in our research and publication of this book. Also, to the Grosse Pointe Foundation for Public Education, for awarding four material grants totaling approximately $25,000. These materials have empowered us to provide rich hands-on learning experiences to holistically treat preschoolers across developmental domains.

To Program Supervisor, Susan Lucchese, at Barnes Early Childhood Center. She provides amazing opportunities to grow and encourages the best in everything her staff does. To the steadfast and generous support of Wayne State University Speech Language Pathology's Clinical Director, Karen O'Leary, and Eastern Michigan's Clinical Director, Audrey Farrugia. Their commitment to university and public school collaboration has resulted in dramatically improved practice for our kiddos over the past 12 years at Barnes Early Childhood Center.

To the graduate students who authentically "put it all on the table," bravely demonstrating newly learned evidence-based strategies on camera to educate parents and for published scrutiny. They never disappoint in creatively incorporating their own unique set of strengths. Each graduate intern has dramatically expanded my skill set. This larger set of strategies to draw from has particularly improved my ability to work effectively with a greater diversity of children.

To the families for the opportunity to work with their children who bring so much joy to life. I have evolved as both a therapist and a person from my valued time with each one. It excites me that so many others will be able to meet these exceptionally wonderful children and learn new strategies to effectively provide therapy, thanks to our families' generosity in sharing their children.

Lastly, thank you to the innovative editors at Thieme. Timothy Hiscock, Kenneth Schubach, Delia DeTurris, Prakash Naorem, and Marcus Laithangbam have envisioned and seen through the development of a book that should provide a comprehensive, up-to-date review of the research with an interactive, hands-on learning experience for the reader. This format empowers readers to seamlessly put research into practice.

It is my goal that this active learning experience not only results in concepts learned more deeply, but also enjoyably. Readers are empowered with knowledge presented multimodally to clearly envision evidence-based therapy strategies. The purpose of this book is not for the reader to copy these strategies. Rather, readers are challenged to incorporate their own theoretical mindsets, prior experiences, and skill set, evolving evidence base and unique talents to improve upon intervention presented in this book.

With this book, my hope is to pay forward all the support and talent that have been generously afforded to me in hopes of changing life-long outcomes for many in need. Good thoughts to you and the important work you do.

Kelly Vess, MA, CCC-SLP

Introduction: Holistic Evaluation and Treatment of Speech Sound Disorders

Kelly Vess

Rationale

It is with great passion that I write this interactive, digital book for you. This book will not serve as a compendium or encyclopedia of every published approach and research article ever written on the topic of speech sound disorders. It will, however, empower you to use research-based practices to effectively diagnose and treat preschoolers with speech sound disorders with or without concomitant developmental delays.

The aim of this book is not to be comprehensive in covering multiple approaches in a cursory manner, which leaves the reader unable to effectively put any of the approaches into practice. I do encourage you to regularly research Google Scholar, the routinely updated www.asha.org/evidence-maps/, and SpeechBITE.com with keywords of specific approaches of interest. My hope is that this book provides the reader with a strong evidence-based methodology and critical thinking skill set. You will continually "stand on the shoulders of giants" by referencing research to make important decisions regarding approaches you choose to abandon, adopt, adapt, or create along the way. I expect you'll improve upon this work.

A Review of Commonly Used Evidence-Based Approaches

Some current evidence-based approaches are promising, yet remain largely inconclusive due to the fact that research in sound speech disorders is overwhelmingly without an alternative intervention or control group. In the absence of a comparison group or an alternative intervention, one must always question if progress simply occurred based on receipt of positive attention, regression toward the mean, placebo effect, maturation, or a combination of all four. For this reason, the Cochrane Systematic Reviews of treatment of dysarthria and childhood apraxia of speech indicate the lack of randomized and quasi-randomized studies, which currently makes it impossible to draw conclusions about efficacy of speech therapy in both behavioral and biofeedback approaches.[1,2]

Some approaches that are developing a promising observational research base in the treatment of childhood apraxia of speech for preschoolers include Integral Stimulation: Dynamic Tactile Temporal Cueing (DTTC), Rapid Syllable Transition Treatment (ReST), Nuffield Dyspraxia Programme-3rd Edition (NDP3), Common Core Vocabulary, and Prompts for Restructuring Oral Muscular Phonetic Targets (PROMPT).[3,4,5,6,7] Additionally, the Cycles Approach, Multiple Oppositions Approach, and Minimal Pair Target Selection Approach have demonstrated efficacy in the treatment of children with multiple speech errors and immature phonological processes.[8,9,10]

Some research provides direction in treatment of children with concomitant conditions. For children with Down's syndrome, a more behavioral approach over a naturalistic modeling approach is indicated with children who are unable to intelligibly repeat a sentence. Conversely, a more naturalistic recasting approach is recommended for children with Down's syndrome who can intelligibly repeat sentences.[11]

In treating children with autism spectrum disorder, Koegel and colleagues found that both discrete trial behavioral teaching and naturalistic teaching were effective in improving speech under stimulus conditions. However, the naturalistic approach resulted in greater generalization to conversational speech.[12] In treatment of childhood dysarthria, which often presents with muscular weakness or paralysis due to neurological damage, a research base is continually developing to support the use of the Lee Silverman Voice Treatment-LOUD (LSVT LOUD) method with preschoolers.[13] Erika Levy's 2014 article in the *International Journal of Communication Disorders* describes how to implement LSVT LOUD.[14]

Adhering to Evidence-Based Practices

Research indicates that early treatment of speech sound disorders is too often overlooked. It is estimated that approximately 8 to 9% of preschool children have speech sound disorders with 5% of children in the first grade continuing to struggle with a persistent diagnosis of speech sound disorders.[15,16] Unfortunately, a number of preschoolers with speech sound disorders remain undiagnosed and are therefore not receiving intervention. This is particularly the case in African American, lower socioeconomic, and English-as-second-language speaking populations.[17,18] Persistent speech errors at the school age to adult level can have damaging effects on social, language, and literacy development.[19,20] Persistence of speech errors could also result in negative discrimination in academic and employment settings.[21,22] As a speech-language pathologist, you are in a unique position to change lives by effectively evaluating and treating speech sound disorders before kindergarten when neuroplasticity is at a greater level.

The stakes are now high more than ever. The current trend appears to be that caseloads are growing as staffing is diminishing.[23] Because more hours cannot be added in a day, time spent with clients, unfortunately, is often decreased in both frequency and total quantity. What to do when the research is unequivocally clear that more therapy sessions equates to greater gains?[24,25,26] I propose we work smarter.

Additionally, according to my privately practicing colleagues, it is not uncommon for insurance companies to require standardized score gains after five sessions or funding is unexpectedly pulled. These colleagues report finding the conversation to be quite awkward when they find out a month later and have to present a $1,000 therapy bill to parents due to insurance not approving coverage in consideration of a lack of standardized testing gains. For this, children in most need, with the most severe limitations, are most likely to not have coverage for therapy.[27]

Standardized testing demands that not only gains be made in therapy but also generalization to testing environments occur over a short period of time. There is a mismatch between our current practice in speech sound intervention and insurance requirements. Our current meta-analytic research indicates that eight sessions, not five, are typically indicated for articulation improvements to occur.[28] Research from my summer speech intervention program, with speech therapy provided by graduate students, however, has consistently indicated that an average of approximately 12 months of gains on standardized articulation scores could be made following five 45-minute individual sessions with preschoolers with speech sound disorders of mixed etiology.[29,30,31]

As a speech-language pathologist, I have diagnosed, treated, and researched preschoolers with speech sound disorders for 18 years in a public school setting. My practice has continually evolved over the years with my consistent research focus on well-designed studies and meta-analytic research as well as annual participation and attendance at American Speech-Language-Hearing Association's (ASHA) national conferences. Importantly, my ongoing research of my diverse caseload within the schools and summer program have challenged my own previously held notions of best practices. The numbers often indicate change in practice and have made me more effective year after year. I expect that your ongoing research with current or future clients will importantly shape your practice as well.

I am additionally an off-campus clinical educator for both Wayne State University and Eastern Michigan University. In collaboration with Wayne State University, I direct a summer speech intervention program annually in which I supervise and teach Wayne State University graduate students. In teaching graduate students, my passion is to help develop speech-language pathologists who are able to explain therapy in terms of "How?," "Why?," and "When?" based on research, critical thinking, and the individual child. Importantly, they must also be able to persuasively explain therapy in layman's terminology to caregivers, our intervention partners. The research is clear that these caregivers, when educated and empowered, make a difference.[28,32]

In this digital interactive book, I'm not advocating the use of a single intervention approach. I support adherence to research-based maxims of best practice that apply to more than just children with speech impairments. These maxims also apply to children with concurrent linguistic, cognitive, attentional, social, and motoric deficits as well as their neurotypical preschool peers. In fact, some of the greatest communication gains during a typical school year and in the summer program are made by preschoolers with autism spectrum disorder, cognitive impairment, and severe language impairment.

Regardless of your therapeutic setting, there's simply no time and funding to waste an evaluation or therapeutic session. If a child is not responding, a therapist has to dynamically change the target, activity, level of prompting, or goal while maintaining positive momentum. A therapist must deeply understand the maxims of best practice and think critically in real time. This book will provide interactive worksheets with videos to learn and practice skills, video analysis to develop critical thinking skills, and challenge the reader to create by always asking, "How can I do this better?"

Some experts surmise that a therapist's level of effectiveness is 75% based on the therapist's ability to build relationships and 25% based on the approach.[33,34] I challenge that notion based on my research and experience of closely supervising approximately 25 graduate interns and being "glued" to their sides during every therapy session. In fact, I've consistently found that graduate students, regardless of interpersonal skills, who closely followed the maxims of best evidence-based practice presented in this book, have clients with the greatest intervention gains.

The most effective graduate intern I've ever worked with was incredibly shy and seemed uncomfortable with children with little prior experience; being that, she was committed to working with geriatric populations. Conversely, the least effective graduate student that I've had was playful, like a living jack-in-the-box, with years of experience working with children. The difference between the two was that the shy intern followed the research-based maxims of best practice very closely, which will be covered within this book, and the gregarious one did not. As Aristotle wrote, "We are what we repeatedly do. Excellence is not an act but a habit." The purpose of this book is to learn effective practices that produce impressive results with habitual adherence.

As a student, I was fortunate to work in research throughout both my undergraduate and graduate studies. I've been blessed with the generous teachings and support of extraordinary people along the way. During my undergraduate studies, Professor Joan Kaderavek, who taught us about speech sound disorders, challenged me to read research asking, "How does this translate to therapy?"

In my graduate studies at Michigan State, Professor Michael Casby taught me how to evaluate research and design studies that control for confounding variables. Professor Mildred Omar afforded me with a doctoral level assistantship as a project manager of a national early intervention grant. These incredible opportunities furthered my love for intervention research with hands-on experience in creating instruments, interventions, and testing interventions under the guidance of great minds.

Currently, I have developed amazing collaborative relationships with Wayne State University's Clinical

Director, Karen O'Leary, and Eastern Michigan's Clinical Director and Assistant Professor, Audrey Farrugia. I also have the ongoing steadfast support of my supervisors, Sue Lucchese and Stefanie Hayes, and educational superintendent, Dr. Jon Dean, who makes both research and "best practice" possible in a public school setting.

Lastly, I am fortunate to present digital clips illustrating best practice assessment and therapy of eight graduate speech-language pathology students working with a diverse population of preschoolers due to the students' and parents' generosity in helping others. I believe these digital clips will change the lives of many.

To pay these opportunities forward, in the final chapter, I will share methods on how to conduct your own research. In the past, there was a research to practice divide, and research primarily occurred in academia. Times have changed. Currently, the expectation for a "highly effective rating," which often equates to job security in the public school system, is that speech-language pathologists minimally perform action research indicating therapy efficacy. I believe that some of our best intervention research will come from therapists in the field, conducted with a diverse caseload in the child's natural preschool environment with the therapist ensuring fidelity occurs in adherence to intervention practices.[35,36,37,38]

In summary, this book with its video accompaniment will guide you as a reader, viewer, and creator, through best practices in the assessment and treatment of speech sound disorders. You will walk with me, my graduate students, and my preschoolers with diverse needs through ten chapters of digital video clips for hands-on practice and analysis. Each of the following chapters will take you through an important aspect in becoming a highly effective therapist: Chapter 1, evaluating speech sound disorders; Chapter 2, establishing a positive working relationship; Chapter 3, selecting complex treatment targets; Chapter 4, selecting linguistic contexts for treatment targets; Chapter 5, developing educationally rich activities; Chapter 6, dynamically providing and fading cues; Chapter 7, treating motor speech disorders; Chapter 8, fostering generalization; Chapter 9, promoting early literacy skills; and Chapter 10, researching your practice.

Finally, to end each chapter, I will share a clinical insight or strategy that I've developed and have qualitatively found to be effective in treating a myriad of preschoolers with speech sound disorders, referred to as "Kelly's Corner." It's my hope that you can learn from both my successes and failures from these past 18 years to further develop your own practice.

Note: Names of videotaped preschoolers are altered throughout this book in protection of confidentiality.

References

[1] Pennington L, Miller N, Robson S. Speech therapy for children with dysarthria acquired before three years of age. Cochrane Database Syst Rev 2009;(4):CD006937

[2] Morgan AT, Vogel AP. Intervention for childhood apraxia of speech. Cochrane Database Syst Rev 2008;(3):CD006278

[3] Strand EA, Stoeckel R, Baas B. Treatment of severe childhood apraxia of speech: a treatment efficacy study. J Med Speech-Lang Pathol 2006;14(4):297–307

[4] Ballard KJ, Robin DA, McCabe P, McDonald J. A treatment for dysprosody in childhood apraxia of speech. J Speech Lang Hear Res 2010;53(5):1227–1245

[5] Williams P, Stephens H. The Nuffield Centre Dyspraxia Programme. In: Williams AL, McLeod S, McCauley RJ, eds. Interventions for Speech Sound Disorders. Baltimore, MD: Brookes; 2010:159

[6] Crosbie S, Holm A, Dodd B. Intervention for children with severe speech disorder: a comparison of two approaches. Int J Lang Commun Disord 2005;40(4):467–491

[7] Dale PS, Hayden DA. Treating speech subsystems in childhood apraxia of speech with tactual input: the PROMPT approach. Am J Speech Lang Pathol 2013;22(4):644–661

[8] Hodson BW, Paden EP. Targeting Intelligible Speech: A Phonological Approach to Remediation. Austin, TX: Pro-Ed; 1991

[9] Williams AL. Multiple oppositions: case studies of variables in phonological intervention. Am J Speech Lang Pathol 2000;9(4):289–299

[10] Dodd B, Crosbie S, McIntosh B, et al. The impact of selecting different contrasts in phonological therapy. Int J Speech-Language Pathol 2008;10(5):334–345

[11] Yoder PJ, Camarata S, Woynaroski T. Treating speech comprehensibility in students with down syndrome. J Speech Lang Hear Res 2016;59(3):446–459

[12] Koegel RL, Camarata S, Koegel LK, Ben-Tall A, Smith AE. Increasing speech intelligibility in children with autism. J Autism Dev Disord 1998;28(3):241–251

[13] Fox CM, Boliek CA. Intensive voice treatment (LSVT LOUD) for children with spastic cerebral palsy and dysarthria. J Speech Lang Hear Res 2012;55(3):930–945

[14] Levy ES. Implementing two treatment approaches to childhood dysarthria. Int J Speech-Language Pathol 2014;16(4):344–354

[15] Law J, Boyle J, Harris F, Harkness A, Nye C. Prevalence and natural history of primary speech and language delay: findings from a systematic review of the literature. Int J Lang Commun Disord 2000;35(2):165–188

[16] Shriberg LD, Tomblin JB, McSweeny JL. Prevalence of speech delay in 6-year-old children and comorbidity with language impairment. J Speech Lang Hear Res 1999;42(6):1461–1481

[17] McLeod S, Harrison LJ, McAllister L, McCormack J. Speech sound disorders in a community study of preschool children. Am J Speech Lang Pathol 2013;22(3):503–522

[18] Morgan PL, Hammer CS, Farkas G, et al. Who receives speech/language services by 5 years of age in the united states? Am J Speech Lang Pathol 2016;25(2):183–199

[19] McCormack J, McLeod S, McAllister L, Harrison LJ. My speech problem, your listening problem, and my frustration: the experience of living with childhood speech impairment. Lang Speech Hear Serv Sch 2010;41(4):379–392

[20] Ha S. The relationship among speech perception, vocabulary size and articulation accuracy in children with speech sound disorders. Commun Sci Disord 2016;21(1):15–23

[21] Overby M, Carrell T, Bernthal J. Teachers' perceptions of students with speech sound disorders: a quantitative and qualitative analysis. Lang Speech Hear Serv Sch 2007;38(4):327–341

[22] Van Dyke DC, Holte L. Communication disorders in children. Pediatr Ann 2003;32(7):436–437

[23] Katz LA, Maag A, Fallon KA, Blenkarn K, Smith MK. What makes a caseload (un)manageable? School-based speech-language pathologists speak. Lang Speech Hear Serv Sch 2010;41(2):139–151

[24] Jacoby GP, Lee L, Kummer AW, Levin L, Creaghead NA. The number of individual treatment units necessary to facilitate functional communication improvements in the speech and language of young children. Am J Speech Lang Pathol 2002;11(4):370–380

[25] Allen MM. Intervention efficacy and intensity for children with speech sound disorder. J Speech Lang Hear Res 2013;56(3):865–877

[26] Kaipa R, Peterson AM. A systematic review of treatment intensity in speech disorders. Int J Speech-Language Pathol 2016;18(6):507–520

[27] Dusing SC, Skinner AC, Mayer ML. Unmet need for therapy services, assistive devices, and related services: data from the national survey of children with special health care needs. Ambul Pediatr 2004;4(5):448–454

[28] Law J, Garrett Z, Nye C. The efficacy of treatment for children with developmental speech and language delay/disorder: a meta-analysis. J Speech Lang Hear Res 2004;47(4):924–943

[29] Vess K, Hansen L, Smith M, Ridella M, Steinberg E. Evidence-based strategies to effectively treat children with speech sound disorders. Poster presented at ASHA Annual Conference, November 2015; Denver, CO

[30] Vess K, Burgess R, Corless E, Discenna T. Selecting consonant clusters: are certain sound combinations more efficacious than others? Poster presented at ASHA Annual Conference, November 2016; Philadelphia, PA

[31] Vess K, Coppielle J, Ingraham B. Targeting /r/ consonant clusters: does generalization occur across phonetic contexts? Poster presented at ASHA Annual Conference, November 2017; Los Angeles, CA

[32] Sugden E, Baker E, Munro N, Williams AL. Involvement of parents in intervention for childhood speech sound disorders: a review of the evidence. Int J Lang Commun Disord 2016;51(6):597–625

[33] Staines GL. The relative efficacy of psychotherapy: reassessing the methods-based paradigm. Rev Gen Psychol 2008;12(4):330–343

[34] Bleile KM. The Late Eight. San Diego, CA: Plural Publishing, Inc.; 2018

[35] Joireman J, Van Lange P. How to Publish High-Quality Research. Washington, DC: American Psychological Association; 2015

[36] Dollaghan CA. Evidence-based practice in communication disorders: what do we know, and when do we know it? J Commun Disord 2004;37(5):391–400

[37] Dodd B. Evidence-based practice and speech-language pathology: strengths, weaknesses, opportunities and threats. Folia Phoniatr Logop 2007;59(3):118–129

[38] Kaderavek JN, Justice LM. Fidelity: an essential component of evidence-based practice in speech-language pathology. Am J Speech Lang Pathol 2010;19(4):369–379

1 Completing a Single Session Speech Evaluation

Children are not things to be molded, but are people to be unfolded.

—Jess Lair

1.1 Background

Starting at the evaluation stage, the child has likely been referred by a parent, teacher, or pediatrician. Ideally, the child's speech would be observed and transcribed in the home or preschool classroom setting. Unfortunately, time and workload demands may not allow for this naturalistic observation. The child should, however, have been referred for a hearing screening before the evaluation.

Articulation intervention is currently recommended at age 3 for children who lack the ability to communicate intelligibly and effectively within their natural environments.[1,2] Research indicates that speech sound disorder therapy at younger ages results in greater functional improvements. This association is likely due to increased brain plasticity and less habituation of speech errors at younger ages.[3] Therefore, it is important that children are evaluated and treated as early as possible. Prior to the evaluation, refer the child for a hearing screening. Direct observation or parent-collected videos of the child communicating in the home, recreational, and/or school environments would also provide invaluable information.

1.2 Ecological Validity: Completing the Speech Evaluation in One Session

The goal of this chapter is to put research into practice. The goal of this chapter is to put research into practice. Clinically relevant research will be reviewed to show how all of the components of a speech evaluation can be completed within the constraints of a single session. Also, evidence-based strategies will be illustrated to active participation in evaluating preschool age children.

In private practice and clinical settings, insurance companies generally provide funding for *one* 45-minute session to complete both the speech and language evaluation. Similarly, in public school settings, typically *one* session is allotted as well.

Regardless of your professional setting, these invaluable evaluation sessions simply cannot be wasted due to funding and time constraints. This is your one opportunity to get a snapshot of both the child's typical and optimal performance. Therefore, it is wise to prepare the testing environment beforehand to establish a positive working relationship.

Digital clips and interactive worksheets referenced in this chapter provide hands-on practice throughout the speech evaluation. I encourage you to make use of these tools as we walk through each stage of the process together.

Moreover, we will cover the American Speech-Language-Hearing Association's (ASHA) recommended components of a speech evaluation in one chapter, keeping true to the single evaluation session constraint in the real world.[4]

The ten components of a speech evaluation are:
1. Obtaining a case history;
2. Establishing compliance;
3. Administering a single-word standardized articulation assessment;
4. Administering a supplemental *consonant cluster screener*;
5. Checking for stimulability with maximum cueing;
6. Collecting a connected speech sample;
7. Calculating Percent Consonants Correct (PCC);
8. Calculating Mean Length of Utterance (MLU);
9. Observing oral muscular structure and speech movements;
10. Obtaining a diadochokinetic (DDK) rate.

Although some therapists may opt to complete the oral mechanism evaluation and DDK rate in the initial stage to guide the speech assessment, I propose we complete these tasks toward the end of the session. At this point, a positive working relationship will likely have developed as the preschooler's comfort level increased due to encouragement received throughout the evaluation. This empowers the therapist to successfully administer the more invasive and challenging tasks of observing the oral mechanism internally and obtaining a DDK rate.

To establish compliance, the evaluation tasks are administered in an easiest to most difficult sequence. This evidence-based strategy of ordering easier tasks to more difficult ones is referred to as demand fading. In demand fading, simpler tasks result in a high rate of compliance. With positive momentum established, more challenging tasks can successfully be faded in.[5] For this, we typically opt to first complete single-word standardized articulation testing. For most pre-schoolers, this would be the easiest task in a speech evaluation.

By the end of this chapter, we'll review generalizations in symptomatology to differentially diagnose speech sound disorders. Speech sound disorders refer to a heterogeneous group of speech disorders. Each has underlying causes, unique speech error patterns, and other aspects of the linguistic system that are developing aberrantly or are delayed for what's expected of a child's chronological age. These can result in errors in articulation, stressing, pausing, intonation, fluency, voicing, and vocal quality.

Differential diagnosis of the following speech sound disorders will be presented:

- Dysarthrias, also referred to as organic motor speech disorders, are neurological motor speech impairments, which present with slow, weak, imprecise, and/or uncoordinated movements of the speech musculature. They may involve respiration, phonation, resonance, and/or oral articulation deficits. Muscular weakness, slowness, or lack of coordination is due to damage to the central and/or peripheral nervous system.[6]
- Childhood Apraxia of Speech (CAS), a neurological childhood speech sound disorder, presents with deficits in planning and programming movement sequences. These deficits result in speech production, pausing, and prosody errors without overt muscular weakness.[7]
- Inconsistent speech sound disorder (ISSD) presents with inconsistent production of words at least 40% of the time. ISSD, unlike CAS, presents with intact prosody and volitional nonspeech movements with improved productions in the contexts of imitation and elicited speech tasks.[7,8]

- Phonological disorders present with speaking patterns in which complex sounds and words are simplified in a predictable manner (e.g., reducing clusters in producing "block," "plane," and "snake" as /bɑk/, /peɪn/, and /seɪk/).
- Articulation impairments present with difficulty in producing individual sounds, often resulting in[1] distortions or substitutions (e.g., frontally lisping /s/ as a /θ/ sound in producing "mouse" as /maʊθ/.

Note: We will address speech perception assessment, an ASHA recommended component of the speech evaluation, in Chapter 9.

1.3 Obtaining a Case History

Ideally, prior to the evaluation, a *Parent Input Form* is completed by the primary caregiver. This form's medical and developmental history questions specifically related to increased risk for concurrent delays. The *Temperament Scale* is included because responses on the right-side column of the form indicate a more reactive temperament, a prognostic indicator of a poorer response to speech therapy.[9]

Additionally, information regarding the child's temperament can also help the therapist arrange the tasks and the testing environment for success using the child's reported motivators (▶ Table 1.1). When evaluating a child who has attentional or behavioral difficulties, or is on the Autism Spectrum Disorder (ASD) continuum, information regarding the child's motivators in ▶ Table 1.1 will be pivotally important in establishing a positive working relationship.[10,11] Research indicates that speech-language therapy not only improves speech and language skills but also behavior, all under the realm of communication.[12,13]

Table 1.1 Parent Input Form

Speech and Language Evaluation: Parent Report	
FAMILY INFORMATION	Name of child:
Child's date of birth:	Today's date:
Person completing form:	Relationship to child:
Mother's name: Complete address:	Father's name: Complete address (if different):
Names and ages of brothers:	Names and ages of sisters:
Contact home phone: Contact cell phone: Contact email:	Primary language spoken in home: Secondary language(s): Language(s) your child speaks/understands:

MEDICAL HISTORY	Please circle	Yes: Please explain or describe.
Were there problems during pregnancy /birth?	yes no	
Has your child ever gone under general anesthesia?	yes no	
Was your child born before due date or at a low birth weight?	yes no	
Has your child been hospitalized at any time?	yes no	
Has your child had his or her vision checked?	yes no	
When has your child had hearing tested?	yes no	
Are there any diagnosed mental, physical, or emotional disabilities?	yes no	
Is there presently or a history of ear, nose, or throat problems? PE tube placement?	yes no	
Does your child have allergies or asthma?	yes no	
Are there any dietary restrictions? Does your child have feeding difficulties?	yes no	
Does your child have dental/oral abnormalities?	yes no	
Is there a family member with a history of speech, language, learning or attention problems?	yes no	
How is your child's fine and gross motor coordination (e.g., drawing, using a fork/spoon, running, walking, jumping)?	poor fair good	
Does your child sleep well?	yes no	
Does your child continue to take naps? If so, when?	yes no	
Did your child experience difficulties potty training? Delay? Difficulties with regularity?	poor fair good	

LANGUAGE
- What concerns you about your child's language?
- When is your child most...
  talkative?
  quiet?
- Who suggested that language be evaluated?
- Has your child received language intervention previously? If yes, when and why?
  Did your child frequently use speech-like babble prior to speaking in words?
  Yes_____No_____
  If no, please explain:
- When did your child first use...
  single words?_____months
  two to three word utterances?_____months
  sentences?_____months
  ○ How many words are in your child's longest utterance (sentence)? About _____words
  please provide an example utterance (sentence):

SPEECH
- What concerns you about your child's speech?
- When is your child's speech...
  most clear?
  least clear?
- Who suggested that speech be evaluated?
- How much of your child's speech do you understand? About _____%
- How much of your child's speech do you think close/immediate family members understand? About _____%
- How much of your child's speech do you think professionals familiar with your child understand (e.g., babysitter, child's teacher)? About _____%
- How much of your child's speech do you think someone unfamiliar with your child would understand? About _____%
- How does your child typically respond ...
  when others do not understand?
  when others correct his speech?
  when others provide a correct model?

○ Do others (e.g., brothers, sisters, classmates) ask/ answer for your child? yes no
If yes, please explain:
○ Does your child often initiate communication with others? yes no
If no, please explain:
○ Does your child often respond to others' questions, requests and comments? yes no
If no, please explain:

• Do others (e.g., brothers, sister, classmates) speak for your child?

TEMPERAMENT	Please circle best/closest response		
• How sensitive is your child to distractions or small changes in/differences in food, clothing, lighting, etc.?	Low sensitivity	Medium	High sensitivity
• How much movement does your child show during the day or night (sleeping, eating, playing)?	Low	Medium	High
• How intense are your child's reactions (positive and negative)?	Low	Medium	High
• How does your child adapt to intrusions, transitions, or changes?	Easily	Medium	With Difficulty
• Does your child become frustrated with obstacles or limits placed on his/her activities?	Not easily frustrated	Variable	Easily frustrated
• How consistent and predictable is your child's daily pattern of hunger, eating, sleeping, and elimination?	Regular	Variable	Irregular
• When upset, how easily can your child be distracted, diverted, and calmed?	Easily soothed	Variable	Hard to soothe
• Does your child initially approach or back away in new situations or from strange people, pets, or objects?	Approach	Variable	Withdraw
• In child group settings, does your child primarily play alone or with other children?	Primarily plays with other children	Variable	Primarily plays alone
• Does your child often use natural gestures when talking for additional clarification?	Frequently	Variable	Rarely
• Does your child engage in pretend play?	Frequently	Variable	Rarely

What motivates your child?
My child's strengths are:
My child needs to work on:
Is there anything your child's teacher or therapist should know about your family's background, religion or faith? If so, please explain.
Does your child currently attend or has attended ...
play group?_____times, _____hrs/week. Was your child successful? Yes No
child care?_____times, _____hrs/week Was your child successful? Yes No
preschool? _____times, _____hrs/week Was your child successful? Yes No

My Child's Favorite....

Books: Activities: TV Shows/Movies: Songs: Toys:

Review the *Parent Input Form* in ▸ Table 1.1. Are there any questions that could be asked that would make the form more useful? If you can't identify any now, you will as your experience and our research base continually evolve. Over the years, I've changed this form several times, and will continue to do so. Consider all forms presented in this book as works in progress for you to improve upon.

1.4 Evaluating the Child at First Sight

Prior to beginning the evaluation, make observations at first glance of how the child moves. The child's bodily movements often times mirror movements in the mouth for children with speech sound disorders.[14,15]

Examine the child's gait coming out of the car or down the hall: Tripping over feet? Moving slowly, clumsily, or toe-walking? Walking with straight legs in a wide gaited shuffle? Excessively using joints in bending knees, possibly to compensate for poor coordination or weak musculature? Dragging feet or toes pointed inwards or outwards, perhaps to increase proprioceptive feedback, which is the body's sense in space?[16,17]

Observations of these immature movements indicate that the child has often not yet achieved differentiation in motor movement. Differentiation is the progression of immature movements to precise, fluid, well-controlled, intentional, complexly coordinated movements. Minimally note these motor observations in your evaluation report to empower the child's intervention team (e.g., the child's preschool teacher).

Also, consider an occupational therapy or physical therapy referral. Children with communication impairments are at significantly higher risk for fine and gross motor impairments. Studies suggest that anywhere between 40 to 90% of children with speech or language impairments have concurrent fine and/or gross motor diiculties.[18]

Additionally, children with motor coordination difficulties in the body may be more likely to demonstrate less oral motor coordination. Oral motor coordination difficulties will be most evident in producing complex speech speech sounds such as consonant clusters, affricates, glides, multisyllabic words, and diphthongs.[19,20] For these children, it will also be important to take note of distorted or centralized vowel errors during standardized testing and in connected speech because vowels are typically not assessed in single word, standardized tests.[21]

At the first sight of the child, make behavioral observations as well. Is the child clinging to the caregiver, bolting across the parking lot, or confidently and compliantly walking at the caregiver's side? If the child appears to have a sensitive temperament, make the decision beforehand to have the caregiver accompany the child.

If the child appears confident, I prefer to have the child come in alone for speech and language testing so that the child does not escape to a caregiver as testing items increase in difficulty. This escape behavior often occurs when the child is reaching a ceiling in which a number of consecutive items must be answered incorrectly prior to completing an assessment.

Note the child's temperament. Is the child sociable or emotionally reactive? Does the child demonstrate a low tolerance for frustration or a seemingly anxious temperament? Reluctance or refusal to enter the room or engage in activities may be the child's attempt to mask underdeveloped skills—in this case, speech.[22]

To assess a child with an emotionally reactive temperament, I use a preferential sequence to establish compliance. A preferential sequence is presenting most rewarding activities first to establish active participation. Then, testing demands can be faded in after positive momentum is established.[23]

Lastly, is the child in "his or her own world," seemingly unaware of the caregiver or others? Is the child unresponsive to the questions and directions? This behavior may indicate social reciprocity difficulties, and require the strongest tangible rewards to complete testing.

Look for sensory seeking or sensory avoidant behaviors. Is the child flapping hands, excessively making sounds, tensing limbs, staring out of the corners of the eyes, humming, or covering ears? These behaviors can elicit a polar purpose of either increasing attention to environmental stimuli or decreasing attention through self-generated distraction.

If the child appears dysregulated, be prepared to bring out the highest engaging toys to establish regulation and attention necessary to complete standardized testing and the full evaluation.

Sensory dysfunction is important to note in the evaluation report. It will play a role in speech therapy outcomes as a generally negative prognostic indicator of response to speech therapy.[9]

Creating Momentum with Preschoolers Who Are Reluctant to Participate or Dysregulated

With children who appear to have sensitive temperaments or are behaviorally dysregulated, begin by giving the highest rewarding toy pieces as a reward for sitting and attending behaviors to establish regulation necessary for participation. Only give preferential directions that you are certain the child will follow: "Here, take a magic toy! What great listening! You are following every direction! What color do you want? Awesome! You're answering every question."[24,25]

After regulation and participation are established in rewarding activities, fade in the test stimulus pictures. Start with only a few pictures and fade in more items over time while maintaining momentum.

I have found children on the ASD spectrum to respond well if a predictable, repetitive response is provided each time, such as a verbal "ding-ding-ding!" for every picture labeled. Interestingly, research in robot-human interaction indicates that the more simple and repetitive the response from robots, the greater the comfort level and playfulness for children with ASD.[26]

Positive momentum established early can carry children with even the most challenging behaviors through an hour-and-half of formal testing by establishing and maintaining compliance.

If the child appears to have attentional issues, you may need to move at a quicker pace in administering items and rewards to maintain attention.[27] For these children, idle hands can be hands swiping a table clear. Conversely, if the child presents with word retrieval deficits, you may need to provide more wait time to allow them to form words while still maintaining engagement.

If you're feeling disengagement is on the horizon, intersperse testing with easier or more preferred tasks to maintain momentum. To avoid rewarding escape behaviors, change the activity, the reward, or increase the reward ratio before the child is under the table, not after.[28]

1.5 Establishing Active Participation and Positive Momentum through Primary Reinforcement of Tangible Rewards

Upon meeting a child for an evaluation, our goal is to quickly establish a positive, prosocial working relationship. Select a variety of toy rewards based on parent-reported interests.[29] The toys should be in the evaluator's reach, not the child's, in an opaque container to prevent visual distraction from the task at hand.[5]

During testing, the child quickly learns that attentive, self-regulated, effortful, responsive, and compliant behavior feels good, with toy rewards distributed on a consistent basis as a primary reinforcer that quickly establishes compliance. These rewards can be referred to as primary reinforcers, which are consequences that strengthen a response with little or no prior learning. Primary reinforcers satisfy a biological need, such as eating and sleeping. For children, they can also include engaging in highly preferred activities and receiving toys as well as pleasurable sensory experiences such as tickling.[30]

Pieces equal practice. In testing, time-efficient primary reinforcers are ones that are quickly disposed of or quickly activated and deactivated. Some examples of quickly disposable primary reinforcers include puzzles, shape sorters, piggy banks, stacking boxes, music blocks, stickers, magnet pick up, and dropping items into containers. Quickly activated turn-taking toys include ball drops, marble shoots, car ramps, car shooters, tops, wind-up toys, and bubbles.

These rewards can be delivered on a continuous schedule of reinforcement, in which each instance of desired behavior is rewarded. They can also be delivered on an intermittent schedule of reinforcement, in which some responses are rewarded, but not everyone.

Note: Unrelated, tangible rewards are only administered during testing. During therapy, however, only naturally occurring, activity-based rewards and objective encouragement are recommended.

Depending on the individual child, the frequency of toy rewards can be on a 1:1 consistent basis or an intermittent basis. At this initial stage of establishing compliance, err on the side of

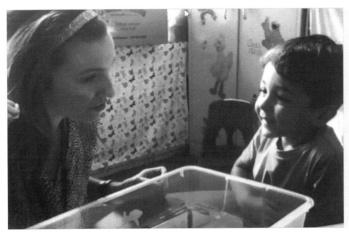

Fig. 1.1 Alyssa establishing compliance with a child with childhood apraxia of speech (CAS) at the initial speech evaluation through preferential activity selection.

reinforcement saturation, which is providing too much of a reward. This is preferable to reinforcement strain, which is providing too little of a reward in response to desired behaviors.[31]

Note in ▶ Fig. 1.1 that intern Alyssa is initially evaluating a preschooler with Childhood Apraxia of Speech (CAS). She quickly established compliance, and a positive working relationship by having the child drop fish into the water during testing as an unrelated, quickly dispensed reward. From the *Parent Input Form* (▶ Table 1.1), Alyssa knew the child loved fishing. As you can see from the picture, the child is highly engaged. Therefore, he performed the difficult task of producing words on demand despite the task's inherent difficulty of directly eliciting speech for a child with CAS.

1.6 Establishing Active Participation and Positive Momentum through Secondary Reinforcement of Verbal Feedback

Additionally, positive verbal encouragement with enthusiasm is provided on an ongoing basis as a secondary reinforcer.[5] A secondary reinforcer is a consequence paired with delivery of a primary reinforcer (toy rewards). The secondary reinforcer of verbal encouragement becomes paired with the child's positive experiences of receiving toy rewards.

The secondary reinforcer of objective encouragement becomes a conditioned reinforcer over time by being associated with the positive feelings of receiving toy rewards. Therefore, the new conditioned reinforcer of objective encouragement can solely be provided at any time. Its efficacy remains even when the child loses interest in the primary reinforcer of receiving toy rewards or engaging in a motivating activity.

Research suggests that feedback in the form of objective encouragement provided 100% of the time results in eliciting optimal performances from preschoolers.[32] Right from the start, the child learns that compliance feels great and associates the therapist with positive experiences. This association is sometimes referred to as the therapist being paired with reinforcers.

Examples of objective encouragement feedback that will serve as a secondary reinforcer in response to a child's participation and emphasize prosocial behavior are as follows: "You pay attention!" "You answer every question!" "You follow every direction!" "You work super hard!"

Remember that word choice is powerful. Renowned linguist William Labov put it best: "Language is a container of thought." I refer to standardized tests not as "tests" but "picture games." Say, "You get to play the picture game." Children should never "have to," but always "get to" participate in testing, therapy, and group activities.[33]

From the get-go, feedback in the form of objective encouragement should always be based on effort (e.g., "Wow! You're almost finished with this whole picture game!"). It should not be subjective praise (e.g., "Good job!"). Research indicates that subjective praise results in children being reluctant to engage in new tasks, such as testing situations.

Conversely, objective encouragement based on effort results in persistence with novel and challenging tasks.[34] Verbal feedback should also be immediate and frequent. In articulation testing, if the child mislabels a picture, you could say, "It's also called a _____. Can you say that word?" During testing, always attend to effort, never accuracy to encourage optimal participation.

Encourage children to be mindful in your objective feedback by paying attention to the details of their efforts. "You finished this whole, big, picture book! Did you work a little hard (pantomiming little muscles) or superhero hard (pantomiming big muscles)?" Provide them with specific feedback, which authentically gives attention to individual efforts and specific actions. Ultimately, it is the child's opinion that counts, not yours. An internal locus of control develops when the child realizes that "the ball is in his or her court." Individual efforts and actions determine success or failure.

1.7 Administering Single-Word Standardized Articulation Tests

n selecting a standardized test for a preschooler, it is important to note that there is a great variability among the single-word speech assessments widely used today. These variations are present in developmental norms referenced, syllabic shape of stimulus items (i.e., syllable structure: CVC, CVCV), polysyllabic words, consonant clusters, and sounds' positions within words.[35]

With preschoolers, it is important to select an instrument that will sensitively detect speech sound errors inherent in a preschool age population. Look for a standardized test that contains the following types of stimulus words[2]:

1. Polysyllabic words (i.e., words containing three or more syllables);
2. The late eight developing sounds (s, z, θ, ð, ʃ, ʒ, ʧ, ʤ, l, ɹ)across positions in a word (i.e., initial, medial, final); and
3. Complex 3-element and 2-element consonant clusters.

Recent research reviewing 12 widely used standardized assessments suggests that most assessments lack 2- and 3-element consonant clusters.[21] In a 2-element consonant cluster, you have two successive consonantal phonemes in a word (e.g., play, fry, sweep, three). In 3-element consonant clusters, there are three successive consonantal phonemes in a word (e.g., scrape, spray, splash). Our replicated research has clearly indicated consonant clusters, particularly 3-element clusters to be the most powerful treatment targets for diverse

groups of preschoolers, underscoring the value in assessing them.

This variability in content can also be seen in poor inter-test reliability in standard scores. We recently researched two popular standardized, single word speech tests. Eight of the 20 preschoolers tested scored a standard score of above 85 on one test. These same eight children scored below 85 on the other within the same calendar week.

If the common practice of an 85 standard score benchmark is implemented as the deciding factor in qualifying for services, the decision would be as arbitrary as a coin toss. For this, clinical judgment must be the deciding factor with particular attention to the quality not quantity of the child's speech errors.

When administering standardized articulation tests, transcribe the child's errors using the International Phonetic Alphabet (IPA) displayed in ▶ Fig. 1.2. The IPA is a system of symbols used to write down sounds, intonations, and words that empower us to globally communicate by transcribing any spoken languages using a universal set of symbols.

It is only by knowing the child's errors that a targeted intervention strategy can be developed that incorporates incompatible cues to these errors. Also, knowledge of the child's errors allows for obvious detection of phonological processes, which can be referred to as simplified speaking patterns of adult speech produced in a predictable manner.

For example, I may transcribe that the child produced /t/ for /k/, /d/ for /g/, and /n/ for /ŋ/ to discover that the child is demonstrating the phonological process of fronting velar sounds.

Also, this knowledge is empowering in developing an incompatible cue to the errored speech, such as teaching the child to have an "open crocodile mouth" to prevent fronting. This is one example of incompatible prompts that are covered in Chapter 6.

1.7.1 Indicating Imitated Words

When testing children with ASD or children with ISSD, also indicate imitated stimulus words (perhaps with an "i" annotation) to indicate that the word was directly imitated. Our recent research suggests that a direct verbal model could inflate testing performance. In studying twelve preschoolers with ASD, we and found that all eleven performed substantially better when provided a direct verbal model to imitate than when independently labeling pictures.[36]

The international phonetic alphabet (revised to 2018)

Consonants (pulmonic)

© 2018 IPA

	Bilabial	Labiodental	Dental	Alveolar	Postaiveolar	Retrodex	Paiatal	Velar	Uvular	Pharyagcal	Gkeal
Plosive	p b			t d		ʈ ɖ	c ɟ	k g	q ɢ		ʔ
Nasal	m	ɱ		n		ɳ	ɲ	ŋ	N		
Tnil	B			r					R		
Tap or Flap		ⱱ		ɾ		ɽ					
Fricative	ɸ β	f v	θ ð	s z	ʃ ʒ	ʂ ʐ	ç j	x ɣ	χ ʁ	ħ ʕ	h ɦ
Lateral fricative				ɬ ɮ							
Approximant		ʋ		ɹ		ɻ	j	ɰ			
Lateral approximant				l		ɭ	ʎ	L			

Symbols to the right in a cell are voiced, to the left are voiceless, shaded areas dencce articulation judged impossible.

Consonants (non-pulmonic)

Clicks	Voiced implosives	Ejectives
⊙ Bilabial	ɓ Bilabial	' Examples
ǀ Dental	ɗ Dental/alveolar	p' Bilabial
! (Post)aiveolar	ʄ Paiatal	t' Dental/alveolar
‡ Postaiveolar	ɠ Vetar	k' Vetar
ǁ Alvester lateral	ʛ Uvutar	s' Alvester tactive

Others symbols

ʍ Voiceless velar lateral fricative
ɰ Veicod lateral-velar approximant
ɥ Veicod lateral-palatal approximant
ʜ Voiceless velar lateral fricative
ʢ Voiced erigloxial examples
ʡ Erigloxial elusive

ɕ ʑ Alvoele-celatal fricatives
ɺ Veicod alvoetae lateral flap
ʃ Simultaneous ʃ and x

Affricates and double articulations can be represented by two symbols joined by a tie bar if necessary. ts k͡p

Vowels

Where symbols appear in pairs, the one so the right replacestate a rounded vowel.

Suprasegmentals

ˈ Primary stress	ˌfoʊnəˈtɪʃən
ˌ Secondary stress	
ː Long	eː
ˑ Half-long	eˑ
˘ Extra-short	ĕ
ǀ Minor (foot) group	
‖ Major (intonation) group	
. Symbol break	ɹiˑækt
‿ Linkung (absence of a break)	

ꟷ Tones and word accents
Level   Contour

e̋ or ꜛ	Extra high	ê or ꜛ	Rising
é	ꜛHigh	ê	ꜜ Falling
ē	ꜛMid	e᷄	ꜛ High rising
è	ꜜLow	e᷅	ꜛ Low rising
ȅ	ꜜExtra low	e᷈	ꜛ Rising-falling
ꜜ	Downstep	ꜛ	Globle rise
ꜛ	Upstep	ꜛ	Globle fall

Diacritics some diacritics may be placed above a symbol with a descender, e.g. ŋ̊

Voiceless	n̥ d̥	Brutality voiced	b̤ a̤	Dental	t̪ d̪
Voiced	s̬ t̬	Creaky voice	b̰ a̰	Apical	t̺ d̺
Aspirated	tʰ dʰ	Linguolabial	t̼ d̼	Laminal	t̻ d̻
More rounded	ɔ̹	Labialized	tʷ dʷ	Nasalized	ẽ
Less rounded	ɔ̜	Palletized	tʲ dʲ	Nasal release	dⁿ
Advanced	u̟	Velarized	tˠ dˠ	Lateral release	dˡ
Retracted	e̠	Phiryngranted	tˤ dˤ	No andlike release	d̚
Centralized	ë	Velarized or phaeyngeaized	ɫ		
Mid-centralized	e̽	Raised	e̝ (ɹ̝ = voiced alveolar fricative)		
Syllabic	n̩	Lowraised	e̞ (β̞ = voiced bilabial approximant)		
Non-syllabic	e̯	Advotcal tosgse root	e̘		
Rhcticky	ɚ a̴	Revdvotcal tosgse root	e̙		

Fig. 1.2 International Phonetic Association, CC BY-SA 3.0, via Wikimedia Commons.

Great caution must be taken when testing children who exhibit echolalia. This is when children imitate your production and even intonation. In these cases, follow-up testing may indicate that the child has regressed because the child is no longer engaging in echolalia. Contrarily, progress may have occurred in that the child is expressing words with a much improved spontaneous production than previously.

Also, when testing children with ISSD, which will be discussed later in the chapter, imitated speech is likely to be clearer than spontaneous speech, so an imitation prompt would likely inflate testing performance. Therefore, imitation prompts should be noted during testing and in reporting results.

1.7.2 Indicating Distortions

Sometimes sounds are produced in a slightly distorted manner instead of being substituted, meaning the child will say "rwing" for ring. It's not "ring" or "wing" but somewhere in the middle. This is referred to as a distorted production.[37]

Diacritic marks, which are phonetic marks indicating a speaker's variation or distortion of a sound, will indicate qualitative changes in production from a sound that is fully errored, to a partially errored sound. Therapy strives toward a fully accurate production. However, diacritics can empower us to see the direction of change in an errored sound. Is it regressing or progressing towards accurate production?

Later developing phonemes /l/, /ɹ/, and /s/ can be tractable to 100% accurate production in preschoolers. Therefore, a measurement detecting qualitative progress is useful for therapeutic decision-making.

This use of diacritics to capture exactly how a sound is produced is called narrow transcription. In IPA, narrow transcription is displayed between brackets instead of slashes (e.g., a frontally lisped bus is transcribed as [bʌs̪]). The following IPA diacritic symbols should be useful as these distortions are common with preschoolers:

- Interdental, or frontal, lisping of /s/ and /z/: The tongue protrudes between the front teeth yet maintains an alveolar sibilant, with a higher-pitched hissing sound. Logically, these errors are transcribed with a tooth directly below the /s/ and /z/: [s̪] and [z̪]
- Lateral lisping of /s/ and /z/: Airflow escapes over the side(s) of the tongue, resulting in a slushy sound. Logically, these errors are transcribed with a small /l/ for lateralized air escaping that can be superscripted next to /s/ and /z/: [sˡ] and [zˡ]
- Lip rounding of /l/ and /ɹ/: Logically, these errors are transcribed with a small /w/ for labial rounding, which can be superscripted next to /l/ and /ɹ/: [lʷ] and [ɹʷ]

What Can Single-Word Articulation Testing Tell Us About Language and Literacy Development?

Performance on single-word speech testing can provide some qualitative information regarding a preschooler's word retrieval skills or expressive vocabulary. A child struggling to label many of the pictures may suggest need for follow-up testing in this area.

Additionally, speech errors that surface during single-word speech testing in themselves can indicate a greater likelihood of a concurrent language impairment. For instance, omissions, or deletions of sounds and syllables at the word level, indicate a greater risk of concurrent language impairment than distorted sounds for children with speech sound disorders.[38,39]

A high rate of atypical speech errors also may be an early indicator of a weaker linguistic system. Atypical speech errors are non developmental errors in that they do not follow the universal rules of typical sound development.

Common examples of atypical speech errors include replacing alveolar consonants with velars, replacing stop sounds with fricatives, replacing fricatives with liquids. In these instances, children are non-developmentally substituting easier sounds for more difficult to produce ones.

The presence of concurrent speech and language impairment places the child at greater risk for literacy difficulties. For instance, difficulty producing polysyllabic words is correlated with poorer phonological awareness skills at the preschool level.[39]

Phonological awareness is a broad skill that refers to a child's ability to identify and manipulate sounds and syllables within a spoken language. Furthermore, research indicates preschoolers with high rates of atypical speech errors at the preschool level to performed more poorly on phonological awareness tasks four years later.[40] See Chapter 7 for a comprehensive list of atypical processes.

1.8 Dynamic Assessment: Assessing for Stimulability

After administering the standardized articulation assessment, the therapist can provide a dynamic assessment, which is observing what the child is capable of when provided with a maximum level of cueing. Here, the therapist's ability to scaffold, or prompt, the child to produce an errored sound correctly will depend on the therapist's level of skill and experience. Prompts in cueing various sounds and sound combinations are covered in Chapter 6.

Stimulability testing has traditionally been defined as a child's ability to imitate a sound immediately following a verbal model. Research indicates that if a child is able to imitate a sound correctly, it will likely naturally develop without intervention. On the other hand, a sound that a child is not able to accurately imitate will require treatment for change to occur.[41]

In dynamic assessment, we assess a child's stimulability when a maximum level of prompting is given. The child's ability to produce errored sounds correctly is interdependent on both the therapist's ability to effectively prompt correct production and the child's ability to produce targets with therapist's support. Stimulability findings, which provide important information regarding selection of treatment targets, are covered in Chapter 3.

1.9 Supplemental *Consonant Cluster Screener*

In stimulability testing, assessing the child's production of consonant clusters is crucially important. Complex consonant clusters are an appropriate and effective treatment target for preschoolers regardless of severity of speech impairment and pervasiveness of their disorder. They will induce the greatest change in both the child's phonological system and articulation.[42]

Therefore, I've developed the *Consonant Cluster Screener* (**Appendix A**). This measures preschoolers' ability to both verbally imitate 2- and 3-element clusters and their ability to produce consonant clusters given the therapist's maximal level of support using the evidence-based strategy of Dynamic, Tactile, Temporal Cueing (DTTC).[43,44]

DTTC is the process of dynamically fading and providing prompts based on the child's moment-to-moment performance to ensure accuracy in production. Tactile refers to touch cues provided externally to the oral structure (e.g., cheeks, jaw, lips), either by the child or therapist, to aid in the accuracy of movement sequences.

With DTTC, a most-to-least level of prompting is used. In the first stages, a maximum level of support is provided with the therapist and child speaking in slowed unison speech. As the child's production improves, speech in unison becomes quicker. With accuracy, unison speech is faded in levels of support to direct imitation, delayed imitation, and lastly spontaneous speech. The level of prompting dynamically changes with fading and increased support provided contingently in response to the child's production, maintaining an accuracy level at or above 80%.[45]

Temporal cueing is exaggerated use of body and mouth movement in space to visually display speech movements. Accurate production, voicing, volume, stress, and prosody can be more easily perceived and produced by the child with temporal cueing.[16] The therapist and child use gestures with fingers, hands, and limbs, and exaggerated oral movements to saliently cue speech.

In this manner, a continuant sound, in which airflow moves with a mild interruption, would have temporal cues that are lengthier in movement and are of greater duration in time. A plosive sound, on the other hand, in which airflow is stopped, would have a temporal (spatial) cue with shorter length of movement and quicker duration.

Please see Video 1.1 of Taylor with Addy, a preschooler with Down's syndrome. Taylor is using cues that I taught her in a half-day training and cues that she herself had created for this particular client. (Cueing techniques are covered in Chapter 6, Dynamically Prompting and Errorless Fading Multimodal Cues.)

With DTTC prompting, verbal preschool age children with speech sound disorders are able to accurately produce many 2- and 3-element consonant clusters regardless of etiology for the speech sound disorder. Whether it is children with speech sound disorder and concurrent autism, Down's syndrome, or dysarthria, consonant clusters are highly effective and appropriate intervention targets as a starting point with prompts provided using a most-to-least prompting hierarchy.[5]

The *Consonant Cluster Screener* (located in **Appendix A**) provides information on production of consonant clusters and the child's stimulability, which will be used for intervention target selection. In this dynamic assessment, children are first asked to repeat each word when shown a picture.

Next, words that children were unable to accurately repeat are reintroduced with a maximum level of DTTC prompting in unison with the examiner's slowed and exaggerated speech. In reintroducing the words with maximal prompting, a picture of the object is *not* displayed so the child can have a blank slate for practicing a new motor speech pattern. Additionally, the child can pay increased attention to the adult's mouth, tactile, and temporal cues.

The *Consonant Cluster Screener* is comprehensive with 36 unique 2- and 3-element English language consonant clusters in the initial position of words assessed to aid in target selection. Consonant clusters are in the initial word position, which research indicates to be more developmentally advanced than clusters in the medial and final positions of words.[46]

Additionally, recent research on of 267 English-speaking preschoolers screened for speech impairment indicates that productions of consonant clusters imitated in the initial position of words are more consistent with the children's spontaneous speech than consonant clusters imitated in the medial and final positions.[47]

Further research, however, will be required to evaluate the consistency in production of a variety of *consonant clusters* in the initial position of words as this study only contained six English consonant clusters.[47]

Importantly, in consideration of realistic time constraints, the direct imitation test condition (e.g., "Say X") took about one-third the time than spontaneous labeling test condition (e.g., "What's that?") in single-word speech testing administration.[47]

Watch the digital clip of intern Taylor completing the *Consonant Cluster Screener* with Jenna in Video 1.2. Transcribe responses in IPA using broad and narrow transcription (as appropriate) on the Examiner Form. (You can compare your transcription to ours in **Appendix B.**)

After completing the *Consonant Cluster Screener* with an imitation prompt, Taylor closes the book and completes a stimulability check with a maximum level of DTTC prompting. Removal of the pictures during stimulability testing with maximum prompting may set the stage for a blank slate in which an errored word can be produced without interference from the child's previous (errored) knowledge of its production.

Inaccurate productions are scored as a "0." Accurate productions are scored as a "1." Mild distortions are scored as a ".5." For mild distortions, I recommend using the recently reviewed IPA diacritics for rounding of /lʷ/ and /ɹʷ/, as well as interdental and lateral lisping of [s̪] and [z̪]. These mild distortions are scored as a ".5" to indicate that they

would be appropriate therapy targets at the preschool level for prevention of habituation due to extensive repetition of inaccurate motor patterns.

Lastly, summarize the results of productions made with maximum prompting using the Score Summary Form in **Appendix A**. The *Consonant Cluster Screener* will provide you with information to select challenging intervention targets that are in the child's reach for maximal therapeutic gains to occur.[48] In Chapter 3, you will reference this summary score sheet to select complex consonant blend targets that maximally improve speech intelligibility.

1.10 Phonological Process Identification

Phonological processes are simplified speaking patterns. These simplified patterns can impact syllable structure, such as deletion of initial/final consonants and weak syllables in words. They can also impact classes of sounds, such as more complex fricative sounds, which require obstructed airflow being replaced by stop consonants, which simply stop airflow. Phonological processes can also be assimilatory in nature in which sounds are impacted by neighboring sounds or syllables (e.g., producing "doggy" /ˈdɔgi/ as /ˈgɔgi/).

To identify phonological processes, please refer to ▶ Table 1.2 for phonological processes exhibited by preschoolers and their typical age of suppression. Phonological processes I have personally found to be most commonly present are in bolded print.

Please see ▶ Table 1.3 for a list of errors that Sampson had on a recent standardized articulation assessment. What phonological processes can you identify in the substitutions and omissions made by Sampson?

For further practice, identify phonological processes based on a list of errors that Landley (▶ Table 1.4) and Kamdyn (▶ Table 1.5) made on recent single-word standardized articulation assessments. (Phonological processes we detected are presented in **Appendix B**.)

Errors can also be assimilatory in nature in that productions are impacted by the surrounding sounds. For instance, in production of s-blends, a child may produce /sneɪk/ for "snake" perfectly; however, the child may produce /fun/ for "spoon" due to coalescence, which is a combination of characteristics from neighboring sounds. Here, the fricative nature of /s/ and labial placement of /p/ combine to form the labial-dental fricative /f/.

Table 1.2 Phonological processes: Description and typical age of suppression[a,b,c]

Phonological Process	Description	Example Correct→Incorrect Orthographic IPA	Typical Age of Suppression (years)
Denasalization	Changing a nasal consonant to a non-nasal	no→dough noʊ→doʊ	2.5
Initial Consonant Deletion	Initial consonant is omitted	cat→at kæt→æt	3
Final Consonant Deletion	Final consonant is omitted	Dog→dah dɔg→dɔ	3
Backing	Posterior velar /k/ and /g/ substitute anterior sounds	bite→bike baɪt→baɪk bus→bug bʌs→ bʌg	3
Fronting	Anterior sounds substitute /k/ and /g/	key→tea ki→ti game→tame geɪm→teɪm	3
Consonant Assimilation	Changing a sound so that it takes on the characteristics of another sound in the word	Dog→gog dɔg→gɔg	3
Reduplication	Repetition of a syllable	water→wawa 'wɔtər→'wɔwɔ	3
Affrication	Substituting an affricate for a nonaffricate	shoe→choo ʃu→ʧu	3
Weak Syllable Deletion	Weak syllables are omitted	banana→nana bə 'nænə→nænə	3
Devoicing; Voiced Errors	Voiced consonants are devoiced; Voiceless consonants are voiced	gate→Kate geɪt→keɪt	3.5
Stopping	Fricative or affricate consonants are replaced by stops: earlier developing sounds suppressed earlier than later developing sounds	van→ban væn→ bæn Cheese→tease ʧiz→diz Them→dem ðɛm→dɛm	3–5
Deaffrication	Replacing an affricate with a stop or fricative	chip→tip ʧɪp→tɪp jam→dam ʤæm→dæm	4
Depalatization	Substituting a nonpalatal for a palatal at the end of the word	fish→fis fɪʃ→fɪs	4
Alveolarization	Substituting an alveolar sound for a nonalveolar one	fan→tan fæn→tæn	4

Table 1.2 (*Continued*) Phonological processes: Description and typical age of suppression[a,b,c]

Phonological Process	Description	Example Correct→Incorrect Orthographic IPA	Typical Age of Suppression (years)
Cluster Reduction (Partial)	Part of the cluster is omitted	*tweet*→*teet* twit→tit *snake*→*nake* sneɪk→neɪk	4.5
Coalescence	Two neighboring sounds are substituted for one sound with shared features	*spoon*→*foon* spun→fun	4.5
Gliding	Liquids /l/ or /r/ are replaced with glide /w/ or /j/ sounds	*lamp*→*wamp* læmp→wæmp *ring*→*wing* rɪŋ→wɪŋ *want*→*yant* wɑnt→jɑnt	6
Epenthesis	Adding a sound between two consonants, typically a schwa ("uh")	*blue*→*buh-lue* blu→bʌlu	8

Sources:

[a]Bleile KM. Manual of Articulation and Phonological Disorders: Infancy through Adulthood. San Diego, CA: Singular Pub. Group; 1995.

[b]Hegde MN. Hegdes Pocket Guide to Assessment in Speech-Language Pathology. San Diego: Singular Publishing Group; 2001.

[c]Peña-Brooks Adriana, Hegde MN. Assessment and Treatment of Articulation and Phonological Disorders in Children: A Dual-Level Text. Austin, TX: PRO-ED; 2007.

Another example of phonetic context impacting intelligibility is consonant harmony, in which two consonants become the same in a CVC syllable. Consonant harmony can be progressive assimilation, in which the left consonant impacts the right (e.g., "dog" becomes /dɔd/), or regressive assimilation, in which the right consonant impacts the left (e.g., "dog" becomes /gɔg/). See ▶ Table 1.2 for phonological processes defined.

It is important to identify phonological processes as these patterns will drive therapy in efficiently improving entire classes of sounds, rather than taking a piecemeal approach to targeting individual sounds. Common phonological processes bolded in ▶ Table 1.2 are the ones that provide the greatest coverage in treating multiple error sounds in a class.

1.11 Connected Speech Sample

Research indicates that performance in connected speech can significantly vary from performance on single word articulation tests.[49] In preschool age children, the common phonological processes of cluster reduction and final consonant deletion are more likely to surface in connected speech than in single word testing. Conversely, the phonological process of epenthesis, insertion of a vowel (typically schwa /ə/) within a consonant cluster, occurs more often in single word testing than connected speech.[50]

In recording a speech sample, you may first decide to gloss the speech sample. To gloss the sample is to transcribe the spontaneous speech sample orthographically (i.e., traditional spelling). Next transcribe the sample with a broad or systematic transcription using IPA consonants and vowels. Lastly, apply narrow transcription to errored sounds to show how distorted sounds are produced.

Commonly used narrow transcription diacritics to indicate prosodic errors include stress diacritics placed before the syllable with primary stress atop [ˈ], with secondary stress on the bottom [ˌ], aspiration indicated by [ʰ], pauses within words indicated by a period [.], and lengthening of sounds indicated by [ː].

Table 1.3 Phonological processes based on Sampson's standardized speech test errors

Stimulus Item *Orthographically* IPA	Sampson's Production *Orthographically* IPA	Phonological Process(es)
teeth /tiθ/	teas /tis/	
rake /ɹeɪk/	wake /weɪk/	
fish /fɪʃ/	fiss /fɪs/	
seal /si/l/	see-awe /siɑ/	
zoo /zu/	sue /su/	
cheese /tʃiz/	tease /tis/	
leaf /lif/	yeaf /jif/	
thumb /θʌm/	fumb /fʌm/	
bathe /beɪð/	bave /beɪv/	
clown /klaʊn/	cown /kaʊn/	
snake /sneɪk/	nake /neɪk/	
thermometer /θər'mɑmətɚ/	mometer /mɑmətɚ/	

[a]Note that /θ, ð/ production varies based on influence of phonetic context.

Table 1.4 Phonological processes based on Landley's standardized speech test errors

Stimulus Item *Orthographically* IPA	Stimulus Item *Orthographically* IPA	Phonological Process(es)
gate /geɪt/	Date /deɪt/	
king /kɪŋ/	Teen /tin/	
ring /ɹɪŋ/	ween /win/	
Van /væn/	Ban /bæn/	
Jar /dʒɑr/	Daw /dɔ/	
watch /wɑtʃ/	Watt /wɑt/	
Them /ðɛm/	Dem dɛm	
bridge /bɹɪdʒ/	bwidge /bwɪdʒ/	
grasshopper /'gɹæs,hɑpɚ/	dwasshooper /'dwæs,hɑpɚ/	
Fish /fɪʃ/	Fis /fɪs/	
Jar /dʒɑr/	Daw /dɔ/	
Rake /ɹeɪk/	Wate /weɪt/	

1.12 Percent Consonant Correct (PCC)

Transcribe 100 consecutive words to evaluate PCC. PCC measures the percentage of consonants accurately produced to gauge conversational speech intelligibility.

At this time in the evaluation, children tend to be more talkative. This is due to the positive experience of standardized speech testing, increased comfort with the evaluator being paired with toy rewards, and positive encouragement provided for on task behavior.

The spontaneous language sample also provides information on diagnostic direction for the selection of appropriate language tests based on strengths and weaknesses that surfaced during the language sample.

To encourage increased verbal expression, the following responsive language elicitation techniques are useful[51,52]:
1. Comment more than question-based on the child's focus of attention or interests.
2. Repeat the child's words with enthusiasm, or a rising intonation with a question format at the end.
3. Prompt elaboration by repeating child's words enthusiastically and adding, "Tell me more."
4. Talk about popular toys, cartoons, or movies you have at home to provide an authentic purpose for the child to share new information from home.

Table 1.5 Phonological processes based on Kamdyn's standardized speech test errors

Stimulus Item *Orthographically* IPA	Stimulus Item *Orthographically* IPA	Phonological Process(es)
Pig /pɪg/	Pid /pɪd/	
Swing /swɪŋ/	Fwin /fwin/	
Knife /naɪf/	Nice /naɪs/	
Fish /fɪʃ/	Fis /fɪs/	
Seal /sil/	Seaw /siɑw/	
Sheep /ʃip/	seep /sip/	
cheese /tʃiz /	Sheeze /ʃiz/	
Weaf /wif/	leaf /lif/	
lemonade /ˈlɛməˈneɪd/	nemonade /ˈnɛməˈneɪd/	
computer /kəmˈpjutɚ/	Puter /ˈpjutɚ/	
Snake /sneɪk/	Sate /seɪt/	
them /ðɛm/	*vem* /vɛm/	
Thermometer /θɚˈmɑmətɚ/	Mometer /ˈmɑmətɚ/	

[a]Note that /θ, ð/ production varies based on influence of phonetic context.

These responsive language strategies create a positive affective domain. This is a learning environment that promotes positive emotions, feelings, and attitudes. This domain creates a setting to observe both a child's typical and optimal level of communication.

By creating a positive affective domain, a child's confidence and comfort level also may increase by limiting direct questions. I have found that asking Wh? questions in a self-talk manner aloud effectively gauges the child's comprehension through the contingency of responses.

Examples include: "I wonder *how* this works? I wonder *why* she doesn't have her shoes? I wonder *when* I'm going to get more presents? I wonder *where* this goes? I wonder *what* this is? I wonder if we have more cars than these (yes/no)? I wonder what this does?

Refer to Landley in Video 1.3 to see intern Maisoun implementing this self-talk technique with Landley. In doing so Maisoun is able to effectively gauge Landley's ability to comprehend Wh? questions without asking one.

1.13 Calculating Percent Consonants Correct (PCC)

First, refer to ▶ Table 1.6. Apply these guidelines throughout to determine whether to count the consonantal phoneme and whether to production as errored or correct.

> ### PCC is calculated by the following steps[53]
>
> Transcribe approximately 100 continuous words in a spontaneous speech sample using gloss (orthographic) transcription initially and then transcribe into broad and narrow (as applicable) transcription using IPA (see ▶ Table 1.7).
>
> Count 100 continuous phonemic consonants (speech sounds that change meaning), not vowels. Refer to ▶ Table 1.6 for guidance.
>
> Find the number of accurate consonantal phonemes and divide that number by total number of consonantal phonemes spoken.
>
> Number of Consonantal Phonemes Correct
> Total Number of Consonantal Phonemes
> = _____% Percent Consonants Correct (PCC)

See ▶ Table 1.7 for both a gloss and IPA transcription of Landley's speech. You can also view her in Video 1.3 to practice transcription of 100 continuous words. Apply criteria given in ▶ Table 1.6 for determining which consonants to count and a consonant's accuracy. Calculate Landley's PCC, and refer to the severity guidelines presented below. Compare your findings to ours in **Appendix B**.

Shriberg and Kwiatkowski proposed PCC to be an effective objective measurement of connected speech to determine the severity of speech impairment.[54] Shriberg et al later researched reliability for PCC and indicated it to be a valid and reliable

Table 1.6 Guidelines for calculating percentage of consonants correct (PCC)

Do not count at all:	Consonants counted as incorrect:	Consonants counted as correct:
All vowels (including rhotic "er" and "ɝ")	Deleted or omitted	Dialectal variations: (e.g., "baf" for "bath" in African-American English)
Repetitions of a syllable (e.g., "po-pony": only score one /p/)	Distorted, substituted, or incorrectly voiced	Casual productions of speech (e.g., "wanna" for "want to")
Consonants in the third repetition of the word	Consonants added to a target consonant (e.g., "pig**t**")	Allophonic variations: "tweny" for "twenty"

Source: Brown R. A First Language: The Early Stages. Cambridge, MA: Harvard University Press; 1973.

Table 1.7 Landley's connected speech sample for percent consonants correct (PCC) analysis (4;1 years)

Orthographically (without speech errors):
Do you think piggies go outside? Here's one. And I wonder where these go. I think their farmer washed them off but not this little piggy. I think needs to put them in here. I think they're gonna go know in here. I think the ladder you. They can go in here. Maybe this should go in here. Um sometimes. Um sometimes the farmer feeds this in a minute. I think cow should go up here. And this cow should go in here. I don't know where he should go. Yeah. But he needs to be in the farm. And where should the mouse go? He's gotta find a ways to sleep. (112 Words)

Phonetically in IPA (without speech errors):
/du ju θɪŋk 'pɪgiz goʊ 'aʊt'saɪd? hɪrz wʌn. ænd aɪ 'wʌndər wɛr ðiz goʊ. aɪ θɪŋk ðɛr 'farmər waʃt ðɛm ɔf bʌt nɑt ðɪs 'lɪtəl 'pɪgi.aɪθɪŋknidztupʊtðɛmɪnhir.aɪθɪŋkðɛr'gɑnəgoʊɪnhir.aɪθɪŋkðə'lædərjunoʊ.ðeɪkæŋgoʊɪnhir.'meɪbɪðɪsʃʊdgoʊɪnhir.ʌm səm'taɪmz. ʌm səm 'taɪmz ðə 'farmər fidz ðɪs ɪn ə 'mɪnət. aɪ θɪŋk kaʊ ʃʊd goʊ ʌp hir. ænd ðɪs kaʊ ʃʊd goʊ ɪnhir. aɪ doʊnt noʊ wɛr hi ʃʊd goʊ. jæ. bʌt hi nidz tu bi ɪn ðə fɑrm. ænd wɛr ʃʊd ðə maʊs goʊ? hiz 'gɑtə faɪnd ə weɪz tu slip./

measurement, particularly for preschoolers aged 3 to 6 years.[53] Shriberg and Kwiatkowski proposed the following PCC guidelines for indicating severity of speech disorder[54]:
- 85–100% PCC: Mild
- 65–85% PCC: Mild-Moderate
- 50–65% PCC: Moderate-Severe
- Less than 50% PCC: Severe

1.14 Calculating Percentage of Intelligible Words (PIW)

If the child is highly unintelligible, thereby making transcription of individual consonants impossible, calculate words intelligible over total words spoken. Try to write at least 100 words. Mark completely unintelligible words as "X" and divide the number of words intelligible by the total number of words (both unintelligible and intelligible) spoken. This measurement of intelligibility in connected speech is referred to as percentage of intelligible words (PIW).[54]

Number of Words Intelligible
Total Number of Words
= _____% Percentage of Intelligible Words (PIW)

Research indicates that when PIW falls below 66% for a child of 4 years and older intervention should be considered.[55] This basic gloss transcription will provide you with baseline data on naturalistic connected speech intelligibility despite inability to broadly or narrowly transcribe it due to unintelligibility.

1.15 Qualitative Judgments of Connected Speech

From the connected speech sample, make qualitative notes regarding the child's volume, pitch, fluency, vocal hoarseness, vocal strain, rate of speech, nasality, use of stress, and intonation to indicate pragmatic intent (e.g., rising intonation for a question, dropping intonation for a statement, and emphatic use of stress for clarification).

Assign a subjective perceived rating of intelligibility, based on percentage of speech understood, with context known and unknown. For example, "This evaluator perceived a child to be 50% intelligible with known context and 30% with an unknown context during connected speech."

Deciding Whether to Select Percent Consonants Correct (PCC) or Percent Consonant Correct Revised (PCC-R)

Percent Consonant Correct-Revised (PCC-R) replicates Percent Consonants Correct (PCC) with an exception that it counts distortions as correct consonants[53]:

Number of Consonantal Phonemes Correct + Distorted Consonants/Total Number of Consonantal Phonemes = _____% PCC-R

I often prefer to use PCC instead of PCC-R. I choose PCC because I target highly frequent /s/, /z/, /l/, and /ɹ/ distortions within consonant clusters at preschool age to prevent habituation. For this, PCC is preferable to measure change in distorted sounds.

PCC-R may be indicated as a more sensitive measurement of speech improvement in a highly unintelligible child. This child would likely produce multiple omission, substitution, or addition errors, which would impact intelligibility more negatively than common distortions. With progress, this child's errors would evolve into distortions, thereby positively impacting intelligibility. In this instance, PCC would less likely detect improvement in overall intelligibility, as all errors are given equal weight.

Table 1.8 Guidelines for segmenting utterances and calculating mean length of utterance (MLU)

Segmenting Utterances

1. Segment language sample into utterances. A sentence, command, compound sentence, and complex sentence each count as an utterance.
2. A run-on sentence with more than one *and* should be separated so that only the initial *and* is used to form a compound sentence with remaining utterances segmented without *and*. *For example*: "I have horses and I have cows and I have goats and I have dogs") is transcribed as 1. /I have horses and I have cows/I have goats/I have dogs/.
3. An utterance's end is indicated by pauses of greater than 2 seconds, rising or dropping intonation indicating a question or statement, or interruption or abandonment of a thought.

Computing MLU

1. Type 50 fully intelligible consecutive utterances (one per line) exactly as the child says them in standard spelling.
2. Delete fillers such as "uh" and repeated words (unless used for emphasis in which every repetition is counted).
3. Count the following as one morpheme: compound words (e.g., birthday), proper names (e.g., Big Bird), ritualized reduplications (e.g., bye-bye), diminutive ending words (e.g., doggy), contractions can't and don't, helping verbs (e.g., is, are, had, were, etc.), irregular past tense words (e.g., went, came, gone).
4. Count as an additional bound morpheme: contracted verbs (e.g., he's, aren't, they're = 2 morphemes), overgeneralized past tense verbs (e.g., goed, comed, costed = 2 morphemes), words containing morphemes (plural-s, possessive-s, third-person present tense verb-s, past tense-ed, verb + ing = 2 morphemes).
5. Add the total number of morphemes in the sample and divide by the total number of utterances.

Source: Paul R, Norbury C, Gosse C. Language Disorders from Infancy through Adolescence: Listening, Speaking, Reading, Writing, and Communicating. St. Louis, MO: Elsevier; 2018.

Also note both the parent's reported intelligibility percentage and parent's perception of unfamiliar individuals' percentage intelligibility of the child. Parent's perception is reported in the *Parent Input Form* (▶ Table 1.1). Research suggests parents, speech-language pathologists, and unfamiliar adults will each likely rate a child's intelligibility dierently.[56]

What is your perceived percentage intelligibility rating of Landley from listening to the connected speech samples with a known context (Video 1.3)? Does it differ from her PCC measurement? If there's a discrepancy, what could explain it?

1.16 Calculating Mean Length of Utterance (MLU)

Please refer to ▶ Table 1.8 for reference while segmenting utterances and calculating MLU. Watch Video 1.4 in its entirety of Sampson with Maisoun to complete a gloss transcription and calculate Sampson's MLU. Gloss transcription is additionally provided for you in ▶ Table 1.9. Refer to Appendix B to compare your MLU calculation with ours. Lastly, refer ▶ Table 1.10 to compare Sampson's MLU with children with and without language impairment.

Table 1.9 Sampson's connected speech sample: Gloss of all utterances transcribed

1. Why
2. Yeah
3. Swimming pool
4. Yeah (take out: imitated)
5. I want to do this one
6. I don't know
7. Yeah (take out: said previously)
8. Why (take out: said previously)
9. Oopsies!
10. From the house maybe
11. What are these
12. I don't know (take out: said previously)
13. Yeah (take out: said previously)
14. Look what is this
15. I don't know (take out: said previously)
16. Oh what is this piece (take out "oh": filler)
17. To wash your hands
18. Yeah (take out: said previously)
19. This is a bathroom
20. There's the bathroom (take out: imitated)
21. I don't know (take out: said previously)
22. I need to go poop
23. Maybe he's too big
24. Nope maybe not
25. Maybe this person
26. Maybe (take out: said previously)
27. Awe no
28. Yeah (take out: said previously)
29. What is this
30. Yeah (take out: said previously)
31. I don't know (take out: said previously)
32. Maybe it's in the house with the big bad wolf
33. Maybe (take out: said previously)
34. I don't know maybe to the bathroom
35. Yeah (take out: said previously)
36. I need to go I need to go potty (take out repeated phrase "I need to go")
37. Oopsies
38. There she goes
39. I don't know (take out: said previously)
40. Maybe this one
41. Yeah (take out: said previously)
42. Big toys (take out: imitated)
43. I never saw big toys before
44. No
45. Nope
46. Yeah (take out: said previously)
47. What is this (take out: said previously)
48. I don't know (take out: said previously)
49. Snake
50. Maybe (take out: said previously)
51. Maybe they're so scary
52. Maybe (take out: said previously)
53. What is this (take out: said previously)
54. Rubber ducky (take out: imitated)
55. Yeah (take out: said previously)
56. Yeah (take out: said previously)
57. I don't know maybe in the bathtub
58. What's this
59. I don't know-maybe a sink
60. Yeah maybe
61. I don't know (take out: said previously)
62. One sink that goes down here
63. And where's the bathroom
64. This is the bathroom
65. I'm putting this sink right right here (take out: word repetition 'right')
66. What's this X (take out: unintelligible word)
67. Maybe (take out: said previously)
68. Somebody's on it
69. I'm just pretending
70. I'm just pretending somebody's under it
71. Why not
72. No
73. How do you do this
74. I'm doing this
75. There we go (take out: imitated)
76. Here's some melon
77. Want this—num-num-num
78. No (take out: said previously)
79. Watermelon (take out: imitated)
80. Watch me spin this
81. Yeah—yeah (take out: said previously)
82. Yeah (take out: said previously)
83. Lamp look
84. Maybe it goes on here
85. This is very X (take out: unintelligible word)
86. Maybe it wiggles
87. Maybe it goes together (take out: imitated)
88. And then this
89. I don't know (take out: said previously)
90. Why (take out: said previously)
91. Baby's going to sleep (take out: imitated)
92. Bye (take out: imitated)
93. Maybe I can play with this next time

To analyze Sampson's MLU using word processing software:

1. Place a space within words to indicate a bound morpheme. Also, take out spaces between words that count as one morpheme, such as proper nouns and reduplications (e.g., Mickey Mouse, nightnight)
2. Make sure to remove utterance numbers (or they will count towards total word count)
3. On Microsoft Word or Google Docs, go to "Tools"→"Word Count"
4. Divide "Word Count" by number of utterances.
5. Refer to ▶ Table 1.3 for typical MLU based on chronological age.

Table 1.10 Mean length of utterance (MLU) for children with specific language impairment and children without language impairment: Group averages (X) and standard deviations (SD)

Age Range	2;6–2;11	3;0–3;5	3;6–3;11	4;0–4;5	4;6–4;11	5;0–5;5	5;6–5;11	6;0–6;5	6;6–6;11
MLU of Children with Language Impairment	X = 2.59 −SD 2.20 + SD 2.98	X = 3.07 −SD 2.59 + SD 3.55	X = 3.36 −SD 2.56 + SD 4.16	X = 3.64 −SD 2.84 + SD 4.44	X = 3.95 −SD 3.25 + SD 4.65	X = 4.09 −SD 3.39 + SD 4.79	X = 4.34 −SD 3.67 + SD 5.01	X = 4.38 −SD 3.63 + SD 5.13	X = 4.63 −SD 3.84 + SD 5.42
n = number sampled	n = 6	n = 15	n = 24	n = 54	n = 72	n = 84	n = 97	n = 108	n = 94
Age Range	2;6–2;11	3;0–3;5	3;6–3;11	4;0–4;5	4;6–4;11	5;0–5;5	5;6–5;11	6;0–6;5	6;6–6;11
MLU of Children without Language Impairment	X = 3.23 −SD 2.52 + SD 3.94	X = 3.81 −SD 3.12 + SD 4.50	X = 4.09 −SD 3.42 + SD 4.76	X = 4.57 −SD 3.81 + SD 5.33	X = 4.75 −SD 3.96 + SD 5.36	X = 4.88 −SD 4.16 + SD 5.60	X = 4.96 −SD 4.26 + SD 5.66	X = 5.07 −SD 4.32 + SD 5.82	X = 5.22 −SD 4.51 + SD 5.93
n = number sampled	n = 17	n = 29	n = 38	n = 49	n = 74	n = 78	n = 77	n = 70	n = 63

Source: Rice ML, Smolik F, Perpich D, Thompson T, Rytting N, Blossom M. Mean length of utterance levels in 6-month intervals for children 3 to 9 years with and without language impairments. Journal of Speech, Language, and Hearing Research. 2010;53(2):333–349.

1.17 Observing Oral Structure and Movement at Rest and in Speech

Lastly, complete an oral mechanism evaluation. This is sequenced toward the end of the evaluation as it can be intrusive for a child to have an oral mechanism evaluation completed by an unfamiliar adult—similar to going to the dentist. By this point, the comfort level between the therapist and child should be well-established.

Please refer ▶ Table 1.11 while watching Video 1.5 in which Torey models a conventional oral mechanism evaluation.

During a typical speech evaluation, I usually do not assess traditional nonspeech motor activities such as puckering lips and smiling on demand, puffing cheeks and holding air, protruding and retracting the tongue, or laterally and vertically moving the tongue on demand. There simply is not enough time. I share the opinion of speech sound disorder experts who have generally found that a cursory observation during speech and at rest provides sufficient information regarding tone, strength, and movement necessary for speaking purposes.[16,57]

An instance however where it would be useful to have a child engage in nonspeech motor acts on demand is in differentially diagnosing CAS from ISSD. Children with CAS will more likely demonstrate difficulty engaging in nonspeech motor movements (such as tongue protrusion, lip retraction/puckering, and blowing) on demand than children with ISSD.[58]

In assessing nonspeech motor activities in preschoolers, CAS expert Edythe Strand recommends having the child engage in naturally rewarding activities such as directing a child to kiss a doll and blow bubbles.[16] Children demonstrate great difficulty with intentional nonspeech oral movements, referred to as nonverbal oral apraxia. Children with CAS are more likely to present with nonverbal oral apraxia.[16]

Observation of the mouth both externally and internally is important. Refer ▶ Table 1.11, Observation of Oral Structure and Speech of Preschoolers. This form will continue to evolve as our research base continues to improve our diagnostic skills. Over the years, I have edited it multiple times with our evolving body of research regarding key characteristics in the differential diagnosis of CAS, ISSD, dysarthria, phonological disorder, and articulation impairment.

Please refer to Video 1.6 and Video 1.7 of Kamdyn and Sampson. Refer ▶ Table 1.11 for guidance on what symptomology to attend to at rest and during speech.

Table 1.11 Observation of oral structure and speech of preschoolers

Name: _____DOB:_____ Eval Date:_____Examiner:_____

Observe the preschooler at rest and during speech. If abnormalities are noted, describe to the right:

Evaluation of the Body
Gait abnormalities: Y_____N___Describe:
Gross motor abnormalities: Y_____N_____ Describe:
Fine motor abnormalities: Y_____N_____Describe:

Evaluation of Face: Indicators of Dysarthria
Symmetrical: Y_____N_____Describe:
Mouth breathing: Y_____N_____Describe:
Tongue Protrusion: Y_____N_____Describe:
Cheeks enlarged/puffy: Y_____N_____Describe:
Lips downturned on corners/frown at rest: Y_____N____Describe:
Involuntary facial spasms/grimaces/wincing: Y____N____Describe:

Evaluation of Connected Speech: Indicators of Phonological Disorder
Individual sound errors are developmental (earlier sounds mastered first): Y_____N____Describe:
Phonological Processes (earlier processes suppressed before later): Y_____N_____ Describe:
Consistency in error patterns (e.g., fronting, stopping, final consonant deletion): Y____N____Describe:
Consistency in simplification patterns based on neighboring sounds: Y____N____Describe:

Evaluation of Connected Speech: Indicators of Childhood Apraxia of Speech
Inconsistency: Saying a word clearly one moment and unintelligibly the next: Y_____N_____
Inconsistency: Speaking clearly spontaneously but not on demand (to answer/imitate): Y_____N_____
Inconsistency in vowel/consonant production: Y_____N____Describe:
Incorrect stress in words/phrases (incorrect syllabic, phrasal stressing): Y_____N____Describe:
Substituting vowels with simpler, central forms such as "uh": Y_____N____Describe:
Are two consonants swapping places with each other in a word (metathesis): Y_____N_____
Inconsistent, abrupt pauses within speech: Y____N____Describe:
Lip pursing groping/mouthing sounds without voice: Y_____N_____Describe:
Lengthened/disrupted co-articulatory transitions between sounds and syllables (e.g., "dah...og" for "dog"; rain...bow):
Y_____N_____Describe:
Articulators & voice uncoordinated (e.g., voicing before lip, jaw movement): Y_____N_____Describe:
Difficulty producing multi-syllabic words: Y_____N_____Describe:

Evaluation of Connected Speech: Indicators of Inconsistent Speech Sound Disorder
Speech is more precise when imitated or elicited than spontaneous: Y_____N_____Describe:
Inconsistency in producing the same word differently greater than 40% of the time over 3 time periods? Y_____N_____

Evaluation of Connected Speech: Indicators of Dysarthria
Limited jaw movement (constrictive): Y_____N____Describe:
Excess jaw movement vertically or laterally when speaking: Y_____N_____Describe:
Struggle/tension in neck to produce vocalizations: Y_____N_____Describe:
Whispered Speech: Y_____N_____Describe:
Hypernasal (whining sounding): Y_____N_____Describe:
Hyponasal (stuffed-up cold sounding): Y_____N_____Describe:
Slow rate of speech: Y_____N_____Describe:
Monotone pitch: Y_____N_____Describe:
Voice:Breathy: Y____N____Harsh: Y___N____Nasal: Y____N____Strained: Y____N____Describe:
Prosody is impacted by muscular weakness: Y_____N_____; Spasticity? Y_____N_____Describe:
Speech errors are generally distortions and consistent: Y____N____Describe:

Dysfluenices
Typical Dysfluencies: Hesitations (pauses): Y____N____Fillers (e.g., um): Y_____N_____
Whole Word Repetitions: Y_____N_____ Phrase Repetitions: Y_____N_____
Stuttering Disfluencies: Part-word Repetitions (e.g., ye-ye-yellow): Y_____N_____
Prolongations (e.g., s.....stop): Y_____N_____**Blocks (struggle w/out speech): Y_____N_____
Note: A high rate of "typical dysfluencies" could be indicative of a fluency or language disorder.

Teeth
"Pacifier" teeth (opening in center of teeth, often from extended pacifier use): Y____N_____
TMJ teeth grinding: Y____N___Describe:
Occlusion (incisor relationship): normal_____overbite_____underbite_____crossbite_____
Location of missing teeth:

Table 1.11 (*Continued*) Observation of oral structure and speech of preschoolers

Name:	DOB:	Eval Date:	Examiner:	

Oral Cavity

Tongue abnormalities: jerky/spasms/writhing/fascilations/aberrant size? Y____N____Describe:

Lingua Frenum: short/normal Describe:

Hard and soft palate height: normal_____high_____low_____

Palate width? Normal_____Narrow_____Wide_____

Hard or soft palate cleft: Y_____N_____Submucousal cleft (dark spot under skin): Y_____N_____

Evaluation of Pharynx: _____ color: normal/abnormal _____ Enlarged Tonsils: Y____N_____

Fistulas (growths/excess tissue): Y____N____Describe:

Other abnormalities noted in structure or movement:

Clinical Challenge: How Did Kamdyn's and Sampson's Oral Movements Differ?

What conclusions could you draw regarding Kamdyn's oral proprioception (i.e., awareness of her jaw, labial, and lingual movements in space) and volitional mouth movements on command in comparison to Sampson's?

Interestingly, Kamdyn additionally points her toes slightly inward while walking, resulting in an added drag of the feet. This feet-inverted gait provides added resistance, thereby increasing her proprioception of her body in space.

Indicating further proprioceptive difficulties in balancing her body in space, Kamdyn naturally resorts to "W" sitting (sitting on her bottom with knees bent and feet positioned outside of the hips like a "W"). She falls over when sitting cross-legged (seated on bottom with legs crossed at the ankles). The addition of a wider base in "W" sitting increases the base for balance to occur with poor proprioception.

Kamdyn's gait and sitting difficulties occur in the absence of known peripheral or central nervous system damage.

Based on your prior experience and knowledge, what therapeutic speech strategies could increase Kamdyn's proprioceptive awareness of her jaw, labial, buccal, and lingual movements? (Evidence based strategies will be demonstrated in Chapter 6.)

1.18 Obtaining a Diadochokinetic Rate

Diadochokinetic rate (also known as DDK rate or AMR [alternating motion rate]) is used to assess motor coordination of lips, jaw, and tongue. It measures how accurately and rapidly one can produce a sequence of connected, alternating sounds.

Traditionally, /pʌ-tʌ-kʌ/ has been used in assessing DDK rate.

I personally can think of very few 3-year-olds with speech impairment who have the attention, compliance, and stamina to complete a /pʌ-tʌ-kʌ/ DDK assessment with an unfamiliar adult. Luckily, researchers with preschool age pop- ulations have found the word "pattycake"(/pætikeɪk/) to have parallel reliability with /pʌ-tʌ-kʌ/ in which they equivalently measure the same skills with similar results.[59,60]

An instance, however, where /pʌ-tʌ-kʌ/ production will likely be poorer in terms of accuracy and consistency in production than the word "patty-cake" /pætikeɪk/ would be for children with CAS. Research indicates that they will be more likely to produce familiar words correctly than novel ones due to increased practice in motor programming and planning of the word, which underlie motor coordination tasks.[61]

1.19 Using Diadochokinetic Rate for Differential Diagnosis

Obtaining a DDK rate is important in that it will provide critical information in differentially diagnosing CAS, ISSD, dysarthria, phonological disorder, and articulation impairment.

Children with CAS will often demonstrate poor accuracy and inconsistency in production of

/pʌ-tʌ-kʌ/. However, their rate is more likely to approximate normal limits than children with dysarthria. Dysarthria often presents with a slow rate of speech with consistent errors that are generally slurred and imprecise distortions. However, in both CAS and dysarthria, the more severe the speech delay, the slower the DDK rate.[62] Finally, articulation impairment can resolve into clear speech.

Unlike dysarthria, CAS, and ISSD, children with phonological speech sound disorders typically produce consistent errors that can be described as phonological processes. These are simplified speaking patterns, often impacting classes of sounds. Errors will likely be substitutions and omissions. In contrast, children with articulation impairment will likely present with a normal rate and consistent production. If individual sounds are errored in the word "pattycake," they will likely present as mild distortions or substitutions of individual sounds with a high level of consistency.[64]

With progress, DDK performance will likely change in terms of consistency and accuracy, reflecting improvement in spontaneous speech.[59] Similarly, speech impairment labels can coexist and evolve over time with improvement. A child's initial CAS diagnosis may evolve into a phonological disorder in which errors present consistently in the form of phonological processes. Likewise, the phonological disorder can continue to evolve into an articulation impairment with only a few residual error sounds remaining. Terminology should similarly change over time to better reflect the speech sound disorder in its evolving state.[65]

1.20 Administering a Diadochokinetic (DDK) Assessment

Refer ▶ Table 1.12 for guidance on how to administer a DDK assessment. For hands-on practice, complete the Diadochokinetic Assessment for Preschoolers Forms for Sampson and Kamdyn. They are shown in Video 1.8 and Video 1.9.

Transcribe the child's productions of each "pattycake" (/pætikeɪk/) in IPA. Time how long it takes to say /pætikeɪk/ 20 times. See ▶ Table 1.8 for guidance on calculating DDK performance in terms of productions per second, percentage of accuracy, percentage of variability, and percentage of consistency.

Compare Sampson's and Kamdyn's DDK performances in terms of rate, accuracy, and

Table 1.12 Diadochokinetic assessment for Preschoolers Form

Child's Name: _____Date: _____ DOB:_____ Examiner:_____
Tell the child, **"We're going to play the pattycake game in which we say the word 'pattycake' 20 times as fast as we can. Let's try five to start."** Breathe in and say 'pattycake' 5 times with the child. **"Okay, now you get to make 20 pattycakes all by yourself as fast as you can. Ready? Take a deep breath."** Put a finger up each time the child says, "pattycake." Write the child's productions over each "pæ-ti-keɪk." (You may need to record for accuracy.) Time how long it takes to say pattycake 20 times.
pæ-ti-keɪk pæ-ti-keɪk pæ-ti-keɪk pæ-ti-keɪk pæ-ti-keɪk
pæ-ti-keɪk pæ-ti-keɪk pæ-ti-keɪk pæ-ti-keɪk pæ-ti-keɪk
pæ-ti-keɪk pæ-ti-keɪk pæ-ti-keɪk pæ-ti-keɪk pæ-ti-keɪk
pæ-ti-keɪk pæ-ti-keɪk pæ-ti-keɪk pæ-ti-keɪk pæ-ti-keɪk
To determine accuracy, divide total number correct by 20 = _____% Accuracy
Total number correct = _____% Accuracy
      20
Number of seconds to produce "pattycake" 20 times = _____(30 seconds is considered average)[a]
To determine rate per second, divide total number of seconds by 20:_____rate per second:
Total number of seconds = _____DDK rate per sec (1.4–1.8 is considered within normal range 3–5 yrs)[a]
      20
To measure consistency, first divide the total number of different inaccurate productions of "pattycake" by 20 to determine % variability:
Number of Different Errored Productions of Pattycake = _____% Variability
        20
Then, subtract %Variability from 100% to establish %Consistency:
100% minus %Variability = _____% Consistency
Observations regarding tongue, lip, cheek, jaw movement:

[a] Robbins J, Klee T. Clinical assessment of oropharyngeal motor development in young children. *Journal of Speech and Hearing Disorders.* 1987;52(3):271.

consistency. How do they differ? What conclusions can you draw based on their DDK performances? Compare your findings with ours in **Appendix B**.

1.21 Contribution of DDK Rate, Accuracy, and Consistency as Indicators of Speech Improvement

DDK rate can be compared to the norms of typically developing children presented by Robbins and Klee in 1987. They essentially found production of "pattycake" at a rate of approximately 1.5 times per second to be typical between 3 and 5 years of age (with a limited range in variability from 1.4 to 1.8 per second). Therefore, an average rate for a typically developing preschooler would be approximately 20 pattycakes produced in 30 seconds. Importantly, however, their findings indicate the DDK rate of typically developing preschoolers does not increase during the preschool years.[66]

Supporting Robbins and Klee's findings of stability of rate despite chronological age maturation in typically developing preschoolers, Williams and Stackhouse also found rate to not increase between the ages of 3 and 5 years.[59] Together, these findings indicate observation of increases in accuracy and consistency of productions in DDK performance over time are likely greater indicators of improvement than a faster rate at preschool age.

1.22 Differential Diagnosis of Speech Sound Disorders

1.22.1 Childhood Apraxia of Speech (CAS)

CAS is a neurological childhood motor speech disorder primarily associated with difficulty in planning and programming movement sequences. CAS is typically characterized by difficulty in producing polysyllabic words, inconsistent speech errors, dysprosody, inappropriately inserted pauses, and breakdowns in coarticulating sounds.

Breakdowns more often occur as words and utterances increase in complexity, taxing motor planning and programming skills.[64] These breakdowns can take the form of prolonged and misplaced pauses, inappropriate stress, substitutions, omissions, additions, repetitions, sound/syllable reversals, and simplification of consonants and vowels.

Children with CAS produce spontaneous speech clearer than when producing speech on demand.[58] Discoordination of the combined activities of respiration, phonation, resonance, and articulation can result in prosodic breakdowns. These prosodic breakdowns present as inappropriate rate, rhythm, stress, pausing, and/or inflection.[67]

Children with CAS also often present with groping behaviors. These are observable struggles to speak that are often accompanied by silence or grunts. The child may mouth words for placement but is unable to coordinate respiration and phonation with articulation. In groping behaviors, phonation may be achieved. However it could be with the absence of jaw, buccal, labial, and lingual movement to shape the voicing into speech.[16]

Recent research indicates that concurrence of two symptoms, namely poor accuracy in DDK assessment and poor production of polysyllabic words, are reliable indicators of the presence of CAS.[64]

1.22.2 Organic Nature of Childhood Apraxia of Speech

A child with CAS is likely to have underlying neurological damage. A plethora of recent research indicates children with CAS to more likely present with concurrent deficits in nonspeech oral motor movements, gross motor, fine motor, speech processing, and expressive language development.[14,15,68,69,70]

Additionally, chromosome abnormalities have recently been discovered that may be attributed to CAS.[71] Recent functional magnetic resonance imaging (MRI) research indicates that in a family with a chromosome mutation linked to CAS, adult members affected with both oral and verbal developmental apraxia of speech presented with 20% less gray matter in the cerebellum than family members unaffected with apraxia. This is similar to the reduction of gray matter reported in adults with ataxia due to cerebellar atrophy who present with similar symptomology.[72]

1.22.3 Inconsistent Speech Sound Disorder

ISSD presents similarly to CAS in its inconsistency of accuracy in verbal production of words. Children with ISSD are more likely to present with appropriate prosody, fluency, and normal rate in speech and diadochokinesis than those with CAS.[8] Another difference is that children with CAS tend to have slightly slower DDK rates and speaking rates than children with ISSD.[63]

Children with ISSD are also more likely to substitute phonemes in words with unrelated phonemes, whereas children with CAS are more likely to use metathesis. This is the transposition in sounds, or syllables switching places within words (e.g., "cab" becomes "back": /kæb/→/bæk/; "baby" becomes "beebay": /ˈbeɪbi/→/bibeɪ/).[73]

Lastly, speech of children with ISSD improves when imitating. Conversely, speech of children with CAS tends to worsen when imitating.[63]

1.22.4 Dysarthria

Unlike symptomology of inconsistencies in CAS and ISSD, dysarthria, also referred to as an organic motor speech disorder, is typically consistent in its speech deficits. Speech tends to be slurred and distorted. Additionally, unlike CAS, speech errors are typically consistent in both spontaneous speech and in on demand contexts.[74]

Unlike CAS, in which vocal quality is spared, vocal quality tends to be negatively impacted according to the type of dysarthria. This could present as inaudible/monotone volume, creakiness, hoarseness, breathiness, or harshness. With dysarthria, speech and vocal quality will be negatively impacted differently by the type of dysarthria: flaccidity, spasticity, paralysis, and ataxia.[75]

Additionally, unlike CAS, children with dysarthria tend to have difficulty with the nonspeech oral motor acts of swallowing and chewing due to muscular weakness and/or incoordination. Children with dysarthria also tend to have less of a discrepancy between receptive and expressive language skills than children with CAS.[74]

During speech of increased length and complexity breakdowns may occur in dysarthria. This is possibly due to the resultant fatigue from increased motor demands. In CAS breakdowns are primarily related to increased demands in planning and programming. However, in dysarthria it is due to increased muscular demands in execution.

One form of dysarthria, ataxic dysarthria, presents with incoordination of motor movement. It is caused by damage to the cerebellum, which plays a key role in planning, programming, and executing speech. Hence, it shares similar speech characteristics as CAS in presenting with inaccuracy of complex coarticulatory movements.

However, ataxic dysarthria can be distinguished from CAS as children with ataxic dysarthria will more likely present with impairment in motor incoordination globally, perhaps resulting in a wider gait or presence of intention tremors.

An intention tremor is an involuntary, rhythmic muscle contraction that presents as a shaking movement in one or more parts of the body, typically extremities such as hands. Additionally, the ataxia can result in uneven breathing patterns in which breath is sporadically held and released unevenly. Lastly, children with ataxia present with more consistency in their errors than children with CAS in connected speech.[16]

1.22.5 Phonological Disorder

Phonological disorder is unlike both CAS and ISSD in that phonological disorder presents with error patterns that are consistent. These error patterns are known as phonological processes, which are rule-based speaking patterns that simplify speech in syllabic complexity or sound production.

Unlike CAS, prosody in rate, rhythm, and stress is typically age appropriate. Children with phonological disorders also tend to present with better vowel production than children with CAS, who tend to centralize vowels or neutralize them as a schwa /ə/.[74]

Unlike dysarthria, children with phonological disorder do not present with overt muscular weakness, incoordination, paralysis of speech musculature, or difficulty with volitional or automatic non speech motor acts of chewing and swallowing inherent to dysarthria.

Children with severe phonological disorder are also more likely to have stronger language comprehension skills than language expression. Whereas, children with dysarthria are more likely to have global receptive and expressive language delays.[74] Omissions of sounds and syllables in phonological processes are prognostic indicators of weaker language skills than sound substitutions for children with phonological disorders.[38,39]

1.22.6 Articulation Impairment

Articulation impairment is difficulty in producing specific speech sounds accurately. Articulation impairment presents with distortions or substitutions of individual sounds. For instance, a labially rounded [lʷ] and [ɹʷ], or inter-dentalized [s̪] and [z̪] are examples of common distortions for children with articulation impairments.

Presence of Weak Muscular Tone and Strength in Functional Speech Sound Disorders

I've worked with many children with functional speech sound disorders (phonological disorder and articulation impairment) who present with weakness in muscular tone (contraction of muscles at rest) and muscular strength (purposeful contraction of the muscle to achieve fluid movements) at the initial evaluation.

Many of these preschoolers have not yet begun to produce more complex speech such as diphthongs, glides, liquids, affricates, consonant clusters, multisyllabic words, and sentences of increasedlength and complexity.

For this, oral motor weakness is observable. Common observations of pre-schoolers with weakness in both muscular tone and strength include mouth breathing, drooling, chubby cheeks, and downturned corners of the lips. Excess jaw movement is also often observed to compensate for labial and lingual weakness in sound formation.

Note intern Jessica with Patty in Video 1.10. Patty is a 3-year-old, who presents with severe phonological disorder with mouth open at rest, downturned corners of the lips, and oversized cheeks.

At 36 months, Patty presented with a small consonantal inventory of /k/, /g/, and the central vowel /ʌ/. Her phonological processes were backing and vowel centralization. Vowel centralization is a reduction of movement in producing a vowel, resulting in a centralized vowel sound. We decided her target request word to be "swap" /swɒp/, which was quickly expanded to "swap it to me" /swɒp ɪtu mi/ after three 45-minute sessions. (Target selection will be is discussed in Chapter 3.)

In Video 1.10, notice the difficulty in both retracting the lips to smile in producing /s/ and protruding the lips in producing /w/ in the word "swap" /swɒp/.

Video 1.10 clearly illustrates the transactional relationship between muscular tone and strength. If the muscle tone is weak, the muscle will not be in an efficient position to purposefully contract, thereby impairing the muscular strength necessary for movement.

To improve Patty's speech, words containing consonant clusters from the sentence to complex sentence level were selected as intervention targets.

Our experience has been that musculature tone and strength quickly improve in children with functional speech sound disorders when treated with complex consonant cluster therapy targets. These cluster targets are additionally embedded in utterances of increased length and complexity, which increases the motoric challenge to further ignite change.

Parents are typically most relieved to see drool disappear with the pursuant increase in both muscular tone and strength.

Between taping Video 1.10 and Video 1.11, Patty received a school year of speech-language therapy as my client, exclusively receiving services in the public school setting. During the school year, she participated in a once weekly speech group with a weekly 30-minute speech-language therapy sessions. She also participated in five 45-minute one-on-one sessions as part of a summer enrichment program with intervention provided by Wayne State graduate students. The students adhered to evidence-based practices (which are covered in this book) under my direct supervision.

Patty's impressive gains over a 12-month period are not unique, but typical, for children with severe phonological impairment using complex treatment targets in our practice.

Notice intern MaryLyn with Patty 12 months later in Video 1.11. Patty is demonstrating significant improvements in both muscular tone and strength with increased speech accuracy, rate, utterance length, and fluidity.

Patty's new target request has increased in both length and syntactical complexity, "Can you dream it to me please? I am a cool girl because I have sparkle teeth."

Table 1.13 Calculating DDK Based on Rate, Accuracy, Variability, and Consistency

1) Divide the total number of seconds by 20 to determine rate in production per second:

$$\frac{\text{Total Number of Seconds to Produce Pattycake 20 Times}}{20} = \_\_\_\_\_ \text{ Productions per second}$$

2) Divide the total number of "Pattycakes" accurately produced by 20 to determine accuracy:

$$\frac{\text{Total Number of Accurate Productions of Pattycake}}{20} = \_\_\_\_\_\% \text{ Accuracy}$$

3a) Divide the total number of different inaccurate productions of Pattycake by 20 to determine variability:

$$\frac{\text{Number of Different Errored Productions of Pattycake}}{20} = \_\_\_\_\% \text{ Variability}$$

3b) Then, subtract % Variability from 100% to establish consistency:

100% minus %Variability = _____% Consistent

1.23 Reporting Results: Diagnosing Speech Sound Disorders

As a speech language pathologist, it is your responsibility to differentially diagnose speech sound disorders with the limited knowledge and tools we currently have. Please refer ▸ Table 1.13 for deficits typically indicated in the differential diagnosis of speech sound disorders.

If uncertain of a diagnosis at the initial evaluation, I may report, "Child presents with the following symptoms that are consistent with dysarthria/ childhood apraxia of speech/inconsistent speech sound disorder/phonological disorder/articulation impairment at this time," with symptomology comprehensively listed both to support and negate impairment indicated.

Speech sound disorders can also co-exist. Motor speech disorders expert Edythe Strand elaborated on the complexity of our field by advocating for the "contribution" level of concomitant disorders in negatively impacting speech. For instance, a child presents with phonological speech sound disorder in predictable phonological processes occurring within CV, CVC, and CVCV word structures in connected speech above 80% of the time. Yet, the child continues to struggle in producing CVCVCV polysyllabic words with inconsistent breakdowns (e.g., "butterfly" [bʌ.bʌ.bʌ] [tʌ.tʌ.tʌ] [ʌ.ʌ.ʌ]) with inappropriately placed pauses between syllables. Here, I could report, "Child primarily presents with phonological speech disorder with a mild contribution of childhood apraxia of speech in production of polysyllabic words, which are inaccurate, inconsistent, and have inappropriately inserted pauses."

1.24 Evaluating a Child Who Is Preverbal or Minimally Verbal

Broome and colleagues, in the *American Journal of Speech Language Pathology* in 2017, provide a thorough review of guidelines in assessing preverbal children with ASD.[76] These recommendations can be applied to all children who are preverbal or minimally verbal. Completion of an oral motor mechanism examination is recommended to observe the oral structure both externally and internally.

Additionally, the following information should be collected from a connected speech sample of vocalizations: jargon, phonetic inventory of vowels and consonants, syllable shape (such as CV, VC, CVCV), stress pattern (e.g., intonation in jargon and stress in words babbled), ability to imitate or produce sounds, level of consistency in vocalizations, and an inventory of core vocabulary words.

For children who are preverbal, I also complete a dynamic assessment, which assesses learnability of a new skill, with an Alternative, Augmentative Communication (AAC) device. I select AAC that capitalizes on the individual child's strengths. I present highly preferred items from the Parent Input Form (▸ Table 1.1). I then work from a most-to-least prompting hierarchy in which the child mands (i.e., requests) highest preferred objects using symbols with hand-over-hand support generally provided at the initial stage.

I gradually fade my cueing using backward chaining. In backward chaining, the last supportive prompt is faded first while consistently maintaining an 80% accuracy rate. First, the child independently completes the last step. Next, support is gradually faded for the child to independently complete the second to last step. Then, support is faded for the third to last step, and so forth.

The benefit in backward chaining is that children can accurately complete complex motor processes with scaffolding. Through repeated practice, the child develops independence in planning, programming, and executing as adults' cues are faded.

The child's response to the AAC device and level of prompting needed is reported in the speech evaluation report. In this engaging, yet structured, back and forth context, note the child's play behaviors, ability to self-regulate, attend, respond to verbal directions, use eye contact, look at faces, imitate motor movements, request, and comment through coordinated eye contact, gestures, or vocalizations. Level of regulation and aberrant response to environmental sensory stimuli (e.g., touch, auditory, visual) are additionally noted.

1.25 Evaluating Children with ASD

Children with ASD are more likely to present with concomitant speech sound disorders.[77,78] Therefore, it is important to assess and treat speech sound disorders with these children.

In my work, I have successfully improved their speech clarity while increasing their sentence length and complexity.

Recent findings indicate diffuse structural and functional abnormalities in the cerebellum in individuals with ASD.[79] The cerebellum occupies only approximately 10% of the brain's weight. However, it contains an estimated 75% of the neuronal cells in the brain. The cerebellum also connects to practically every area of the brain through approximately 200 million mossy fibers.[80]

The cerebellum plays a key role across developmental domains in both perception and production: gross motor, fine motor, oculomotor, speech, language, emotion, behavior, tactile, visual, auditory, balance, proprioception, and executive functioning skills.[79]

Targeting the cerebellum with complex treatment targets that the cerebellum is responsible for could ignite optimal neuronal connections when neuroplasticity is at a high level.

Improving neuronal connection within the cerebellum could have a cascading impact on children who are preverbal or minimally verbal with ASD in improving speech, language, and socialization outcomes.

Comprehensive therapy techniques to specifically target the cerebellum through focused stimulation with complex therapy targets are covered in Chapter 7.

1.26 Evaluating Children Who Are Verbal with ASD

As previously mentioned, in assessment of verbal preschoolers with ASD, the recommendations are similar to that of typically developing children outlined in this chapter.

It is important to note imitated versus spontaneous production. As reported earlier in the chapter, I've found many preschoolers with ASD are able to imitate intonation and articulation clearly using echolalia with speech breaking down at the spontaneous production level.

It is important to note imitated versus spontaneous production. As reported earlier in the chapter, I've found many preschoolers with ASD are able to imitate intonation and articulation clearly using echolalia with speech breaking down at the spontaneous production level.

Breakdowns at the spontaneous speech level may partially be due to the child not yet having a lexical representation of the word. This is not fully understanding its meaning, perception, and production.[73] Lastly, the provision of tangible reinforcement during standardized testing is a recommended modification for children with ASD as they will be less likely to actively participate for the reward of social interaction.[81,82]

1.27 Evaluating Children Who Are Multilingual

In evaluating a multilingual child, it is recommended that you work with an interpreter and the child's parents. Here, transcription in IPA will truly come in handy. Ask parents what words the child says incorrectly by saying the errored words exactly as the child says them. To the best of your ability, transcribe how the parents report the child to say errored words. Also transcribe the parent-reported accurate production of each word using IPA to help determine distortions, substitutions, phonological processes, or omissions of sounds that the child is making.

Realize that you may not hear meaningful phonemic differences in non-English languages, which can be based on a sound's length, aspiration, tone, or stress. Your ears simply will likely not hear a distinction. For target selection, your goal is to attempt to discover phonological processes or errors that occur in both the child's native language and English.

For instance, the child may delete final consonants, front velar sounds, stop fricatives, and reduce clusters in both languages. By working on suppression of these phonological processes in English, positive gains may generalize to the child's native language due to a researched phenomenon of generalization occurring to non targeted sounds. However, generalization across languages currently has a limited research base.[83,84,85]

The following phonological processes are evident across multiple languages: reduplication, weak syllable deletion, initial/final consonant deletion, voicing errors, consonant harmony assimilation, fronting, backing, stopping, cluster reduction, and gliding.[73]

For further information, a 2017 tutorial by McLeod and Verdon titled *Speech Assessment for Multilingual Children Who Do Not Speak the Same Language(s) as the Speech-Language Pathologist* in the *American Journal of Speech Language Pathology* reviews best practices in assessing speech of multilingual children.[86]

1.28 Chapter Summary

In this chapter, we completed every ASHA recommended component of a speech evaluation: (1) Obtaining a case history; (2) Establishing compliance; (3) Administering a single-word standardized articulation assessment; (4) Administering a supplemental *Consonant Cluster Screener*; (5) Checking for stimulability with maximum cueing (Kelly's Corner Video 1.12); (6) Collecting a connected speech sample; (7) Calculating Percent Consonants Correct (PCC); (8) Calculating Mean Length of Utterance (MLU); (9) Observing oral muscular structure and speech movements; and (10) Obtaining a DDK rate.

We additionally reviewed symptomology to differentially diagnose CAS, dysarthria, ISSD, severe phonological disorder, and articulation impairment. Lastly, we looked at considerations in evaluating populations who are with ASD, multilingual, minimally verbal, and preverbal.

The aim of this book is to empower readers with effective evidence-based practice in the evaluation and treatment of speech sound disorders. It is my hope that this chapter sufficiently covered the basics for you to conduct a thorough, yet ecologically valid, speech evaluation in consideration of realistic time and funding constraints.

References

[1] American Speech Language Hearing Association. Speech Sound Disorders Practice Portal Website. https://www.asha.org/PRPSpecificTopic.aspx?folderid=8589935321. Accessed October 14, 2018

[2] Bernthal JE, Bankson NW, Flipsen P. Articulation and Phonological Disorders: Speech Sound Disorders in Children. 7th ed. Boston: Pearson; 2017

[3] Jacoby GP, Lee L, Kummer AW, Levin L, Creaghead NA. The number of individual treatment units necessary to facilitate functional communication improvements in the speech and language of young children. Am J Speech Lang Pathol. 2002; 11(4):370–380

[4] American Speech Language Hearing Association. Ad Hoc Committee on Apraxia of Speech in Children. Website. http://www.asha.org/TR2007-00278/. Published 2007. Accessed October 14, 2018

[5] Duker PC, Didden R, Sigafoos J. One-to-One Training: Instructional Procedures for Learners with Developmental Disabilities. Austin, TX: Pro-Ed; 2004

[6] Institute of Medicine. Disability in America: Toward a National Agenda for Prevention. Washington, DC: The National Academies Press. https://doi.org/10.17226/1579. Published 1991. Accessed October 14, 2018

[7] Bowen C. Terminology, classification, description, measurement, assessment and targets. In: Bowen C, ed. Children's Speech Sound Disorders. 2nd ed. Hoboken, NJ: Wiley Blackwell; 2015

[8] Dodd B. Differential diagnosis of pediatric speech sound disorder. Curr Dev Disord Rep. 2014; 1(3):189–196

[9] Tung L-C, Lin C-K, Hsieh C-L, Chen CC, Huang CT, Wang CH. Sensory integration dysfunction affects efficacy of speech therapy on children with functional articulation disorders. Neuropsychiatr Dis Treat. 2013; 9:87–92

[10] Gopin CB, Berwid O, Marks DJ, Mlodnicka A, Halperin JM. ADHD preschoolers with and without ODD: do they act differently depending on degree of task engagement/reward? J Atten Disord. 2013; 17(7):608–619

[11] Baker MJ, Koegel RL, Koegel LK. Increasing the social behavior of young children with autism using their obsessive behaviors. Res Pract Persons Severe Disabl. 1998; 23(4):300–308

[12] Law J, Garrett Z, Nye C. Speech and language therapy interventions for children with primary speech and language delay or disorder. Cochrane Database Syst Rev. 2003(3): CD004110

[13] Donaldson AL, Stahmer AC, Team collaboration. Team collaboration: the use of behavior principles for serving students with ASD. Lang Speech Hear Serv Sch. 2014; 45(4):261–276

[14] Nip IS, Green JR, Marx DB. The co-emergence of cognition, language, and speech motor control in early development: a longitudinal correlation study. J Commun Disord. 2011; 44(2):149–160

[15] Nijland L, Terband H, Maassen B. Cognitive functions in childhood apraxia of speech. J Speech Lang Hear Res. 2015; 58(3):550–565

[16] Strand EA. Diagnosis and management of CAS: Dynamic Temporal and Tactile Cueing. Video presentation hosted by University of Texas at Dallas, Callier Center, sponsored by Once Upon A Time Foundation. 2007. Website: https://www.utdallas.edu/calliercenter/events/CAS/. Accessed October 14, 2018

[17] Missiuna C, Gaines BR, Pollock N. Recognizing and referring children at risk for developmental coordination disorder: role of the speech-language pathologist. J Speech Lang Pathol Audiol. 2002; 26(4):172–179

[18] Hill EL. Non-specific nature of specific language impairment: a review of the literature with regard to concomitant motor impairments. Int J Lang Commun Disord. 2001; 36(2):149–171

[19] And AB, Dodd B. Do all speech-disordered children have motor deficits? Clin Linguist Phon. 1996; 10(2):77–101

[20] Carr CW, Moreno-De-Luca D, Parker C, et al. Chiari I malformation, delayed gross motor skills, severe speech delay, and epileptiform discharges in a child with FOXP1 haploinsufficiency. Eur J Hum Genet. 2010; 18(11):1216–1220

[21] Macrae T. Stimulus characteristics of single-word tests of children's speech sound production. Lang Speech Hear Serv Sch. 2017; 48(4):219–233

[22] Minahan J. The Behavior Code Companion: Strategies, Tools, and Interventions for Supporting Students with Anxiety-Related or Oppositional Behaviors. Cambridge, MA: Harvard Education Press; 2014

[23] Morgan PL. Increasing task engagement using preference or choice-making. Remedial Spec Educ. 2006; 27(3):176–187

[24] Matheson AS, Shriver MD. Training teachers to give effective commands: effects on student compliance and academic behaviors. School Psych Rev. 2005; 34(2):209–212

[25] Hester PP, Hendrickson JM, Gable RA. Forty years later—the value of praise, ignoring, and rules for preschoolers at risk for behavior disorders. Educ Treat Child. 2009; 32(4):513–535

[26] Kozima H, Nakagawa C, Yasuda Y. Interactive robots for communication-care: a case-study in autism therapy. ROMAN 2005 IEEE International Workshop on Robot and Human Interactive Communication. 2005.

[27] Zanolli K, Daggett J, Pestine H. The influence of the pace of teacher attention on preschool children's engagement. Behav Modif. 1995; 19(3):339–356

[28] Koegel LK, Koegel BL, Koegel RL, Vernon TW. Pivotal response treatment. In: Luiselli JK, ed. Children and Youth with Autism Spectrum Disorder (ASD): Recent Advancements and Innovations in Assessment, Education, and Intervention. New York, NY: Oxford University Press; 2014:134–144.

[29] Fisher WW, Piazza CC, Bowman LG, Amari A, Owens JC, Amari A. Integrating caregiver report with systematic choice assessment to enhance reinforcer identification. Am J Ment Retard. 1996; 101(1):15–25

[30] Mason SA, McGee GG, Farmer-Dougan V, Risley TR. A practical strategy for ongoing reinforcer assessment. J Appl Behav Anal. 1989; 22(2):171–179

[31] Gable RA, Hester PH, Rock ML, Hughes KG. Back to basics. Intervention Sch Clin. 2009; 44(4):195–205

[32] Sullivan KJ, Kantak SS, Burtner PA. Motor learning in children: feedback effects on skill acquisition. Phys Ther. 2008; 88(6):720–732

[33] Cimpian A, Arce H-MC, Markman EM, Dweck CS. Subtle linguistic cues affect children's motivation. Psychol Sci. 2007; 18(4):314–316

[34] Corpus JH, Lepper MR. The effects of person versus performance praise on children's motivation: gender and age as moderating factors. Educ Psychol. 2007; 27(4):487–508

[35] Flipsen P, Jr, Ogiela DA. Psychometric characteristics of single-word tests of children's speech sound production. Lang Speech Hear Serv Sch. 2015; 46(2):166–178

[36] Vess K, Szczembara R. Testing speech of preschoolers with autism spectrum disorder: impact of imitated versus spontaneous productions. Poster presented at: Annual American Speech, Language and Hearing Association Convention; November, 2019; Ft. Lauderdale, FL

[37] Bleile KM. The Late Eight. 3rd ed. San Diego, CA: Plural Publishing; 2018

[38] Macrae T, Tyler AA. Speech abilities in preschool children with speech sound disorder with and without co-occurring language impairment. Lang Speech Hear Serv Sch. 2014; 45 (4):302–313

[39] Masso S, Baker E, McLeod S, Wang C. Polysyllable speech accuracy and predictors of later literacy development in preschool children with speech sound disorders. J Speech Lang Hear Res. 2017; 60(7):1877–1890

[40] Preston JL, Hull M, Edwards ML. Preschool speech error patterns predict articulation and phonological awareness outcomes in children with histories of speech sound disorders. Am J Speech Lang Pathol. 2013; 22(2):173–184

[41] Miccio AW, Elbert M, Forrest K. The relationship between stimulability and phonological acquisition in children with normally developing and disordered phonologies. Am J Speech Lang Pathol. 1999; 8(4):347–363

[42] Storkel HL. Implementing evidence-based practice: selecting treatment words to boost phonological learning. Lang Speech Hear Serv Sch. 2018; 49(3):482–496

[43] Strand EA, Stoeckel R, Baas B. Treatment of severe childhood apraxia of speech: a treatment efficacy study. J Med Speech-Lang Pathol. 2006; 14(4):297–307

[44] Murray E, McCabe P, Ballard KJ. A systematic review of treatment outcomes for children with childhood apraxia of speech. Am J Speech Lang Pathol. 2014; 23(3):486–504

[45] Rosenbek JC, Lemme ML, Ahern MB, Harris EH, Wertz RT. A treatment for apraxia of speech in adults. J Speech Hear Disord. 1973; 38(4):462–472

[46] McLeod S, van Doorn J, Reed VA. Normal acquisition of consonant clusters. Am J Speech Lang Pathol. 2001; 10(2):99–110

[47] McLeod S, Masso S. Screening Children's Speech: The Impact of Imitated Elicitation and Word Position. Lang Speech Hear Serv Sch. 2019; 50(1):71–82

[48] Storkel HL. The complexity approach to phonological treatment: how to select treatment targets. Lang Speech Hear Serv Sch. 2018; 49(3):463–481

[49] Ertmer DJ. Relationships between speech intelligibility and word articulation scores in children with hearing loss. J Speech Lang Hear Res. 2010; 53(5):1075–1086

[50] McLeod S, Hand L, Rosenthal JB, Hayes B. The effect of sampling condition on children's productions of consonant clusters. J Speech Hear Res. 1994; 37(4):868–882

[51] Girolametto L, Weitzman E. Responsiveness of child care providers in interactions with toddlers and preschoolers. Lang Speech Hear Serv Sch. 2002; 33(4):268–281

[52] Haebig E, McDuffie A, Ellis Weismer S. The contribution of two categories of parent verbal responsiveness to later language for toddlers and preschoolers on the autism spectrum. Am J Speech Lang Pathol. 2013; 22(1):57–70

[53] Shriberg LD, Austin D, Lewis BA, McSweeny JL, Wilson DL. The percentage of consonants correct (PCC) metric: extensions and reliability data. J Speech Lang Hear Res. 1997; 40(4):708–722

[54] Shriberg LD, Kwiatkowski J. Phonological disorders III: a procedure for assessing severity of involvement. J Speech Hear Disord. 1982; 47(3):256–270

[55] Gordon-Brannan M, Hodson BW. Intelligibility/severity measurements of prekindergarten children's speech. Am J Speech Lang Pathol. 2000; 9(2):141–150

[56] Flipsen P, Jr. Speaker-listener familiarity: parents as judges of delayed speech intelligibility. J Commun Disord. 1995; 28 (1):3–19

[57] Bleile K. Evaluating articulation and phonological disorders when the clock is running. Am J Speech Lang Pathol. 2002; 11(3):243–249

[58] Dodd B. Differential Diagnosis and Treatment of Speech Disordered Children. 3rd ed. Hoboken, NJ: Wiley; 2013

[59] Williams P, Stackhouse J. Diadochokinetic skills: normal and atypical performance in children aged 3–5 years. Int J Lang Commun Disord. 1998; 33 Suppl:481–486

[60] Zamani P, Rezai H, Garmatani NT. Meaningful words and non-words repetitive articulatory rate (oral diadochokinesis) in Persian speaking children. J Psycholinguist Res. 2017; 46 (4):897–904

[61] Case J, Grigos MI. Articulatory control in childhood apraxia of speech in a novel word-learning task. J Speech Lang Hear Res. 2016; 59(6):1253–1268

[62] Ziegler W. Task-related factors in oral motor control: speech and oral diadochokinesis in dysarthria and apraxia of speech. Brain Lang. 2002; 80(3):556–575

[63] Dodd B, Holm A, Crosbie S, McIntosh B. Core vocabulary intervention. In: Williams AL, McLeod S, McCauley RJ, eds. Interventions for Speech Sound Disorders in Children. Baltimore, MD: Paul H. Brookes: 2010:117–136

[64] Murray E, McCabe P, Heard R, Ballard KJ. Differential diagnosis of children with suspected childhood apraxia of speech. J Speech Lang Hear Res. 2015; 58(1):43–60

[65] Strand EA, McCauley RJ. Differential diagnosis of severe speech impairment in young children. ASHA Lead. 2008; 13(10):10–13

[66] Robbins J, Klee T. Clinical assessment of oropharyngeal motor development in young children. J Speech Hear Disord. 1987; 52(3):271–277

[67] ASHA Ad Hoc Apraxia Committee American Speech-Language Hearing Association. Childhood Apraxia of Speech. https://www.asha.org/practice-portal/clinical-topics/childhood-apraxia-of-speech/. Published 2007. Accessed October 14, 2018

[68] Shriberg LD, Strand EA, Fourakis M, et al. A diagnostic marker to discriminate childhood apraxia of speech from speech delay: III. theoretical coherence of the pause marker with speech processing deficits in childhood apraxia of speech. J Speech Lang Hear Res. 2017; 60(4):S1135–S1152

[69] Watkins KE, Vargha-Khadem F, Ashburner J, et al. MRI analysis of an inherited speech and language disorder: structural brain abnormalities. Brain. 2002; 125(Pt 3):465–478

[70] Highman C, Leitão S, Hennessey N, Piek J. Prelinguistic communication development in children with childhood apraxia of speech: a retrospective analysis. Int J Speech Lang Pathol. 2012; 14(1):35–47

[71] Argyropoulos GPD, Watkins KE, Belton-Pagnamenta E, et al. Neocerebellar Crus I abnormalities associated with a speech and language disorder due to a mutation in FOXP2. Cerebellum. 2019; 18(3):309–319

[72] Dayan M, Olivito G, Molinari M, Cercignani M, Bozzali M, Leggio M. Impact of cerebellar atrophy on cortical gray matter and cerebellar peduncles as assessed by voxel-based morphometry and high angular resolution diffusion imaging. Funct Neurol. 2016; 31(4):239–248

[73] McLeod S, Baker E. Children's Speech: An Evidence-Based Approach to Assessment and Intervention. Boston, MA: Pearson; 2017

[74] Stoeckel R. 2014. Childhood apraxia of speech: from research to practice. Paper presented at presentation at Minnesota Speech Language Hearing Association Annual Conference; April 11, 2014; Rochester, MN

[75] Duffy JR. Motor Speech Disorders: Substrates, Differential Diagnosis, and Management. 3rd ed. St. Louis, MO: Mosby; 2013

[76] Broome K, McCabe P, Docking K, Doble M. A systematic review of speech assessments for children with autism spectrum disorder: recommendations for best practice. Am J Speech Lang Pathol. 2017; 26(3):1011–1029

[77] Shriberg LD, Paul R, Black LM, van Santen JP. The hypothesis of apraxia of speech in children with autism spectrum disorder. J Autism Dev Disord. 2011; 41(4):405–426

[78] Tierney C, Mayes S, Lohs SR, Black A, Gisin E, Veglia M. How valid is the checklist for autism spectrum disorder when a child has apraxia of speech? J Dev Behav Pediatr. 2015; 36 (8):569–574

[79] Salman MS, Tsai P. The role of the pediatric cerebellum in motor functions, cognition, and behavior: a clinical perspective. Neuroimaging Clin N Am. 2016; 26(3):317–329

[80] Poretti A, Huisman TA. The pediatric cerebellum. Neuroimaging Clin N Am. 2016; 26(3):xiii–xiv

[81] Koegel LK, Koegel RL, Smith A. Variables related to differences in standardized test outcomes for children with autism. J Autism Dev Disord. 1997; 27(3):233–243

[82] Lord C, McGee JP. Educating Children with Autism. Washington DC: National Academy Press; 2001

[83] Gildersleeve-Neumann CE, Kester ES, Davis BL, Peña ED. English speech sound development in preschool-aged children from bilingual English-Spanish environments. Lang Speech Hear Serv Sch. 2008; 39(3):314–328

[84] Gierut JA, Morrisette ML, Ziemer SM. Nonwords and generalization in children with phonological disorders. Am J Speech Lang Pathol. 2010; 19(2):167–177

[85] van der Merwe A, Steyn M. Model-driven treatment of childhood apraxia of speech: positive effects of the speech motor learning approach. Am J Speech Lang Pathol. 2018; 27(1):37–51

[86] McLeod S, Verdon S, International Expert Panel on Multilingual Children's Speech. Tutorial: Speech assessment for multilingual children who do not speak the same language(s) as the speech-language pathologist. Am J Speech Lang Pathol. 2017; 26(3):691–708

2 Setting the Stage for Success: Establishing a Positive Working Relationship

What a child can do in cooperation today, can be done alone tomorrow.

—Lev Vygotsky

2.1 Reviewing the Research: The Pervasive Nature of Communication Disorders

By second grade, children with speech sound disorders are more likely to be rated negatively in academic, behavioral, and social competence by teachers.[1] It is estimated that 34% of children with speech sound disorders additionally present with language impairment.[2]

The outlook is dismal for preschool age children with speech sound disorder and concurrent language impairment. Preschool children with speech and concurrent receptive language impairment are more likely to be rated poorly by their peers compared to typically developing peers. The more severe the level of impairment, the more negative the rating.[3]

Additionally, parents and teachers rate preschoolers with a speech sound disorder and concurrent language impairment as having poorer task orientation, poorer social skills, and a lower frustration threshold. These children are also rated as lacking assertiveness and being more dependent and isolated in the classroom.[4]

The pervasive nature of having a concurrent language impairment is underscored by these children with language impairments demonstrating a greater number of problem behaviors than their nonimpaired peers.

Additionally, children who present with both speech sound disorder and concurrent language impairment are more likely to present with attentional deficit disorder.[5] A recent meta-analytic review indicates that children with attentional deficit disorder are at greater risk for off task and disruptive behavior in the classroom at school age.[6]

Recent meta-analytic research indicates these problem behaviors increase with every year of age.[7] As adults, they are at greater risk for persistent social skill challenges, mental health disorders, and increased unemployment. The more severe the receptive language impairment, the poorer the outcome.[8,9,10]

In Law and colleagues' 29-year follow-up study, 5-year-old children with the most significantly delayed receptive language vocabulary testing performance were more likely as 34-year-old adults to self-report poorly on scales of self-efficacy. Self-efficacy is the belief in an individual's ability to achieve goals. Instead, these adults report having an external locus of control, reporting to have little influence over personal life outcomes.[10]

2.2 Fine Motor, Gross Motor, and Sensory Differences

The pervasive nature of having a speech sound disorder with a concurrent language impairment extends beyond being at higher risk for social, emotional, and attentional difficulties.

Compared to typically developing peers, children who present exclusively with persistent speech sound disorders[11] as well as those who present with concurrent language impairment are at higher risk for fine and gross motor delays.[12,13,14,15,16,17,18,19]

Considering these deficits, meta-analytical research indicates speech language pathologists may be able to indirectly positively impact fine and gross motor skill development. This can be accomplished by providing task-oriented activities within speech language therapy sessions and in home practice projects.[20]

Task-oriented activities have a cause-effect, meaningful, goal achievement component. Examples include a gross motor activity of shooting a basketball or a fine motor activity of putting a coin in a piggy bank. Refer to graduate student Christina's lending library for examples of task-oriented fine and gross motor activities in Video 2.1.

Creative Challenge

Can you create five engaging fine motor and five engaging gross motor activities that are task-oriented having a cause-effect component? Ensure they are developmentally appropriate for preschoolers of diverse etiologies and ability levels. These will serve as engaging activities for speech and language therapy.

Recent research suggests that the presence of speech and language impairments may also correlate with increased sensory system difficulties in the following areas: (1) vestibular, maintaining balance and spatial organization; (2) proprioception, sensing body position, motion, and equilibrium; and (3) tactile, sensing pressure, vibration, movement, pain, and temperature through touch.[21]

Research indicates that children with speech sound disorders and sensory system differences will additionally respond less efficiently to articulation therapy than children with intact sensory systems.[22]

2.3 Pragmatic Communication Deficits

Law and colleagues' 2004 meta analysis indicates that speech language therapy accomplishes more than improvement in speech clarity and expressive language skills. This review indicates that it can also positively impacts behavior.[23]

An emphasis on developing prosocial communication behaviors cannot be overstated. Children with communication disorders are more likely to demonstrate pragmatic difficulties both inside and outside of the classroom environment. These pragmatic challenges specifically include difficulties with attending,[24] following directions,[25] and answering questions.[26]

Research infers that grit, an ability to persist when faced with difficult tasks or adversity, serves as a protective factor in helping children overcome the challenges of having a communication disorder.[27]

Considering the challenges aforementioned, children with communication impairments will likely have to work harder in the classroom than their typically developing peers. For this, speech language pathologists should provide objective encouragement that emphasizes the child's efforts.

Developmental psychologist Carol Dweck explains that emphasizing efforts promotes a growth mindset instead of a fixed one. She defines a fixed mindset as one in which children believe that their abilities, intelligence, and talent are fixed traits like eye color. Conversely, children with a growth mindset believe that talents and abilities can be developed through effort and persistence.[28]

2.4 Impact of Encouragement versus Praise

A powerful tool in helping the child develop a growth mindset is the ongoing provision of objective encouragement. We define verbal encouragement as objective statements highlighting the child's efforts (e.g., "You worked super hard on this!") or specific behaviors (e.g., "You made the snake sound!").

Conversely, receiving praise can contribute to children having a fixed mindset. Praise statements are judgmental of the work (e.g., "Good job!") or the child (e.g., "You're so smart!"). Research indicates that children receiving praise will less likely attempt novel activities. On the other hand, they will more likely attempt novel activities after receiving objective encouragement.[29]

Children who received praise are more likely to develop a fixed mindset regarding their ability. Research indicates this fixed mindset can negatively impact academic engagement and performance throughout their school years.[30,31,32]

2.5 Sensory Processing Deficits

The greater likelihood of having sensory processing deficits indicates that emphasis on children "keeping hands to self" prevents impulsively grabbing materials and touching peers. This creates an environment more conducive to learning.

A replacement behavior is a desirable behavior that replaces an undesirable one. Having children engage in an incompatible replacement behavior, such as interlacing fingers together, effectively eliminates touching peers during group times.

2.6 Primary Goal: Child Develops an Internal Locus of Control

Intervention strategies presented in this chapter propose combining three evidence-based approaches to optimally improve social communication skills while helping the child develop an internal locus of control. *Locus* is Latin for place. Locus of control literally refers to the place of control. A child with an internal locus of control sees himself or herself as an active and effective agent of change in his or her environment.

The ultimate goal of therapy is for the child to develop a strong internal locus of control in which the child believes that success is based on the child's own efforts. This conviction contrasts with a child with a stronger external locus of control who believes failure or success in learning is a result of forces outside of his or her control.

Realistically, both internal and external factors affect a child's ability to learn and achieve goals. However, the child with a strong internal locus of control is better equipped to overcome life's challenges. These challenges can be neurological, such as having concurrent attentional deficits, dyslexia, or motor impairments. These challenges can also be environmental, such as having negligent caregivers, ineffective teachers, and living in poverty.

2.7 Evidence-Based Practice for Optimal Improvement in Behavior

Recent meta-analytic research of over 33 behavioral intervention approaches used in the classroom for elementary age children with attentional deficit disorder indicates three approaches to be the most effective based on both teacher ratings and direct observation. Gaastra and colleagues found these three approaches to be most effective[10,33]:

1. Antecedent-based intervention: Interventions that manipulate antecedent conditions, such as environment, task, or instructional methodology to prevent or decrease problem behavior;
2. Consequence-based interventions: Interventions that use reinforcement, planned ignoring, or discipline to increase desired behavior while decreasing problem behavior;
3. Self-regulation intervention: Interventions aimed at the children's development of self control and problem-solving skills to independently direct behavior toward achieving goals.

These behavioral intervention approaches will be reviewed along with how to effectively implement them singly or in combinations within a therapeutic setting. Doing so establishes an effective working relationship and improves prosocial communication behaviors.

2.7.1 First Approach: Antecedent-Based Intervention by Learning Prosocial Communication Rules

At the initial evaluation and in the beginning stages of therapy, enthusiastically provide objective and specific verbal feedback focused on prosocial behaviors.

Five pivotal areas of pragmatic success are paying attention, answering every question, following every direction, working super hard, and keeping hands to self. Visually model these rules with accompanying gestures.

These proactive behaviors not only set the stage for an effective learning relationship in therapy but also encourage prosocial behaviors for current and future classroom placements.

In teaching prosocial rules during group therapy sessions, I routinely have children state rules, paired with a physical gesture. This review is done in chorus with each other, along with the therapist, considering that research indicates that children learn better when they are actively participating.[25,33]

Pairing gestures with rules not only aids children in actively learning the rules, but also provides for a visual reminder known as a pre-corrective prompt.

A pre-corrective prompt reminds children of a rule prior to activities or contexts that are at high risk for a misbehavior. For example, if I know a child has difficulty keeping "hands to self," we begin the session rehearsing the prompt in choral speech with the accompanying gesture of interlaced fingers. I'll prompt, "What are we going to do?" The children respond with interlaced fingers, "Keep our hands to ourselves."

Pictures instead of gestures can be used as visual reminders. I personally find it difficult to have five pictures on hand at all times. Yet, my hands are always available.

If you are organized and coordinated, having pictures laminated and hung around your neck or within reach in therapeutic or group setting environments would be beneficial. This is considering that it is estimated that more than a third of children with speech sound disorders present with concurrent language impairment.[2]

The five social communication rules are paired with engaging gestures as a checklist to actively review across settings.

See Video 2.2 of intern Maisoun with Sampson going through prosocial rules with accompanying gestures. She is using a cloze procedure in which the last words are omitted for the child to independently fill in the blank to increase active participation in learning.[34]

You'll see a small group demonstrating these same prosocial rules on their last day of summer speech camp in Video 2.3. Their graduation diploma, further emphasizing the rules, is in **Appendix D.**

We routinely review these rules within a group of about 20 preschoolers in our weekly speech and language groups. After reviewing the rules, we reward the group by raining bubbles over them for "following every direction" by both nonverbally and verbally participating in reviewing all of the rules.

In group settings, calling a child's name with a gestural reminder empowers the child to efficiently self-reflect and self-correct. This sole use of a gestural cue lessens the auditory processing demands and distraction to the group's momentum.

The child and I model these rules for caregivers. Caregivers have also reported success in being able to encourage prosocial behaviors using these gestures within the natural environment, such as the grocery store.

Creative Challenge

Can you create three to five prosocial rules for working with preschoolers with communication impairments? What engaging and memorable gestures would you pair with each of the rules? What would a visual representation with pictures demonstrating the desired behavior (never the undesired one) look like? What would your graduation diploma, further emphasizing the rules, look like?

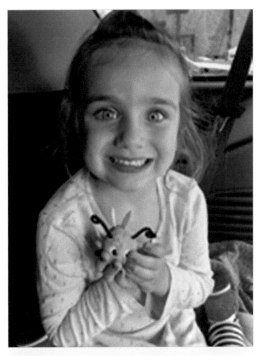

Fig. 2.1 Practicing speech to complete a fine motor-based homework activity, "present."

Lastly, in referring to behaviors with the child, it is important to always present the desired behavior positively. For instance, instead of stating, "no running" or "stop running," say, "walking feet." Stating the behavior positively prevents a preschooler from inadvertently hearing directions to engage in the undesired behavior.[35]

2.7.2 Consequence-Based Interventions: Rewarding Prosocial Behaviors

At the end of each speech therapy session, the child gets a "present," which is a hands-on, home practice activity to be completed with a caregiver. A simple example is making a spider with a small ball of playdough, eight pipe cleaners for legs, and two button eyes.

The child is to request each body part with a carrier phrase, such as "Can you scrape or drop it to me please?" This target request phrase is written on a card for the caregiver to reference in having the child produce it accurately for each toy piece.

▶ Fig. 2.1 displays a picture of Jenna completing a bumblebee with her mother after requesting, "Can you scrape it to me please because I'm a cool girl?" for each bumblebee body part. In producing her target sentence, she is meeting her goals in suppressing phonological processes of fronting /k/ and /g/, cluster reduction, and gliding of /l/ and /r/.

Beyond reinforcing prosocial learning behaviors, these home activities (i.e., "presents") additionally provide guided practice for caregivers in manding. Manding is a verbal behavior used to accomplish goals. In this case, the child is manding, or requesting, natural rewards from the parent during home practice activities.

In 1982, Hart and Risely defined incidental teaching as a four-step process: (1) arranging the setting that contains materials (or activities) of interest to the child; (2) waiting for the child to initiate communication for the object or activity; (3) asking for more elaborate language or advanced speech; and (4) providing the object (or access to the activity) for which the child has initiated communication.[36] Mastering this simple, well-researched process is empowering for both caregivers and therapists in accelerating communication gains across natural environments.[37,38,39,40,41,42,43,44,45,46,47]

Caregivers providing incidental teaching opportunities in the natural environment have been shown to expedite speech and language gains.[48] Caregivers are instructed to have the child mand for toys, foods, drinks, and activities. The child requests for these naturally occurring rewards using a target phrase accurately throughout the daily routine across different settings and with different people to encourage generalization.

Encourage caregivers to participate in selecting natural rewards to encourage a partnership in the therapy process. By having the parents complete the *Interest Inventory Form* shown in ▶ Table 2.1, parents can play a central role in individualizing activities for their children.

Caregivers' participation in the homework process expedites intervention gains.[49]

With preschool age children, research indicates a continuous schedule of reinforcement (1:1 ratio of production of target to reward) to be most effective at the teaching (establishment) stage.

However, an intermittent schedule of reinforcement may be used at the generalization stage depending on the individual child. At the generalization stage, the target is being produced across environments, people, and activities at an 80% accuracy level or higher.[50]

2.8 Meeting the Needs of a Large and Diverse Caseload with Hands-on Activities

During a typical school year, I have a caseload of about 50 preschoolers. Research indicates this to be typical for a public school speech language pathologist. A majority of speech language pathologists unfortunately report caseload sizes as "unmanageable."[51]

For myself, a typical preschool caseload is diverse with preschoolers with autism spectrum disorder, pervasive developmental disorders, language impairment, speech sound disorders, and expressive language impairment. Regardless of impairment, every week I send the same, developmentally appropriate, fine motor, hands-on activities (i.e., "presents") home for preschoolers to practice their unique communication goals.

These hands-on activities are meant to be process-oriented experiences, not product oriented. Process-oriented activities are open-ended in that the child is free to create whatever the child pleases, with the emphasis being on exploration in learning.

Table 2.1 Interest Inventory

Loving Learning: What Makes Learning Memorable and Meaningful ?
We try to individualize your child's learning experience as much as possible in improving communication skills. Your input is invaluable in creating a special and effective learning experience for your child. Please provide your input so we can provide a rich learning experience for your child.

1-What are your child's favorite toys?

2-What are your child's favorite books?

3- What are your child's favorite TV shows?

4-What are your child's favorite movies?

5-What are your child's favorite songs?

6-What are your child's favorite activities or sports?

7-What are your child's favorite places?

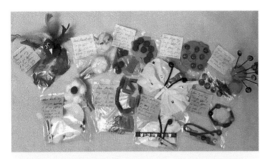

Fig. 2.2 Examples of weekly caregiver home activities for manding within activity-based intervention.

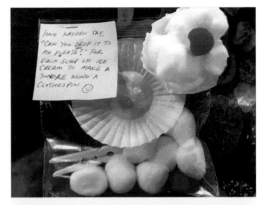

Fig. 2.3 Making a sundae with a clothespin: "Can you drop (give) it to me please?"

These activities are not to be product oriented, in which the emphasis is on recreating a product that is envisioned by a model produced by an adult. For instance, the child may take the spider parts of pipe cleaners and buttons to make a birthday cake with candles or a shining sun after requesting each piece.

Parent or community volunteers can help by making play dough and donating craft items to lessen the financial burden. Keep projects simple, with 8 to 12 pieces for hands-on repetitions for each child. Please see ▶ Fig. 2.2 and ▶ Fig. 2.3 for examples of weekly activities. These activities should be developmentally appropriate and provide for fine motor practice considering the elevated risk of fine motor delays for children with communication disorders.

Additionally, these activities provide an increase in exposure to various textures in consideration of the elevated risk of sensory processing differences for children with communication impairments. Lastly, the variety of home practice projects increases the repertoire of play activities for children with autism spectrum disorder.[52]

Creative Challenge

Can you come up with a simple, engaging, developmentally appropriate fine motor activity that would provide for approximately 8 to 12 pieces to request?

Consider financial and time constraints. (My current budget for materials is $100 for each school year.) Use recycled or nearly free objects that can be purchased in bulk at a local discount store. You could realistically create about 50 simple, hands on activities to send home to each child on a weekly basis.

Another option is developing a lending library for gross and fine motor activities which can be sent home on a rotational basis, such as Christina's lending library in Video 2.1. Each week, when the child returns a toy, the child can receive a new toy. Many children with speech sound disorders have gross motor impairments.[15] These activities provide for additional opportunities to efficiently ignite change in both speech and gross motor systems. Sample activities include the child manding with a target phrase to take turns in activities such as ring toss, bull's eye ball throw, bean bag toss, golfing, bowling, fishing, and the Velcro mitt catch game.

It is important to note that children may not always receive "presents" (i.e., task-oriented homework practice). At the end of each therapy session, the five rules are reviewed. If a child had not "followed every direction" by refusing to participate in an activity, then no present is provided with a clear explanation why.

Reviewing the therapy session by going through the checklist at the end of every session encourages the child to self-monitor. This is a self-management strategy in which a child thinks about his or her own behavior and decides whether it is appropriate. The child then chooses an appropriate replacement behavior.[53] When going through the checklist, children will often self-monitor by honestly answering "no" to a behavioral rule that was not adhered to.

After the child decides that his or her behavior was inappropriate, he or she plans to follow the target rule and is assured that a "present" will be available to earn at the next session, thereby promoting a growth mindset. Research suggests that self-monitoring is an effective strategy for pre-schoolers in increasing on task behavior.[54,55] It has been my experience that typically one instance of not receiving a "present" serves as a strong deterrent to noncompliance. This memorable consequence will likely occur no more than once during a school year for a few children on my caseload.

Not receiving a present is a negative consequence. A negative consequence is an unpleasant result that decreases the probability of a behavior from occurring. In this case, removal of a privilege, which is receipt of a present at the end of therapy, is the negative consequence. Other common negative consequences include ignoring an undesired behavior, such as a tantrum, in which the child is left to experience the emotional and physical discomfort of dysregulation for noncompliance. Another negative consequence is the removal of attention in which the child is in time away for disruptive behavior, such as hurting another child.

Logical negative consequences are consequences directly related to the behavior. They can also serve as an effective teaching tool in deterring problem behavior. Examples of logical negative consequences would be for the child to pick up toys that were dumped from a bucket, dispose of toys that are broken due to misuse, pick up thrown objects, and clean up poured drinks on the floor.

According to Positive Behavior Interventions Support researcher Robert Horner, negative consequences for noncompliance are necessary in that they serve the four important functions: (1) preventing a problem behavior from escalating; (2) preventing a problem behavior from being rewarded; (3) preventing a problem behavior from interrupting instruction; and (4) providing a teaching opportunity to learn which behaviors are inappropriate.[56]

If the child has many behavioral areas to improve upon (e.g., lack of attention, noncompliance, nonresponsive to questions/directions, impulsively grabbing materials/touching others), focus on the single rule that will have the most pivotal impact on the child's pragmatic communication skills.

For instance, "Keeping hands to self" may be a good starting point. This is due to the increased likelihood that a child seeking touch (sensory seeking) will likely come into contact with a child who is avoiding it (sensory avoidant). Considering the increased risk for these sensory differences in preschoolers with communication impairment, touching others could be quite disruptive to learning.[21]

Effective behavior intervention focuses on prevention of misbehavior.[57,58] In preventing noncompliance, it is recommended that therapists select highly engaging activities, deliver natural rewards consistently and swiftly. On-task behavior should be nonverbally (e.g., thumbs up) and verbally acknowledged while ignoring off-task behavior. Working at an accelerated pace also ensures density of practice while maintaining attention.

Rewarding activities are not freely available, but are delivered based upon compliance and accurate production of targeted behavior. The therapist must additionally ensure not to accidentally reward undesired behavior or nonparticipation with attention, removal of undesired tasks, or provision of rewards to a child when disengaged or dysregulated.[59]

2.9 Prevention of Undesired Behavior through Pacing and Change of Activity to Prevent Boredom

With sensory-motivated behaviors (such as verbal clicking or visually staring out of the corner of the eye), attentional deficits, and escape-motivated behaviors, research indicates that maintaining a quick pace and changing activities before boredom occurs can additionally maintain attention and on-task behavior.[60]

See Video 2.4 as intern Alicia engages Ronnie in a fine motor activity of making camouflage binoculars. To help him produce his target, she gains his attention and participation using a cloze procedure (e.g., "Ready, set, _____") to request each feather, and note how she changes the activity to maintain Ronnie's attention.

2.10 Increasing On-Task Behavior through a Token Economy System

In our next video, Video 2.5, you will see intern Taylor using a token economy system with Maria. A token economy system is a form of behavior modification designed to increase desirable behavior and decrease undesirable behavior with tokens. Tokens are symbols representing currency that can be readily delivered, such as stamps, stickers, check marks, poker chips, pretend money, picture cards, and tickets. Tokens are immediately provided to the child for demonstrating a desired behavior and can be exchanged for a desired object or privilege at a later time.[61]

Our social communication goal for Maria is to increase her attention to tasks. Usually, Maria wants to move quickly to the next "party station" (i.e., activity station) after 1 to 2 minutes. (Each station is designed to last around six minutes.) To lengthen the duration of Maria's attention to task, Taylor provides a sticker for completing each activity on the checklist. When all activities are complete, Maria can receive her privilege to proceed to the next party station.

We are also looking to improve Maria's nonverbal communication skills in gross motor activities. Notice Maria's low level of motor imitation. This has also been noted by her preschool teacher. Maria's teacher reports a lack of nonverbal participation in gross motor activities such as yoga, music n' movement, or use of hand gestures within fingerplay songs such as the Eensy, Weensy, Spider.

The most effective token symbols that we've developed use pictures of the child's favorite television or movie characters, which are easily downloaded and printed from the internet. When the child collects all the popular television show or movie characters, the rewarding object or privilege is earned. Another example of a token system is a picture of the child's favored icon cut up into a simple puzzle for the child to earn each piece to connect. Here, token systems serve as both a primary reinforcer, as being rewards in themselves, and a secondary reinforcer as currency to be exchanged later for a reward or privilege.

Creative Challenge

Think of a challenging behavior of a preschool age client. State the appropriate replacement behavior positively and simply with an accompanying gesture and picture. Develop a token system based on the child's unique interests for both the tokens and the reward (object or privilege earned at a later time).

For both Alicia's and Taylor's videos (Video 2.4 and Video 2.5), analyze their use of evidence-based strategies by completing Therapist's Use of Evidence-Based Behavioral Practices Likert Scale (▶ Table 2.2). A Likert scale is a psychological measure that gauges attitudes, values, and opinions by indicating extent of agreement to a series of statements. Use the scale in conjunction with therapy videos to reflect on areas of strength and weakness. Complete the Likert scale for simple visual inspection of areas of strength and weakness. Use your evaluations to envision how practice can be improved upon.

I encourage you to additionally view videos of your own therapy sessions with parent per mission. Complete this scale for objective analysis of your practice. Through the years, we've always found the most beneficial question to ask is "How can we do this better?" For this, I believe "Suggestions for Improvement" in ▶ Table 2.2 will be of most value to you in continually evolving your practice.

2.11 Self-Regulation Intervention: The Child Becomes the Teacher

Over time, the locus of control for the child's behavior is transferred from the adult to the child. A most-to-least prompting hierarchy is used to teach the rules. In a most-to-least prompting hierarchy, prompts are delivered in a sequence of highest level of support provided in the initial stages to prevent errors. Supports are faded over time while maintaining an 80% accuracy level until, eventually, prompts are completely faded.

When first learning prosocial rules, the highest level of support is provided as the therapist, with gestures, provides direct explicit verbal instruction regarding what to do and say. The therapist speaks and moves with the child, and visually models the behavior. The therapist is providing a maximum level of support (scaffolding) which enables the child to work within a child's zone of proximal development.[62] The zone of proximal development is the distance between what the child can independently achieve to the level that is possible for the child with an adult or a more capable peer's assistance.

Vygotsky referred to this assistance as scaffolding, which is prompting that ensures success for the child. Scaffolding provides support for the child to learn at his or her highest level while considering what the child already knows. In therapy, over time, the therapist fades scaffolding gradually to ensure that the child is positively participating verbally and gesturally with the least level of prompting necessary at a minimal 80% accuracy level.

The process of fading scaffolding is the passing of the locus of control externally from the adult to

Table 2.2 Therapist's use of evidence-based behavioral practices

Therapist & Child:					
Please indicate your level of agreement to the following statements. The therapist....	Strongly Disagree	Disagree	Neutral	Agree	Strongly Agree
1. Ensures child's attention is obtained prior to speaking.	1	2	3	4	5
2. States tasks in positive language (e.g., "You get to" instead of "You have to").	1	2	3	4	5
3. Presents tasks/ask questions that the child can answer and models responses as necessary.	1	2	3	4	5
4. Has a 100% response rate to all questions and directions (i.e., "No low-offs).	1	2	3	4	5
5. Uses facial expressions and gestures to convey enthusiasm and/or warmth.	1	2	3	4	5
6. Has rewards in therapist's reach and not the child's reach to elicit requests.	1	2	3	4	5
7. Works at a quick enough pace to maintain attention and ensure frequency of production.	1	2	3	4	5
8. Provides sufficient prompting to ensure 80% accuracy.	1	2	3	4	5
9. Provides specific feedback regarding targeted speech behavior.	1	2	3	4	5
10. Provides specific feedback regarding targeted pro-social behaviors and effort.	1	2	3	4	5
11. Provides objective encouragement instead of praise.	1	2	3	4	5
12. Illustrates prosocial behavioral rules or executive function processes with gestures.	1	2	3	4	5

Strengths:
Weaknesses:
Suggestions for Improvement:

the child internally. This process of transfer is critical in the child's development of an internal locus of control, which is the child being self-efficacious and in control of individual success.[62,63]

2.12 Creating Your Own Eiffel Tower

I likened this process of developing an internal locus of control to constructing the Eiffel Tower. Therapy at its best begins with high expectations of the child's capabilities. Think big and outside of the box. Gustave Eiffel's vision to create the tallest structure in the world was inspired by the Egyptian pyramids.

Also think efficiently like Gustave Eiffel. Knowing that wind was the tower's greatest threat, he spent his limited resource of iron weight primarily on the foundation. Therefore, the tower is able to withstand five times the highest winds ever reported.

Your resource is time, which is very limited. Like Gustave Eiffel, you must use your time judiciously in developing a strong foundation. This strong foundation is the development of an internal locus of control. We are doing so because we understand developing a strong foundation can help the child withstand the "wind." The wind represents the ongoing external forces that children with communication impairments will continually have to overcome.

In building the Eiffel Tower, Gustav used his materials efficiently by paying attention to the details of his work. He incorporated only the most efficient techniques of using a triangular, crisscross design and hollowed the weight of the iron with holes inserted throughout. Both of these strategies resulted in an ability to increase height with every pound of weight optimally used. Take a close look at any bridge today and you'll likely see these details.

Like constructing Gustave's Eiffel Tower, in therapy, details matter. You must cut the fat by only incorporating highly effective evidence-based strategies that produce optimal gains. Our limited therapy time is even more valuable considering neuroplasticity is higher at younger ages. Therefore, absolutely no time should be spent in using ineffectual therapy strategies, such as auditory bombardment. (In auditory bombardment a child is passively engaged in therapy by being "bombarded" with hearing a sound produced accurately numerous times.)

When the Eiffel Tower was being built in 1887, engineers criticized that it would not withstand the wind and would blow over. In 1889, at its tallest height, the scaffolds were meticulously removed. The tower withstood the wind as the tallest structure in the world for the next 40 years. Today, it is equally appreciated for its efficient construction and artistic beauty in being one of the most visited monuments in the world.

In transferring the locus of control to the child, there's the meticulous process of removing the scaffolds while ensuring an 80% success rate. This is when the child becomes his or her own teacher and in doing so will be better able to withstand the on-going "winds" of life in all the challenges that lie ahead. It is in overcoming these challenges that children with communication impairments will develop and reveal their exceptional gifts.

As a therapist, I'm inspired by Gustave Eiffel. I believe we too should have high expectations, look outside of our realm of practice for innovation, adhere to only the most effective of evidence-based strategies, involve in creating new practices, and, most importantly, focusing our efforts on building a strong foundation.

Refer ▶ Fig. 2.4, a photo of the Eiffel Tower in 1889 at its tallest height, yet in a highly scaffolded position with workers and beams ensuring its stature during construction. That year, the workers and beams disappeared and the structure poetically and independently stood on its own. Similarly, the child will be released of assistance and scaffolds with growth, majestically shining on his or her own as in ▶ Fig. 2.5.

Refer to the two video clips of graduate student Christina working with John (Video 2.6 and Video 2.7). In the first clip, John is receiving a maximum level of prompting throughout his first therapy

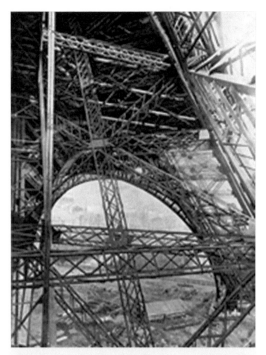

Fig. 2.4 A highly scaffolded Eiffel Tower in 1889.

session. In the second clip, four therapy sessions later, he has taken the role as his own teacher and is independently cueing himself with no assistance.

On a side note, with preschoolers fronting /t/ and /d/ for /k/ and /g/ sounds, we reward approximations such as the glottal stop /h/ in initial stages of therapy. Successive approximations, productions closer to the target, will be differentially rewarded as lingual strength develops with chronological age maturation.

2.13 Positive Behavior Intervention Support to Establish Positive Self-Image and Relationships

*The 1997 Amendment of the Individuals with Disabilities Act (IDEA)*stated that Positive Behavior Interventions and Supports (referred to as PBS formerly and PBIS currently) should be implemented with any child whose behavior "impedes his or her learning or the learning of others."[64] Key components of PBIS intervention are as follows[65]:

1. Positive feedback (e.g., objective encouragement) from the adult to the child 80% of the

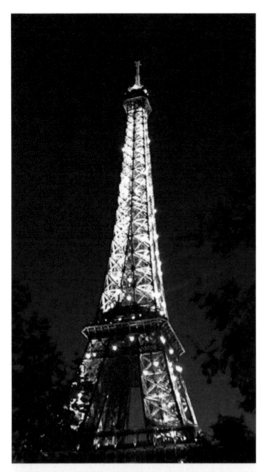

Fig. 2.5 The majestic Eiffel Tower currently.

bank) for later access to an object or privilege (adopted at the school's discretion).

Currently, PBIS has a plethora of studies at the elementary and preschool age levels. Research indicates it to be effective in improving children's self-regulation, concentration, social-emotional functioning, prosocial behaviors, and even possibly mathematical performance.[66,67,68,69]

Research indicates that self-regulation and prosocial problem solving in children with developmental disabilities are of crucial importance for peer rejection occurring more often to children with weak emotional regulation and problem-solving skills.[70] Additionally, research indicates that improvements in self-regulation in preschool is directly linked to improvements in emergent literacy, vocabulary, and math skills at the preschool level, thereby improving kindergarten preparedness.[71]

PBIS suggests three to five rules to be universally adopted at a school-wide level that emphasize safety, respect, and responsibility.[65] PBIS researcher and curriculum developer Elizabeth Steed suggests the following school-wide rules to adapt PBIS concepts to the preschool level[58]: (1) Listen to others; (2) be a good friend; and (3) be a team player.

Creative Challenge

Use Steed's recommended preschool rules to create a *Behavior Matrix*. Simply state rules in positive language appropriate to each routine. For an extra challenge, include pictures demonstrating desired behaviors for visual support.

time with negative feedback (e.g., corrections, redirections) occurring no more than 20% of the time.

2. Explicit teaching and rehearsal and practice of prosocial rules in positive terminology (e.g., "walking feet" not "no running"), using consistent language and visual supports (e.g., posters to serve as visual reminders of school rules).

3. Immediate and consistent response to prosocial behavior with explicit feedback naming the behavior (e.g., "I see you're sharing!").

4. Rules are reinforced by use of common language across staff members and settings (e.g., "Keeping hands to yourself" on the playground, in the classroom, and in the hallway).

5. Inclusion of a token system in which a student receives currency (e.g., play money to go in a

In schools with PBIS implemented, teachers report a decrease in stress, burnout, and increased levels of self-efficacy.[72] Direct observation research of elementary teachers has also found students in PBIS classrooms to receive higher rates of encouragement from teachers and demonstrate fewer behavioral disruptions. Conversely, teachers who provided a lower rate of positive encouragement and a higher rate of negative feedback had significantly more behavioral disruptions in their classrooms.[73]

Additionally, research indicates PBIS results in school staff reporting a higher rate of organizational health.[74] Organizational Health Survey author Wayne Hoy refers to an organizationally healthy school as one "in which the institution, administration, and teachers are in harmony. The school meets functional needs as it successfully copes with disruptive external forces and directs its energies towards its mission."[75]

Similar to PBIS's emphasis on positive encouragement provided to students 80% of the time in establishing prosocial behavior, I adhere to the principle of errorless learning for 80% of the time in speech and language therapy. Errorless learning is ensuring that the child is accurate minimally 80% of the time through gradually fading prompts.[59] Being successful approximately 80% of the time encourages a positive self-image, positive relations, and positive momentum, which have demonstrated efficacy in teaching children with developmental disorders.[76]

Be mindful that encouraging verbal input is at 80% or more and redirection is limited to 20% or less in your interactions with children. If you need to find a way to increase encouragement to 80% in the absence of overt prosocial behaviors, catch the child "being good" by providing positive encouragement for neutral behaviors. For example, "All right! You're keeping your hands to yourself!" when the child is inactively standing.

Another example is providing a verbal direction to a behavior that the child has already begun to engage in, such as "I need you to sit down (as the child is already beginning to sit)."[77,78] Positive behavior and intervention strategists refer to these as "gotchas," which are capturing incidental moments to increase the ratio of positive interactions to negative ones.[65]

Directions can also be provided within the context of naturally reinforcing activities. Naturally reinforcing activities directly reward the child's behavior because they are preferential to the child. By pairing verbal directions with these rewarding activities, "following directions" becomes associated with naturally occurring positive consequences.

Additionally, capitalizing on demonstrating prosocial communication behaviors such as following directions or answering questions during naturally rewarding activities provides more opportunities for positive learning experiences to occur. For example, giving directions to "shoot the ball" to a child who loves basketball allows for feedback on how well she or he follows directions. Asking preferential questions, such as "What color would you like?" enables feedback for consistently answering questions.

2.14 Strategies to Effectively Intervene with Difficult Behaviors

As I stated earlier, I believe 99.99% of improving behavior is based on prevention of off-task and disruptive behavior by emphasizing the prosocial rules previously stated and using evidence-based strategies that establish and maintain momentum.

According to Rappaport and Minahan at the Child Mind Institute (ChildMind.org), inappropriate behaviors often serve to mask underdeveloped skills in children with impairments.[79] For instance, if a child fears embarrassment related to poor articulation, the child may refuse to talk in groups or therapy.

2.15 Discovering the Function of the Behavior

Keep a log of the preceding factors prior to the behavior (antecedents), the child's behavior, and resultant consequences.

This is referred to as an ABC log. The ABC log empowers the therapist with data to effectively change the behavior through discovery of its intent. See ▶ Table 2.3 for an example of an ABC log.

With data from the ABC log, the therapist can then determine what the function of a challenging behavior is to teach an appropriate replacement behavior. This can be done by completing a Functional Behavior Assessment.

A Functional Behavioral Assessment (FBA) is identifying factors, actions, or events in the environment that consistently precede and follow challenging behavior.

According to Neilsen and McEvoy's research, the use of FBA has increased significantly following reauthorization of the Individual with Disabilities Act in 1997, which mandated that an FBA be conducted when children with disabilities demonstrate challenging behaviors.[80]

Two functional behavior assessments, the Motivation Assessment Scale (MAS)[81] and Questions About Behavior Function (QABF),[82] are commonly used by teachers and therapists.[83] Currently, they are both free and publicly accessible on the Internet.

However, research indicates both assessments to have mixed construct validity, which is assessing what they claim to be: functions of maladaptive behaviors.[39,83,84,85,86,87]

Table 2.3 ABC log

Specific behavior of concern					
Date, time, activity, place, people (teacher/peer)	Antecedent: What occurred before the behavior?	Behavior: What was the child's behavior and severity (e.g., duration & frequency)?	Consequence: What happened after the behavior?	Child's Response: How did child respond to the consequence?	Possible Function of the behavior?
Date : Time: Activity : Place : People :					
Date : Time: Activity : Place : People :					
Date : Time: Activity : Place : People :					

Research additionally indicates inconsistencies in inter-rater reliability, which is the level of agreement in judging observed behaviors across raters. These challenges in validity and reliability have been indicated for both MAS[88,89,90] and QAFB[83,91] assessments.

2.16 A Multistep Process to Improve Disruptive Behaviors

Minahan and Rappaport's book *The Behavior Code: A Practical Guide to Understanding and Teaching the Most Challenging Students* presents a multistep process known as FAIR, which stands for creation of a functional hypothesis for the challenging behavior, accommodations, interaction strategies, and response strategies.[92] The four components are:
1. Functional hypothesis: Manage the antecedents or environmental variables that tend to set off the inappropriate behaviors.
2. Accommodations: Reinforce desired behaviors through errorless learning to guarantee success minimally at an 80% level.
3. Interaction strategies: Teach a replacement behavior, such as requesting a break, while strengthening underdeveloped skills that are causing frustration with a level of prompting that ensures success.

4. Response strategies: Respond to an inappropriate behavior in a way that deters it, while avoiding accidentally rewarding it with attention, removal of environmental/tasks demands, or provision of rewards to soothe or calm the child.

A more detailed explanation of the FAIR process and numerous evidence-based articles on how to effectively intervene in a variety of challenging behaviors and mental health conditions are currently available at Childmind.org. Childmind.org is developed by the nonprofit Child Mind Institute with a mission to educate parents and professionals to transform lives of children with mental health and learning disorders.

2.17 Working with a Child Who Refuses to Participate

Lastly, what do with the child who refuses to participate or talk? Nothing. In my professional experience, I have had to sit with a child and do nothing for an entire 30-minute therapy session. It is important to learn that "Nothing begets nothing." Sitting and doing nothing is incredibly boring. I sit alongside the child and refrain from giving him or her attention. I'll have a favorite toy nearby that the child does not get access to unless the child decides to participate. When time is up, the session is over. The child is told that he or she can play with the favored toy or activity the next time. I have effectively used this technique in one-on-one therapy and in group settings when a child has refused to participate. Typically, one session of "nothing begets nothing" has been a memorably boring experience that encourages participation in the future.

When Is "Time Away" Appropriate?

Children put in time away unfortunately are likely the ones who need positive interactions, attention, and time to develop secure relationships with adults the most.[93] Secure, positive relationships cannot be created by spending less time with children. However, if a child has physically or verbally harmed another child or adult, time away is an appropriate option that should be consistently and quickly administered.

2.17.1 Bullying

Children deserve a safe environment free of teasing (i.e., being put-down), and bullying (i.e., repetitive physical, verbal, or relational bullying through exclusion). This is important for both the deliverer and receiver of harm. A clear, zero tolerance message, of hurting others must be salient. It is not appropriate to respond to bullying using planned ignoring. Ignoring bullying can send a message of acceptance of this behavior.[94]

Bullying not only impacts the well-being of the child being bullied but also the child doing the bullying. Even into adult age, negative repercussions impact income level, and mental and physical health for both the victims and victimizers.[95,96]

Prevent bullying through exclusion of peers at the preschool level. Stopbullying.gov, a website managed by the U.S. Department of Health and Human Services, recommends having a firm stance that "everyone can play," to help create an inclusive learning environment.[97] Refer to Stopbullying.gov for further reference.

2.18 Developing Executive Function Skills

Executive function can be defined as the ability to plan and coordinate willful action in the face of alternatives, monitor and update action as necessary, and suppress distracting material by focusing attention on the task at hand.[98]

Research indicates that impairment in executive function skills has a negative impact across social, academic, and motor domains.[99] Executive function can be defined by three primary functions[100]:

1. Inhibitory control: Ability to plan and coordinate a willful action in the face of alternatives;
2. Cognitive flexibility: Ability to monitor and update action as necessary;
3. Working memory: Ability to suppress distracting material by focusing attention on the task at hand to take a task to completion.

What would breakdowns in each area look like in a preschool setting? Suppose it is recess time on a snowy day. The teacher gives a four-step verbal instruction to a group of 4- to 5-year-olds to put on their hat, coat, boots, and gloves.

The child with inhibitory control difficulties may demonstrate difficulties initiating the dressing routine. This child seems to lack a plan on how to get dressed. The child may simply sit in the cubby. The child may also wander off, not appearing to know where or how to begin.

The child with cognitive flexibility difficulties may have a hat and coat on but stop dressing or become dysregulated in an all-out tantrum because of a roadblock. This roadblock could be as simple as not being able to zip a jacket independently. The child does not ask for assistance or proceed to put boots until help is available. This child would likely benefit from focusing on how to identify problems, plan a solution, and perform an action to solve problems.

The child with working memory deficits may put on a hat and coat, and then physically wander off. The child may also abandon an action midway by taking one shoe off and stop due to becoming distracted by another child's actions. Special attention to teaching the child to self-monitor in taking tasks to completion would be of great benefit for this child.

Populations of children who are at greater risks for executive function deficits include children with attention deficit disorder,[101] autism spectrum disorder,[102] cognitive impairment,[103] developmental coordination disorder,[104] Down's syndrome,[105] language impairment,[106] low birthweight,[107] and Smith-Magenis syndrome.[108]

Meta-analytic research indicates that improvement in one of these three areas of executive function (inhibitory control, cognitive flexibility, and working memory) will not likely generalize to improvement in the other areas.[109]

For this, we incorporate a multistep approach that holistically addresses all three major areas of executive function. In improving executive function skills, we use multi-modal cueing with a most to least prompting hierarchy to teach these complex processes. Lastly, we remove scaffolds and transfer the locus of control to the child while ensuring an 80% accuracy level.

After learning this process, the child will be challenged to independently use executive function skills to solve problems, initiate, and complete tasks across situations. A visual checklist is invaluable for the child to independently self monitor in planning, initiating, executing, and taking tasks to completion.

In Chapter 5, Developing Educationally Rich Activities, we review proven methods to improve executive function.

2.19 Chapter Summary

In this chapter, we reviewed the pervasive nature of communication disorders and how they often concurrently present with attentional, social, fine motor, gross motor, sensory, and executive function deficits. We discussed comprehensively treating children by concurrently treating multiple developmental domains.

Also, we reviewed how social-emotional well being at adult age can be negatively impacted by language impairment. These can be indicated by poorer employment outcomes, a more negative self-perception, poorer self-efficacy, and an external locus of control.[8]

This knowledge empowers us to proactively work to change these outcomes. We can make a difference for children with communication impairments by fostering an internal locus of control through emphasis on effort, teaching prosocial communicative behaviors, and providing rich learning experiences that treat the whole child. See Kelly's Corner Video 2.8 for further explanation of teaching prosocial behaviors.

Importantly, we can intelligently provide scaffolds to help preschoolers perform at their highest levels across developmental domains. In doing so at an early age, with neuroplasticity at a high level, optimal neuronal change can transpire.

We can gradually remove these scaffolds after building a strong foundation. Lastly, scaffolding can be entirely removed as the child "becomes the teacher" which will empower the child to develop the self-efficacy necessary to overcome the adversities of having a communication impairment.

References

[1] Overby M, Carrell T, Bernthal J. Teachers' perceptions of students with speech sound disorders: a quantitative and qualitative analysis. Lang Speech Hear Serv Sch. 2007; 38 (4):327–341

[2] Eadie P, Morgan A, Ukoumunne OC, Ttofari Eecen K, Wake M, Reilly S. Speech sound disorder at 4 years: prevalence, comorbidities, and predictors in a community cohort of children. Dev Med Child Neurol. 2015; 57(6):578–584

[3] Gertner BL, Rice ML, Hadley PA. Influence of communicative competence on peer preferences in a preschool classroom. J Speech Hear Res. 1994; 37(4):913–923

[4] McCabe PC. Social and behavioral correlates of preschoolers with specific language impairment. Psychol Sch. 2005; 42 (4):373–387

[5] McGrath LM, Hutaff-Lee C, Scott A, Boada R, Shriberg LD, Pennington BF. Children with comorbid speech sound disorder and specific language impairment are at increased risk for attention-deficit/hyperactivity disorder. J Abnorm Child Psychol. 2008; 36(2):151–163

[6] Gaastra GF, Groen Y, Tucha L, Tucha O. The effects of classroom interventions on off-task and disruptive classroom behavior in children with symptoms of attention-deficit/hyperactivity disorder: a meta-analytic review. PLoS One. 2016; 11(2):e0148841

[7] Curtis PR, Frey JR, Watson CD, Hampton LH, Roberts MY. Language disorders and problem behaviors: a meta-analysis. Pediatrics. 2018; 142(2):e20173551

[8] Marton K, Abramoff B, Rosenzweig S. Social cognition and language in children with specific language impairment (SLI). J Commun Disord. 2005; 38(2):143–162

[9] Beitchman J, Wilson B, Johnson C. et al. Fourteen-year fol low-up of speech/language-impaired and control children: psychiatric outcome. J Am Acad Child Adolesc Psychiatry. 2001; 40(1):75–82

[10] Law J, Rush R, Schoon I, Parsons S. Modeling developmental language difficulties from school entry into adulthood: literacy, mental health, and employment outcomes. J Speech Lang Hear Res. 2009; 52(6):1401–1416

[11] Redle E, Vannest J, Maloney T, et al. Functional MRI evidence for fine motor praxis dysfunction in children with persistent speech disorders. Brain Res. 2015; 1597:47–56

[12] Cheng H-C, Chen H-Y, Tsai C-L, Chen Y-J, Cherng R-J. Comorbidity of motor and language impairments in preschool children of Taiwan. Res Dev Disabil. 2009; 30(5):1054–1061

[13] Webster RI, Majnemer A, Platt RW, Shevell MI. Motor function at school age in children with a preschool diagnosis of developmental language impairment. J Pediatr 2005;146(1) 80–85

[14] Müürsepp I, Ereline J, Gapeyeva H, Pääsuke M. Motor performance in 5-year-old preschool children with developmental speech and language disorders. Acta Paediatr. 2009; 98(8):1334–1338

[15] Newmeyer AJ, Grether S, Grasha C, et al. Fine motor function and oral-motor imitation skills in preschool-age children with speech-sound disorders. Clin Pediatr (Phila). 2007; 46 (7):604–611

[16] Hill EL. Non-specific nature of specific language impairment: a review of the literature with regard to concomitant

motor impairments. Int J Lang Commun Disord. 2001; 36 (2):149–171

[17] Visscher C, Houwen S, Scherder EJ, Moolenaar B, Hartman E. Motor profile of children with developmental speech and language disorders. Pediatrics. 2007; 120(1):e158–e163

[18] Iverson JM, Braddock BA. Gesture and motor skill in relation to language in children with language impairment. J Speech Lang Hear Res. 2011; 54(1):72–86

[19] Rechetnikov RP, Maitra K. Motor impairments in children associated with impairments of speech or language: a meta-analytic review of research literature. Am J Occup Ther. 2009; 63(3):255–263

[20] Smits-Engelsman BC, Blank R, van der Kaay AC, et al. Efficacy of interventions to improve motor performance in children with developmental coordination disorder: a combined systematic review and meta-analysis. Dev Med Child Neurol. 2013; 55(3):229–237

[21] Takarae Y, Luna B, Minshew NJ, Sweeney JA. Patterns of visual sensory and sensorimotor abnormalities in autism vary in relation to history of early language delay. J Int Neuropsychol Soc. 2008; 14(6):980–989

[22] Tung LC, Lin CK, Hsieh CL, Chen CC, Huang CT, Wang CH. Sensory integration dysfunction affects efficacy of speech therapy on children with functional articulation disorders. Neuropsychiatr Dis Treat. 2013; 9:87–92

[23] Law J, Garrett Z, Nye C. The efficacy of treatment for children with developmental speech and language delay/disorder: a meta-analysis. J Speech Lang Hear Res. 2004; 47 (4):924–943

[24] McCabe PC, Marshall DJ. Measuring the social competence of preschool children with specific language impairment: correspondence among informant ratings and behavioral observations. Topics Early Child Spec Educ. 2006; 26 (4):234–246

[25] Gill CB, Klecan-Aker J, Roberts T, Fredenburg KA. Following directions: rehearsal and visualization strategies for children with specific language impairment. Child Lang Teach Ther. 2003; 19(1):85–103

[26] Deevy P, Leonard LB. The comprehension of wh-questions in children with specific language impairment. J Speech Lang Hear Res. 2004; 47(4):802–815

[27] Harrison LJ, McLeod S. Risk and protective factors associated with speech and language impairment in a nationally representative sample of 4- to 5-year-old children. J Speech Lang Hear Res. 2010; 53(2):508–529

[28] Dweck CS. Mindset: The New Psychology of Success. New York, NY: Ballantine Books; 2016

[29] Cimpian A, Arce H-MC, Markman EM, Dweck CS. Subtle linguistic cues affect children's motivation. Psychol Sci. 2007; 18(4):314–316

[30] Gunderson EA, Gripshover SJ, Romero C, Dweck CS, Goldin-Meadow S, Levine SC. Parent praise to 1–3 year-olds predicts children's motivational frameworks 5 years later. Child Dev. 2013; 84(5):1526–1541

[31] Ginsburg GS, Bronstein P. Family factors related to children's intrinsic/extrinsic motivational orientation and academic performance. Child Dev. 1993; 64(5):1461–1474

[32] Dweck CS, Walton GM, Cohen GL. Academic tenacity: mindsets and skills that promote long-term learning. Bill & Melinda Gates Foundation. Website. http://k12education. gatesfoundation.org/resource/academic-tenacity-mindsets-and-skills-that-promote-long-term-learning/ Published 2014. Accessed August 16, 2018

[33] Feldman K, Denti L. High-access instruction: practical strategies to increase active learning in diverse classrooms. Focus Except Child. 2017; 36(7)

[34] Bellon-Harn ML, Credeur-Pampolina ME, Leboeuf L. Scaffolded-language intervention: speech production outcomes. Comm Disord Q. 2012; 34(2):120–132

[35] Trussell RP. Classroom universals to prevent problem behaviors. Intervention Sch Clin. 2008; 43(3):179–185

[36] Hart BM, Risley TR. How to Use Incidental Teaching for Elaborating Language. Austin, TX: Pro-ed; 1982

[37] Koegel RL, Camarata S, Koegel LK, Ben-Tall A, Smith AE. Increasing speech intelligibility in children with autism. J Autism Dev Disord. 1998; 28(3):241–251

[38] Yoder PJ, Warren SF. Relative treatment effects of two prelinguistic communication interventions on language development in toddlers with developmental delays vary by maternal characteristics. J Speech Lang Hear Res. 2001; 44 (1):224–237

[39] Ganz JB, Simpson RL. Effects on communicative requesting and speech development of the picture exchange communication system in children with characteristics of autism. J Autism Dev Disord. 2004; 34(4):395–409

[40] Camarata S. Naturalistic intervention for speech intelligibility and speech accuracy. In: Williams AL, McLeod S, McCauley RJ, eds. Interventions for Speech Sound Disorders in Children. Baltimore, MD: Paul H. Brookes; 2010:381–405

[41] Scherer N, Kaiser AP. Enhanced milieu teaching with phonological emphasis: application for children with CLP in treatment of sound disorders in children. In Williams AL, McLeod S, McCauley RJ, eds. Interventions for Speech Sound Disorders in Children. Baltimore, Md: Paul H. Brookes; 2010:427–452

[42] Thiemann-Bourque KS. Instruction using the Picture Exchange Communication Systems (PECS) appears to enhance generalization of communication skills among children with autism in comparison to Responsive Education and Prelinguistic Milieu Teaching (RPMT). Evid Based Commun Assess Interv. 2010; 4(4):192–195

[43] Roberts MY, Kaiser AP. The effectiveness of parent-implemented language interventions: a meta-analysis. Am J Speech Lang Pathol. 2011; 20(3):180–199

[44] Kaiser AP, Roberts MY. Parent-implemented enhanced milieu teaching with preschool children who have intellectual disabilities. J Speech Lang Hear Res. 2013; 56(1):295–309

[45] Dale PS, Hayden DA. Treating speech subsystems in childhood apraxia of speech with tactual input: the PROMPT approach. Am J Speech Lang Pathol. 2013; 22(4):644–661

[46] Bauer SM, Jones EA. Requesting and verbal imitation intervention for infants with Down syndrome: generalization, intelligibility, and problem solving. J Dev Phys Disabil. 2014; 27(1):37–66

[47] Roberts MY, Kaiser AP, Wolfe CE, Bryant JD, Spidalieri AM. Effects of the teach-model-coach-review instructional approach on caregiver use of language support strategies and children's expressive language skills. J Speech Lang Hear Res. 2014; 57(5):1851–1869

[48] Günther T, Hautvast S. Addition of contingency management to increase home practice in young children with a speech sound disorder. Int J Lang Commun Disord. 2010; 45 (3):345–353

[49] Bowen C, Cupples L. PACT: parents and children together in phonological therapy. Adv Speech Lang Pathol. 2006; 8 (3):282–292

[50] Kazdin AE. Behavior Modification in Applied Settings. Belmont, CA: Wadsworth/Thomson Learning; 2013

[51] Katz LA, Maag A, Fallon KA, Blenkarn K, Smith MK. What makes a caseload (un)manageable? School-based speech-language pathologists speak. Lang Speech Hear Serv Sch. 2010; 41(2):139–151

2

47

[52] Yoder P, Stone WL. A randomized comparison of the effect of two prelinguistic communication interventions on the acquisition of spoken communication in preschoolers with ASD. J Speech Lang Hear Res. 2006; 49(4):698–711

[53] Rafferty LA. Step-by-step: teaching students to self-monitor. Teach Except Child. 2010; 43(2):50–58

[54] Haas-Warner SJ. Effects of self-monitoring on preschoolers' on-task behavior. Top Early Child Spec Educ. 1991; 11(2):59–73

[55] McFarland L, Saunders R, Allen S. Reflective practice and self-evaluation in learning positive guidance: experiences of early childhood practicum students. Early Child Educ J. 2009; 36(6):505–511

[56] Sailor W, Dunlap G, Sugai G, Horner R. Handbook of Positive Behavior Support. New York: Springer; 2009

[57] Carter DR, Norman RK. Class-wide positive behavior support in preschool: improving teacher implementation through consultation. Early Child Educ J. 2010; 38(4):279–288

[58] Steed EA. Adapting the behavior education program for preschool settings. Beyond Behav. 2011; 20(1):37–41

[59] Duker PC, Didden R, Sigafoos J. One-to-One Training: Instructional Procedures for Learners with Developmental Disabilities. Austin, TX: Pro-Ed; 2004

[60] Roberts-Pennell D, Sigafoos J. Teaching young children with developmental disabilities to request more play using the behaviour chain interruption strategy. J Appl Res Intellect Disabil. 1999; 12(2):100–112

[61] Reitman D, Murphy MA, Hupp SDA, O'Callaghan PM. Behavior change and perceptions of change: evaluating the effectiveness of a token economy. Child Fam Behav Ther. 2004; 26(2):17–36

[62] Vygotsky LS, Cole M. Mind in Society: The Development of Higher Psychological Processes. Cambridge, MA: Harvard University Press; 1978

[63] Bandura A. Self-Efficacy in Changing Societies. 2nd ed. Cambridge, UK: Cambridge University Press; 2010

[64] U.S. Department of Education. Individuals with Disabilities Education Act Amendments of 1997

[65] OSEP Technical Assistance Center on Positive Behavioral Interventions and Supports. Positive Behavioral Interventions & Supports. Website: http://www.pbis.org. Accessed August 19, 2018

[66] Bradshaw CP, Waasdorp TE, Leaf PJ. Effects of school-wide positive behavioral interventions and supports on child behavior problems. Pediatrics. 2012; 130(5):e1136–e1145

[67] Jolstead KA, Caldarella P, Hansen B, Korth BB, Williams L, Kamps D. Implementing positive behavior support in preschools: an exploratory study of CW-FIT Tier 1. J Posit Behav Interv. 2016; 19(1):48–60

[68] Muscott HS, Mann EL, LeBrun MR. Positive behavioral interventions and supports in New Hampshire: effects of large-scale implementation of schoolwide positive behavior support on student discipline and academic achievement. J Posit Behav Interv. 2008; 10(3):190–205

[69] Steed EA, Pomerleau T, Muscott H, Rohde L. Program-wide positive behavioral interventions and supports in rural preschools. Rural Spec Educ Q. 2017; 32(1):38–46

[70] Odom SL, Zercher C, Li S, Marquart JM, Sandall S, Brown WH. Social acceptance and rejection of preschool children with disabilities: a mixed-method analysis. J Educ Psychol. 2006; 98(4):807–823

[71] McClelland MM, Cameron CE, Connor CM, Farris CL, Jewkes AM, Morrison FJ. Links between behavioral regulation and preschoolers' literacy, vocabulary, and math skills. Dev Psychol. 2007; 43(4):947–959

[72] Ross SW, Romer N, Horner RH. Teacher well-being and the implementation of school-wide positive behavior interventions and supports. J Posit Behav Interv. 2011; 14(2):118–128

[73] Reinke WM, Herman KC, Stormont M. Classroom-level positive behavior supports in schools implementing SW-PBIS. J Posit Behav Interv. 2012; 15(1):39–50

[74] Bradshaw CP, Koth CW, Thornton LA, Leaf PJ. Altering school climate through school-wide positive behavioral interventions and supports: findings from a group-randomized effectiveness trial. Prev Sci 2009;10(2):100–115

[75] Hoy WK. Educational Administration: Theory, Research, and Practice. 9th ed. New York, NY: McGraw-Hill; 2013

[76] Mueller MM, Palkovic CM, Maynard CS. Errorless learning: review and practical application for teaching children with pervasive developmental disorders. Psychol Sch. 2007; 44(7):691–700

[77] Walker HM, Ramsey E, Gresham FM. Antisocial Behavior in School: Evidence-Based Practices. Belmont, CA: Thomson/Wadsworth; 2004

[78] Lewis TJ, Hudson S, Richter M, Johnson N. Scientifically supported practices in emotional and behavioral disorders: a proposed approach and brief review of current practices. Behav Disord. 2004; 29(3):247–259

[79] Rappaport N, Minahan J. Breaking the behavior code: how teachers can read and respond more effectively to disruptive students. Child Mind Institute: Childmind.org. Website: https://childmind.org/article/breaking-behavior-code. Accessed August 18, 2018

[80] Neilsen SL, McEvoy MA. Functional behavioral assessment in early education settings. J Early Interv. 2004; 26(2):115–131

[81] Durand VM, Crimmins DB. The Motivation Assessment Scale (MAS) Administration Guide. Topeka, Kan.: Monaco & Associates; 1992

[82] Paclawskyj TR. Questions about Behavioral Function (QABF): A Behavioral Checklist for Functional Assessment of Aberrant Behavior. LSU Historical Dissertations and Thesis. 6855; 1998

[83] Koritsas S, Iacono T. Psychometric comparison of the motivation assessment scale (MAS) and the Questions About Behavioral Function (QABF). J Intellect Disabil Res. 2013; 57(8):747–757

[84] Bihm EM, Kienlen TL, Ness ME, Poindexter AR. Factor structure of the motivation assessment scale for persons with mental retardation. Psychol Rep 1991;68(3 Pt 2):1235–1238

[85] Matson JL, Bamburg JW, Cherry KE, Paclawskyj TR. A validity study on the Questions about Behavioral Function (QABF) scale: predicting treatment success for self-injury, aggression, and stereotypies. Res Dev Disabil. 1999; 20(2):163–175

[86] Paclawskyj TR, Matson JL, Rush KS, Smalls Y, Vollmer TR. Questions About Behavior Function (QABF): a behavioral checklist for functional assessment of aberrant behavior. Res Dev Disabil. 2000; 21(3):223–229

[87] Paclawskyj TR, Matson JL, Rush KS, Smalls Y, Vollmer TR. Assessment of the convergent validity of the Questions About Behavior Function scale with analogue functional analysis and the motivation assessment scale. J Intellect Disabil Res. 2001; 45(Pt 6):484–494

[88] Zarcone JR, Rodgers TA, Iwata BA, Rourke DA, Dorsey MF. Reliability analysis of the motivation assessment scale: a failure to replicate. Res Dev Disabil. 1991; 12(4):349–360

[89] Sigafoos J, Kerr M, Roberts D. Interrater reliability of the motivation assessment scale: failure to replicate with aggressive behavior. Res Dev Disabil. 1994; 15(5):333–342

[90] Newton JT, Sturmey P. The motivation assessment scale: inter-rater reliability and internal consistency in a British sample. J Ment Defic Res. 1991; 35(Pt 5):472–474

[91] May ME, Sheng Y, Chitiyo M, Brandt RC, Howe AP. Internal consistency and inter-rater reliability of the Questions About Behavioral Function (QABF) rating scale when used by teachers and paraprofessionals. Educ Treat Child. 2014; 37(2):347–364

[92] Minahan J, Rappaport N. The Behavior Code: A Practical Guide to Understanding and Teaching the Most Challenging Students. Cambridge, MA: Harvard Education Press; 2013

[93] Williford AP, Vick Whittaker JE, Vitiello VE, Downer JT. Children's engagement within the preschool classroom and their development of self-regulation. Early Educ Dev. 2013; 24(2):162–187

[94] Gini G, Pozzoli T, Borghi F, Franzoni L. The role of bystanders in students' perception of bullying and sense of safety. J Sch Psychol. 2008; 46(6):617–638

[95] Vlachou M, Andreou E, Botsoglou K, Didaskalou E. Bully/victim problems among preschool children: a review of current research evidence. Educ Psychol Rev. 2011; 23(3):329–358

[96] Wolke D, Copeland WE, Angold A, Costello EJ. Impact of bullying in childhood on adult health, wealth, crime, and social outcomes. Psychol Sci. 2013; 24(10):1958–1970

[97] U.S. Department of Health and Human Services. Stop Bullying on the Spot. Website: http://www.stopbullying.gov. Accessed August 13, 2018

[98] Miller EK, Wallis JD. Executive function and higher-order cognition: definition and neural substrates. In: Squire LR, ed. Encyclopedia of Neuroscience, Volume 4. Oxford, England: Academic Press; 2009:99–104

[99] McClelland M, Cameron C. Developing together: the role of executive function and motor skills in children's early academic lives. Early Child Res Q. 2019; 46:142–151

[100] MacDonald M, Lipscomb S, McClelland MM, et al. Relations of preschoolers' visual-motor and object manipulation skills with executive function and social behavior. Res Q Exerc Sport. 2016; 87(4):396–407

[101] Sjöwall D, Thorell LB. A critical appraisal of the role of neuropsychological deficits in preschool ADHD. Child Neuropsychol. 2019; 25(1):60–80

[102] Stephens RL, Watson LR, Crais ER, Reznick JS. Infant quantitative risk for autism spectrum disorder predicts executive function in early childhood. Autism Res. 2018; 11 (11):1532–1541

[103] Alloway TP. Working memory and executive function profiles of individuals with borderline intellectual functioning. J Intellect Disabil Res. 2010; 54(5):448–456

[104] Biotteau M, Chaix Y, Blais M, Tallet J, Péran P, Albaret JM. Neural Signature of DCD: a critical review of MRI neuroimaging studies. Front Neurol. 2016; 7:227

[105] Daunhauer LA, Fidler DJ, Hahn L, Will E, Lee NR, Hepburn S. Profiles of everyday executive functioning in young children with down syndrome. Am J Intellect Dev Disabil. 2014; 119 (4):303–318

[106] Yang HC, Gray S. Executive function in preschoolers with primary language impairment. J Speech Lang Hear Res. 2017; 60(2):379–392

[107] Miller SE, DeBoer MD, Scharf RJ. Executive functioning in low birth weight children entering kindergarten. J Perinatol. 2018; 38(1):98–103

[108] Wilde L, Oliver C. Brief report: Contrasting profiles of everyday executive functioning in Smith–Magenis syndrome and Down syndrome. J Autism Dev Disord. 2017; 47(8):2602–2609

[109] Kassai R, Futo J, Demetrovics Z, Takacs ZK. A meta-analysis of the experimental evidence on the near- and far-transfer effects among children's executive function skills. Psychol Bull. 2019; 145(2):165–188

3 Selecting Complex Treatment Targets

Act as if what you do makes a difference. It does.
—William James

There isn't enough time for inefficient practice. In 2018 an ASHA survey of 279 speech-language pathologists serving preschool age populations throughout the US ranked high caseload as the second most pressing challenge to effectively treating preschoolers. The related burden of excessive paperwork ranked first.[1]

In the private sector, insurance companies often require standardized test score improvements for continuation of therapy within a month, after only four to five therapy sessions. Also, recent research indicates that most children are largely receiving a total of 30 to 60 minutes of speech therapy weekly, regardless of severity level.[2]

There is currently a mismatch in realistic time limitations in the services we provide and the speech sound disorder efficacy research we reference, which is based on about twice as much intervention time. Speech intervention efficacy studies are largely based on a schedule of two or three 30- to 60-minute sessions weekly.[3] Additionally, current meta-analytic research suggests that speech therapy gains typically become evident after 8 weeks of therapy, not four or five.[4]

Your current hurdle could be a high caseload which could limit direct therapy time or loss of insurance coverage, which would preemptively cease services. Either way, the solution remains the same: work smarter with the limited time provided.

My public preschool caseload of preschoolers has doubled from 25 preschoolers to about 50 in the past 18 years. Necessity has forced me to attend to the details. These details are in providing only the best evidence-based practices for gains to develop efficiently.

This chapter will specifically cover how to select the most complex treatment targets for optimal gains. The most complex treatment targets that we will select will result in improvement in both simpler and complex untreated sounds.

I will present evidence-based maxims to select treatment targets that optimally induce change. These recommendations are evidence based strategies implemented over four to five 45-minute therapy sessions over a 6 weeks' time period with 82 preschoolers.

A four to five, 45-minute session time constraint for gains to occur is reported by my private practicing colleagues to be a common expectation from insurance companies. Losses of coverage could easily occur from lack of measurable progress in a month.

For this, I present to you how I have implemented, adapted, and applied the complexity approach to select targets. The approach is not new. It has been developed and researched over the past two decades.[5,6,7,8,9] I will incorporate this research with current findings from our summer preschool speech intervention program.

For five consecutive years our impressive speech gains, after four to five 45-minute sessions, were consistently replicated each year. This consistency in results suggests that these outcomes should not be attributed to chance.

Please see ▶ Table 3.1 for a visual picture of how sounds universally develop.[10] Gierut has extensively researched and advocated for integration of these universals into our field to effectively evaluate and treat speech sound disorders. She advocates for the selection of complex targets to ignite optimal change across developmental domains.[11]

Understanding these universals helps in selecting complex targets. It also illustrates the trajectory of growth during therapy. Regardless of intervention approach in selecting simple or complex treatment targets, sounds on the lower steps will uniformly develop before higher ones.

Our research demonstrates that with the complexity approach, the higher you aim, the more quickly the child will traverse the staircase, demonstrating improvement on simpler sounds and phonological processes before more complex ones.

Each stair step cannot exist without the one below it. In selecting a complex treatment target, assume the step below will spontaneously develop before the step atop with requiring direct treatment for simpler sounds on the bottom steps.

This is due to a cascading effect that is unidirectional in that it only moves in a downward

Table 3.1 Implicational universals for phonological development: a stair step progression

3-Elements Clusters (require presence of 2-element clusters)
2-Element Clusters (require presence of affricates)
Affricates (require presence of fricatives)
Fricatives (require presence of stops)
Stops (voiceless stops generally require voiced stops)

direction. More complex sounds result in natural remediation of less complex ones. On the other hand, less complex treatment sounds do not result in spontaneous development of more complex ones.

Cognates are consonant minimal pairs produced in the same place and manner but differ in voicing. Generally, when selecting between cognates, select the voiced cognate as a treatment target. In the English language voiced cognates typically imply the presence of their voiceless pair.

The exception in English to voiced cognates being more complex than voiceless cognates is in the developmental order of oral stops. Voiced cognates /b, d, g/ generally develop before voiceless cognates /p, t, k/. This exception may possibly be due to /p, t, k/ typically being aspirated in the initial position of words and in the beginning of stressed syllables (e.g., volunteer → /ˌvɑlənˈtʊ/).

With this background regarding the hierarchy of the complexity of our speech sound system, we can more easily discuss complexity levels and maxims to select the most effective treatment targets.

3.1 Maxim #1: Select 3-Element Consonant Clusters over 2-Element Clusters

In our intervention, graduate students had the option of selecting a 3-element or 2-element consonant cluster treatment target based on a combination of factors. Graduate students considered the individual child's error sounds, phonological processes, and stimulability. We define stimulability as the child's ability to produce targets correctly given a maximum level of prompting.

Our detailed error analysis of 82 preschoolers after four to five 45-minute therapy sessions indicated that the selection of 3-element treatment targets (e.g., /spl/) resulted in substantially greater gains than selection of 2-element clusters (e.g., /sl/).

Single-word standardized testing results indicated that those treated with 3-element clusters had greater improvements in untreated sounds. The 3-element consonant cluster group improved in producing an average of 10 sounds correctly. Whereas, the 2-element consonant cluster group improved in producing an average of only six sounds correctly.

Furthermore, detailed item analysis of sound improvement for 82 preschoolers indicated that the preschoolers treated with 3-element consonant clusters made substantially greater gains.

The 3-element consonant cluster treatment targets resulted in not only production of a greater number of consonants correct, but also greater improvement in both more complex affricate and 2-element cluster sounds.

The 3-element group averaged 39% improvement in affricates versus only an average of 5% improvement for the 2-element consonant cluster group.

The 3-element consonant cluster group also made greater gains producing untreated 2-element consonant clusters with a 13% average improvement versus only a 7% improvement for the 2-element consonant cluster group.

Skeptically, we can ask, "Which came first: the chicken or the egg?" Perhaps graduate students selected 3-element clusters for children better able to produce 3-element clusters with a maximum level of cueing at baseline. In this case, these children would have had naturally better speech motor skills, thereby predicting greater gains regardless of the target selected. Unfortunately, the graduate students' specific reasoning for selecting 2-element or 3-element targets was not recorded and therefore remains unknown.

It is known that the 3-element consonant blend group averaged a baseline of 32 errors on the Clinical Assessment of Articulation and Phonology-2. Whereas, the 2-element consonant blend averaged slightly better at baseline with 28 errors. This suggests speech ability at baseline was not likely the determining factor of improved gains for the 3-element consonant cluster treatment group.

3.2 Maxim #2: Select More Complex Treatment Targets to Expeditiously Target Simpler Ones

Our research for the past 5 years describes how the complexity approach ignites change in the sound system. Gains are not initially made on the complex treatment targets themselves or even on untreated sounds of the same place and manner. For example, the treatment target "clean" would not result in immediate improvement of the similar word "glove."

Rather, gains are initially made in a downward, cascading fashion, with dramatic improvements on earlier developing sounds and sound combinations.

Supporting this downward, cascading impact over a lateral impact were limited lateral gains for both an affricate blend treatment target group and a 2-element consonant treatment target group.

For both treatment groups, gains were not made laterally. Progress on affricates occurred maximally if the treatment target was a 3-element cluster. Moderately, when a 2-element cluster was selected and very minimally if an affricate was selected.

Similarly progress on 2-element clusters was substantial when a 3-element cluster was selected and very minimally evident when a 2-element cluster was selected. The consistent message is to aim higher in therapy to make progress on your goals.

This research clearly indicates that the complexity approach does not change the universal developmental trajectory of sound development. Simpler sounds develop before more complex ones. Select 3-element treatment targets to effectively treat earlier developing singleton sounds as well as later developing affricates and 2-element consonant clusters.

3.2.1 Selecting a Consonant Cluster Treatment Target

At this point, we have completed the speech evaluation and possibly the *Supplemental Complex Consonant Blend Screener* (▶ Table 3.2) for important information regarding the child's ability to produce sounds accurately given a maximal level of prompting. Follow the steps outlined in ▶ Table 3.2 to select the most effective consonant cluster.

When selecting intervention targets, do *not* select initial consonant clusters that the child can already accurately imitate. Research indicates that these sounds will naturally develop[12] or are already produced accurately by the child if accurately imitated in the initial position of words.[13]

Table 3.2 How to select a consonant cluster for optimal gain

In selecting a treatment target, focus on four pivotal questions:
1) What are the child's phonological processes?
2) What sounds does the child distort?
3) What is/are the most complex blend or blends that the child can accurately produce with maximum cueing (that also contain immature phonological processes or error sounds)?
4) What complex cluster blends would directly impact simpler sounds?

3.2.2 Selecting a Treatment Target for Carter, a Child with Mild Speech Sound Disorder

Let's start with Carter, a 48-month-old child with an educational eligibility of Articulation Impairment. He presents with later developing phonological processes. His baseline Percent Consonants Correct (PCC) was 72% in spontaneous conversation. Please refer ▶ Table 3.3.

With this standardized testing information, we can answer the following first two questions in consonant cluster treatment target selections:

1. What phonological processes emerged in errors presented?
2. What sound(s) are distorted or errored?

Answering Question 1: Phonological processes that emerged include gliding of /l/ and / ɹ / (lif→ wif; ɹɪŋ → wɪŋ); deaffrication of /ʧ/ and /ʤ/ (ʧiz → ʃiz; ʤɑɹ →ʒɑɹ); and, labialization of /θ/ (fʌm→ θʌm; ðɛm → vɛm).

Answering Question 2: The /s/ and /z/ are produced with lateral airflow escaping twice during testing, which is referred to as a lateral lisp and can be a persistent speech sound error. Generally, we want to encourage greater maxillary (cheek) and labial (lip) retraction to reduce airflow through the selection of retracted neighboring sounds, which we'll discuss in Chapter 4, *Selecting LinguisticContext for Treatment Targets.*

Table 3.3 Carter's baseline performance on single word standardized speech testing

Orthographic spelling: IPA → Carter's Production
Teeth: tiθ → tiv
Cage: keɪʤ → keɪʒ
Ring: ɹɪŋ → wɪŋ
Zoo: zu→ lzu (lateralized)
Jar: ʤɑr→ ʒɑr
Cheese: ʧiz → ʃiz
Rake: ɹeɪk → weɪk
Leaf: lif→ wif
Watch: wɑʧ → wɑʃ
Thumb: fʌm→ θʌm
Them: ðɛm → vɛm
Clown: klaʊn→ kwaʊn
Flag: flæg → fwæg
Glove: glʌv → gwʌv
School: skul → sku
Bridge: bɹɪʤ → bwɪʒ
Treasure: ʧɹɛʒər → twɛʒər
Fingernail: fɪŋgərneɪl → fɪŋgərneɪ
Lemonade: lɛməneɪd → wɛməneɪd
Thermometer: θərmɑmətər→ mɑmɑmətər

3

We now want to select a treatment target that addresses the phonological processes of gliding of /l/ and / ɹ /, deaffrication of /ʧ/ and /ʤ/, and labialization of /θ/. We'll also want to focus on suppression of the lateral lisp of /s/ and /z/. We can only focus on what the child is able to *accurately* produce given a maximum level of cueing, which brings us to our next question:

3. What sounds can the child accurately produce with a maximum level of cueing?

There are three reasons for only selecting sounds that the child *can* produce with a maximum level of cueing. First, we want to work within the child's *zone of proximal development*, a level in which the child can accurately perform with a more capable person's assistance. Second, we do not want to frustrate the child by placing demands that are not currently in the child's reach. Third, we do not want to reinforce speech errors with natural rewards.

Minimal accuracy level of 80% is our standard baseline to expedite speech gains in reinforcing accurate productions while avoiding negative practice.[14] Therefore, the child must be able to produce the target correctly with a therapist providing a level of cueing needed to ensure 80% accuracy.

Avoiding Negative Practice

I recall clearly a child who did *not* make gains following five intervention sessions. The graduate intern had selected treatment targets of /sl/ and /fl/ by manding with "Can you slide it or fly it?" However, the child was unable to produce the treatment targets accurately with a maximum level of prompting.

Given a maximum level of cueing, he continually reduced clusters in producing "/kæn ju saɪd ɪt ɔrfaɪ ɪt?/" throughout the five therapy sessions with the provision of natural rewards after every errored request.

The intern was determined to achieve accurate production and would not change the target to a simpler cluster. She felt that the child would feel as if he had failed if a different cluster was selected. Thus, cluster reduction was reinforced instead of being suppressed through dense production with ongoing provision of natural rewards.

I have also made this mistake by believing that I could achieve accuracy through creative cueing and hard work. This commitment to an errored target results in wasting valuable therapy time and reinforces errors.

Now, we will need to know what sounds are stimulable with a maximum level of cueing. Please view Video 3.1 and complete *Consonant Blend Screener's* second column labelled "**Stimulable**" (**in Appendix A at the end of this book**). Alicia is demonstrating prompting for all consonant clusters in this video for demonstration purposes. In standard practice, Alicia would only assess stimulability with maximum cueing for clusters that the child was unable to accurately imitate.

Develop Prompts That Make Sense to You and the Individual Child

You'll notice Alicia's prompts differ from Taylor's in the second chapter. They are cues that Alicia has developed for Carter's specific errors. She selects cues that are incompatible with his speech errors, such as a big smile to suppress air escaping in a lateral lisp. She also saliently cues sounds that are most difficult for Carter through the use of extended time and exaggerated movements.

Alicia, like every graduate intern I've mentored, has been taught a variety of prompts and has also developed unique prompts on her own. You, like Alicia, will learn a variety of prompts throughout this book. Some you will copy, others you will adapt, and many you'll invent along the way. Enjoy this learning process as your skillset will continually evolve with every child you treat.

With the *Supplemental Consonant Cluster Screener* completed, we are now able to answer question 3: What sounds can Carter accurately produce with a maximum level of cueing?

Carter was both able to suppress all phonological processes provided there was a maximum level of cueing and produce laterally distorted /s/ and /z/ accurately. Therefore, all phonological processes and distorted sounds would be appropriate targets.

Progressing to our fourth and final question:

4. *What complex cluster blends would directly impact simpler sounds?*

Select the most complex 3-element consonant clusters over 2-element consonant clusters. Select clusters over affricates and singletons. In this way, we can make greater gains in both quantity and complexity of sounds produced correctly.

Because speech is a continuous motor movement, we want to place these targets in a phrase or sentence in which all sounds can be accurately produced to avoid reinforcement of errored speech. (Note: In Chapter 4, *Selecting Linguistic Context for Treatment Targets* we'll discuss exceptions to the rule in requiring accuracy for every word spoken in a carrier phrase.)

For Carter, the intern selected: "Can you scrape it to me please?" /kæn ju skɹeɪp ɪt tu mi pliz?/

The intern selected this treatment target to work with Carter to suppress the phonological process of gliding /ɹ/ and /l/, correct the lateral lisp of /s/, and produce the voiced cognate /z/. Carter can produce all sounds in the sentence accurately with a maximum level of cueing.

3.2.3 Could Multiple Treatment Targets Be Selected Over One?

Could another treatment target be selected that would more directly address the deaffrication of /tʃ/ and /dʒ/? Perhaps Alicia could have added another treatment target, such as: "Can you scrape it or *drop* (/dʒɹɑp/) it to me please?"

Our current research indicates that selection of either one or two treatment targets results in generally the same outcome in terms of improvement in both a decrease in the number of errors and complexity of errors improved upon.

Specifically, we compared outcomes of 28 preschoolers with one 3-element treatment target selected (e.g., scrape → skɹeɪp) to 20 preschoolers who had one 3-element cluster (e.g., "scrape") and an additional cluster treatment target selected (e.g., both "scape" and "drop"). We found no difference in improvement in terms of total number of sounds improved upon. Both groups averaged 32% improvement in number of errors. There were very minimal differences in affricates and 2-element cluster improvements between the groups (38–39% improvement in affricate production and 12–14% in 2-element consonant cluster production). Put simply, our current research indicates adding an additional cluster to a 3-element treatment target does not likely impact outcomes.

Putting Research into Action

Why would you favor selection of one treatment target to be appropriate in Carter's case?

Why would you select two or more treatment targets to be appropriate in Carter's case?

In my reasoning, selection of one treatment target would be appropriate because of the downward cascading effect of 3-element consonant clusters to both untreated 2-element consonant clusters and affricates. However, it is important to note that these untreated, later developing 2-element consonant clusters and affricates will demonstrate improvements at a slower rate than the earlier developing sounds. For this, perhaps adding an affricate blend would have more directly addressed the projection of cheeks, lips, and the palatal placement of affricates that is motorically dissimilar to the retraction of articulators and placement in the word "scrape"→/skɹeɪp/. Please see Video 3.2 in which Carter mands with this treatment target.

After completing four 45-minute therapy sessions using this carrier phrase across activities, Carter's number of single-word standardized testing errors decreased from 27 to 18. This is an impressive 33% improvement in speech sound production. His PCC within spontaneous conversation improved from 72% to 80%.

3.2.4 Benefit in Selecting Two Treatment Targets to Improve Affricate Production

A primary benefit in selecting two treatment targets when affricate blends are present is that the affricate blend /dʒɹ/ is a motor movement produced quite differently than /skɹ/. With affricates, the maxillary and labial (cheek and lip) muscles are protracted with lips rounded in a forward pursing motion. When producing /skɹ/, oppositional to /dʒɹ/, the maxillary muscles are retracted with lips in a smile motion.

Coarticulation is the impact of neighboring sounds on the production of a phoneme. Because of coarticulation the /ɹ/ is produced quite differently in the words "scrape" and "drop." The IPA indicates that /ɹ/ is alveopalatal in placement. When you produce the /ɹ/, notice how the /ɹ/ in "scrape" is produced more posteriorly in the mouth, whereas the /ɹ/ in "drop" is produced more bilaterally on the alveolar ridge.

Please see Video 3.3, Alyssa with Harrison manding, "Can you scrape or drop it to me please?" /kæn ju skɹeɪp ɔrdɹɑp ɪt tu mi pliz?/.

To get a glimpse of the continuous use of the same treatment target across activities, see Video 3.4.

Alyssa is with Harrison on a different therapy day with a different activity. Note that the request treatment target remains the same across activities, time, and people so that deeper learning occurs. Hence, the target can be produced independently by the child. Across all settings, the treatment target remains: "Can you scrape or drop it to me please?" /kæn ju skɹeɪp ɔrdɹɑp ɪt tu mi pliz?/.

The Questionable Efficacy of /θɹ/ as a Treatment Target

Notice that we did not select a /θɹ/ blend to suppress the phonological process of labialization of /θ/. In the first year of our summer program, we studied seven preschoolers who had the /θɹ/ consonant cluster treatment target verb "throw" selected. We selected /θɹ/ for three reasons. (1) It is a later developing consonant cluster. (2) /θ/ and /ɹ/ are maximally distinct sounds. (3) Both were errored phonemes that the child could correctly produce given a maximum level of prompting.

Despite our solid theoretical reasoning based on the complexity approach, we found /θɹ/ to be largely ineffectual in improving both singleton and cluster sounds. The seven preschoolers assigned to the /θɹ/ treatment target made dismal gains. After four or five, 45-minute therapy sessions, their group average was only three less singleton sound errors with no improvement in producing consonant clusters on single-word standardized speech testing. Hence, we currently opt not to select /θɹ/ as a treatment target when other consonant cluster errors are present.

What could explain the relative lack of efficacy of /θɹ/? Perhaps it is the placement of /θ/. The tongue protruded from the mouth with /θ/ may be too distinct of a speech motor behavior to directly impact the development of other sounds, which are produced labially or interorally. Because of the unique interdental placement of /θ/ (and its voiced cognate ð), I refer to them as "the outsiders" in that they are less likely to have an impact on others.

Of course, these dismal gains could be attributed to chance in that only seven children were studied. Further research with a larger, randomly distributed population is needed to reveal the true value of /θɹ/ as a primary treatment target. We currently add /θɹ/ as a secondary target to preemptively plant a seed for accurate production but have ceased using it as a primary target unless it is the sole error sound remaining.

3.3 Maxim #3: Select One or a Few Exemplars as Treatment Target(s) to Foster an Internal Locus of Control

Research regarding the efficacy of using nonwords indicates that nonword treatment targets generalize to other untreated words and have an initial benefit in that there is not a history of reinforcement for errored production. For example, a child fronting /k/ would have history of frequently producing "can" as "tan" /kæn/→ /tæn/.[15]

We can put this useful research into practice in its generalization of nonsense words to improvements in both conversational speech and untreated words. We do so by using the same or a limited number of treatment targets in a single sentence, sentences, or a paragraph context for an extended length of time, possibly an entire school year. Three reasons for the use of the same target over time are outlined below.

First, using one or only a couple of treatment target exemplars empowers the child to focus on how the target is produced rather than on recalling a variety of words. We want the child to think of the targeted motor movement. For example, the child thinks, "Is my tongue in the back of my mouth?" when producing "can." The child is not concerned with the semantics (meanings) of 20 different words containing the /k/ sound in a variety of positions within a word.

Second, the use of the same treatment target sentence, sentences, or paragraph enables the child and the caregivers to practice it across different people and environments, thereby expediting gains and generalization. Parents enlist grandparents, babysitters, and caregivers to follow through with the child's request sentence(s) as well. We typically ask parents to place the child's treatment target on their refrigerator and elicit minimally one natural request daily.

Lastly, and most importantly, we use the same target so the child can develop an internal locus of control in becoming his or her own teacher. This is the number one goal of speech and language therapy. There are, and always will be, external forces that we cannot control. Children with communication impairments often present with concurrent neurological differences that will require self-efficacy and grit to succeed. For this, even more than their typically developing peers, they need to develop a strong

3

internal locus of control in believing that they can ultimately determine their own successes or failures.

Why Select Real Words Instead of Nonsense Words?

Recent research indicates that selection of nonsense words versus real words did not significantly impact intervention outcomes.[16] Also, nonsense words would have intrinsic limited acceptability and would have to explicitly be taught, requiring time and effort to learn. People would have to "buy in" to using nonsense words across natural settings. Though nonsense words may expedite gains in the initial stages of therapy, opt to select real words to improve acceptability of the treatment target across settings and people outside of the clinical setting from day one of therapy.

Additionally, 3-element and 2-element treatment target verbs that we select (e.g., *swap, scrape, spray, stretch*) are typically not frequently occurring in a child's vocabulary. As you will see in videos 3-5 and videos 3-6, Patty requests with the uncommon verbs "swap" and "sweep." These infrequent verbs have similar benefits as nonsense words in that there is a limited or nonexistent reinforcement history of errored production. This provides a blank slate in which new speech motor movements can be more easily learned.

3.4 Maxim #4: Select Consonant Cluster Treatment Targets to Treat Syllable Structure Phonological Processes

What treatment target would be appropriate to treat phonological processes impacting syllable structure, such as phonological processes of initial consonant deletion, final consonant deletion, weak syllable deletion, and cluster reduction?

Once again, our five consecutive years of research findings encourage us to think big. Treat the child at the highest level of the staircase (▶ Table 3.1) with a maximum level of cueing to ignite change on earlier developing phonological processes. Our research indicates that, after only four to five sessions over a 6-week period, selection of either a 2-element or

3-element consonant clusters in the initial position of words will generalize to improvement in producing (untreated) polysyllabic words. By treating the more advanced structural processes of cluster reduction we can impact earlier structural phonological processes of consonant and syllable deletion.

3.4.1 Selecting a Treatment Target for Jacob, a Child with Syllable Structure Phonological Processes of Final Consonant Deletion

Let's now look at Jacob, a 42-month-old child with an educational eligibility of Articulation Impairment, who presents with severe speech impairment. He produced final consonant deletion at baseline on single-word standardized testing. Please see ▶ Table 3.4.

We'll now go through our four questions in determining treatment targets for Jacob.

1. *What phonological processes emerged in errors presented?*

Final consonant deletion, fronting of velars, cluster reduction, labialization of /f/, /v/, and /θ/, stopping of fricatives /s/, /z/, and /ʒ/, gliding /l/ and /ɹ /, and deaffrication.

Note: Syllable deletion only presented once (kəm 'pjutər → pjutʌ) and assimilation errors only presented twice (swɪŋ → fin; ðɛm → wɛm). Therefore, natural remediation of these processes is expected.

2. *What sound(s) are distorted or errored?*

Not applicable. Phonological processes are present in which entire classes of sounds are impacted with substitutions.

3. *What sounds can Jacob accurately produce with a maximum level of cueing?*

Jacob was able to produce all consonant cluster combinations accurately on the *Supplement Complex Consonant Cluster Screener* with a maximum level of cueing.

4. *What complex cluster blends would directly impact simpler sounds?*

Jacob had difficulty producing /ʃ/, /ʒ/, /tʃ /, and /dʒ/. All of these sounds could directly be impacted by selecting the most complex sound /dʒ/ in a consonant cluster, such as drop (/dʒɹɑp/).

Table 3.4 Jacob's baseline performance on single-word standardized speech testing

Orthographic spelling: IPA → Jacob's Production
Pig: pɪg → pɪt
Bed: bɛd → bɛt
Teeth: tiθ → ti
Dog: dɔg → dɔ
Cage: keɪʤ → teɪ
Gate: geɪt → te
Mouse: maʊz → maʊ
Knife: naɪf → naɪ
King: kɪŋ → tin
Ring: ɹɪŋ → win
House: haʊs → haʊ
Hive: haɪv → haɪ
Fish: fɪʃ → fɪt
Van: væn → bæn
Seal: sil → sioʊ
Zoo: zu → ju
Sheep: ʃip → sip
Jar: ʤɑr → dɑr
Cheese: ʧiz → ti
Rake: ɹeɪk → weɪ
Leaf: lif → jiv
Watch: wɑʧ → wɑ
Thumb: θʌm → fʌm
Bathe: beɪð → beɪ
Them: ðɛm → wɛm
Clown: klaʊn → waʊn
Glove: glʌv → dwʌb
School: skul → tul
Snake: sneɪk → seɪk
Swing: swɪŋ → fin
Bridge: bɹɪʤ → bwɪd
Computer: kəm'pjutər → pjutʌ
Dinosaur: 'daɪnəˌsɔr → 'daɪnəˌsoʊ
Grasshopper: 'gɹæsˌhɑpər → 'gwæsˌhɑpər
Lemonade: 'lɛmə'neɪd → wɛmə'neɪd
Thermometer: θər'mɑmətər → fermometər

Alyssa, Jacob's intern, decided that he needed a lot of repetition to suppress fronting and wanted to address all of his phonological processes. She therefore selected: "Can you scrape or dream it to me please? I am a cool guy because I have sparkle teeth." /kæn ju skɹeɪp ɔr dɹim ɪt tu mi pliz? aɪ æm ə kul gaɪ bɪ'kɔz aɪ hæv 'spɑrkəl tiθ/.

What could you see as benefits to selecting a simpler intervention target for Jacob such as "Can you scrape it to me please?" /kæn ju skɹeɪp ɪt tu mi pliz?/.

What could you see as the benefits to selecting multiple intervention treatment targets for Jacob, as Alyssa chose? What could you see as benefits in using multiple sentences as a linguistic context? "Can you scrape it to me please? I am a cool guy because I have sparkle teeth?" (/kæn ju skɹeɪp ɔr dɹim ɪt tu mi pliz? aɪæm ə kulgaɪbɪ'kɔzaɪhæv 'spɑrkəltiθ?/)?

After completing five 45-minute therapy sessions using these carrier sentences across activities, Jacob's number of single-word standardized testing errors decreased from 54 to 39, a 28% improvement in speech sound production.

Notice that Alyssa's treatment targets for Jacob were placed in the context of two sentences, one being a complex sentence. He used this sentence combination throughout the five intervention sessions. His gains were impressive, which brings us to our next maxim.

3.5 Maxim #5: Place Treatment Targets in Sentences of Increased Length and Complexity to Improve Production of Polysyllabic Words

Our research suggests that children benefit more in the production of polysyllabic words if their treatment target word is placed in carrier sentences instead of produced at the single word level. For instance, requesting with a treatment target in a sentence such as "Can you *scrape* it to me please because I'm a cool guy?" instead of having a child to request simply using the word "*scrape*" resulted in greater improvements in polysyllabic word production.

A possible explanation is that the continuity of motor movement involved in producing utterances of increased length and complexity provides for increased motor coordination practice, thereby indirectly improving polysyllabic word production. This newly found analysis of our data supports Alyssa's intuitive selection of multiple sentences with a complex sentence to treat Jacob.

It is important to note that in our research polysyllabic words were not used as a treatment target or included in any of the carrier sentences for any of the 82 preschoolers participating in the speech intervention program. However, substantial gains in production of polysyllabic words were made after only four to five 45-minute therapy sessions for children with polysyllabic errors at baseline.

These improvements in polysyllabic word production when only clusters were targeted further illustrate how the complexity approach ignites change in simpler developmental phonological processes of consonant and syllable deletion before later ones of cluster reduction. Our research shows that these earlier developing phonological processes will be suppressed before later developing processes, such as cluster reduction, which we are directly targeting.

3.6 Maxim #6: Select Consonant Cluster Treatment Targets with Maximally Distinct Sounds

Some children present with only primarily centralized vowels, such as /ʌ/, and early consonants, such as stops (located at the bottom of ▶ Table 3.1). Once again, to expedite gains we'll want to focus on going to the highest level of the staircase with a maximum level of adult prompting provided to the child.

Complex consonant clusters not only induce the greatest level of change but can also improve oral motor coordination by selecting pairs that are *maximally distinct*. Clusters that are *maximally distinct* are neighboring sounds that are maximally different in placement and manner to improve oral motor coordination required for continuous speech. In explaining this method of cluster selection to parents, I describe it as creating "acrobatics in the mouth" to improve oral motor coordination for increased speech clarity.

For instance, if we select the /s/ to begin a cluster as a target with restricted airflow, we'll want to select a neighboring liquid or glide to improve oral motor coordination by moving from a constricted airflow to open airflow.

It is important to note that the /s/ is an advanced sound that is both an alveolar and a fricative, indicating that it can directly impact many untreated alveolar and fricative sounds. Our research reveals that both 3-element and 2-element /s/ blend consonant clusters, produce greater gains than non-/s/ blend consonant clusters, such as "glide" (/glaɪd/). The /s/ also plays a pivotal role in expressive morphological (i.e., grammatical) development.

Children with a limited consonantal inventory and centralized vowels often present with oral muscular weakness, possibly exacerbated by underuse in their limited production of sounds, particularly coordinated sounds of diphthongs, glides, affricates, and clusters. As a result, they are often unable to produce later developing blends containing /l/ and /ɹ/ to be combined with /s/.

Therefore, we often blend /s/ with the open airflow, earlier developing glide /w/ instead in that it is also maximally distinct from /s/. The treatment target cluster blend that we often use with children who primarily communicate with centralized vowels and a few stop consonants is /sw./ The /sw/ blend has consistently indicated substantive gains after only four to five therapy sessions.

3.6.1 Selecting a Treatment Target for a Child with a Limited Phonetic Inventory

Let us now select a treatment target for Patty, a 36-month-old child with severe speech impairment who presents with a limited consonant inventory of oral stops /p, b, t, m, n, k, g/, the fricative /ʃ/, and glide /w/. Please see ▶ Table 3.5.

1. *What are her phonological processes?* Initial consonant deletion, final consonant deletion, syllable deletion, cluster reduction, stopping, and assimilation errors.
2. *What can she produce with a maximum level of cueing?* With a maximum level of prompting, Patty can produce /s/, but not with a simple imitation prompt.
3. *What sounds are errored or distorted?* The /s/ and /z/ are produced as a /ʃ/ as the cheeks and

Table 3.5 Patty's baseline performance on single word standardized speech testing

Pig: pɪg → pɪ
Teeth: tiθ → tit
Dog: dɔg → gɔg
Cage: keɪdʒ → geɪ
Gate: geɪt → geɪk
Mouse: maʊs → maʊt
Knife: naɪf → naɪt
King: kɪŋ → tɪn
House: haʊs → aʊ
Zoo: zu → ʃu
Sheep: ʃip → ʃik
Jar: dʒɑr → bɑr
Cheese: tʃiz → ʃi
Rake: ɹeɪk → weɪk
Leaf: lif → **ti**
Web: wɛb → **g**ɛ
Yo-Yo: joʊ-joʊ → doʊ-doʊ
Bathe: beɪð → peɪk
Them: ðɛm → pɛm
Clown: klaʊn → kaʊn
School: skul → ku
Grasshopper: ˈgɹæsˌhɑpər → gwʌ
Fingernail: ˈfɪŋgərˌneɪl → gʌ
Lemonade: ˈlɛməˈneɪd → weɪd
Basketball: ˈbæskətˌbɔl → kə

lips are not retracted during production and air escapes laterally and the tongue is in a centralized position.

4. *What complex cluster blends would directly impact simpler sounds?*

By selecting the 2-element consonant cluster /sw/, we can encourage gains by a downward cascading effect in developing both affricate and singleton fricative sounds (see ▸ Table 3.1).

At the time of working with Patty, we hadn't yet discovered the significant improvement that 3-element cluster targets made over 2-element cluster targets. Otherwise, we would have checked for the stimulability of /skw/ with this newly learned information and selected a 3-element consonant cluster word such as "squash." Can you think of another 3-element consonant cluster that we could use, keeping in mind that she is unable to produce /l/ and /ɹ/ given a maximum level of prompting?

Patty was unable to produce the carrier sentence "Can you swap it to me please?" (/kænjuswɑpɪttu mi?/). Therefore, intern Jessica chose "swap" as a starting point and quickly expanded the utterance to "Can you sweep it to me?" to encourage labial and maxillary retractions with the neighboring impact of the tense (long) /i/ vowel.

After completing four 45-minute therapy sessions using this carrier phrase across activities, Patty's number of single-word standardized testing errors decreased from 55 to 49, an 11% improvement in sound production.

3.7 Maxim #7: Treat Individual Sound Errors with Consonant Cluster Targets

3.7.1 Selecting a Treatment Target for a Child with Distorted /l/, /ɹ/, and /s/

In this next scenario, we'll select a target for 47-month-old Haisley. She is rounding /l/ and /ɹ/ and interdentally lisping /s/. Taylor, her intern, had selected "Can you scrape it or spray it to me please?" to address all errors deeply through distinct phonetic contexts provided in "scrape" (with lips and cheeks retracted) and "spray" (with lips and cheeks protruding forward).

In Video 3.7, you will see Haisley, using three consonant cluster treatment targets to suppress gliding of /l/ and /ɹ/ and lisping of /s/ in her initial therapy session with a maximal level of prompting.

In Video 3.8, you will see Haisley in her third 45-minute session manding, provided a moderate level of prompting. The intern's verbal model has been faded with only temporal cues provided.

After completing five 45-minute therapy sessions using this request sentence target across activities, Haisley's number of single-word standardized testing errors decreased from 26 to 18, a 31% improvement in sound production.

3.8 Maxim #8: "Please" Is Not a Magic Word: Include it Judiciously

Should the child *always* say "please"? Our research of 82 preschoolers who had 3-element and 2-element consonant cluster targets hints that, after completing four to five sessions.

Whether or not children say "please" (/pliz/) in their target sentences does not differentially impact their production of /l/ or /z/ on post testing.

Our research indicated that regardless of /l/ or /z/ directly being in the request sentence, both post-intervention groups averaged a 22% improvement in producing /l/, and a 26% improvement in producing /z/ on single-word standardized testing.

For this, we recommend generally not adding "please" to a child's treatment target request sentence unless the child can produce the word correctly given a maximum level of prompting. This is to avoid reinforcing errors, such as gliding of [lʷ] and lateral lisping of [zˡ]. Manners can also be addressed by encouraging, "Thank you," for natural rewards.

3.8.1 Putting Research into Practice: Selecting Consonant Cluster Treatment Targets

In selecting consonant cluster treatment targets, look for a cluster that addresses multiple phonological processes and error sounds. In this way, you'll get maximum value for your target. For instance, if the child presents with phonological processes of stopping of fricatives, fronting velars, and gliding, an /skɹ/ mand would be a valuable target in that it addresses all three phonological processes simultaneously.

Refer to ▸ Table 3.6. What single treatment target verb would you pick for the following phonological

Table 3.6 Selecting cluster treatment targets to suppress phonological processes

1. Deaffrication of /ʧ / and gliding of /l/ and / ɹ /: drop /dɹɑp/
2. Stopping, fronting velars, and gliding (but unable to produce /l/ and /ɹ/ with maximum prompting): squash /skwɑʃ/
3. Cluster reduction: scrape /skɹeɪp/
4. Stopping, fronting velars (but unable suppress fronting with maximum prompting), gliding: stretch /stɹɛʧ /
5. Stopping, cluster reduction, and producing /w/ for /l/: splash /splæʃ/
6. Stopping, fronting velars, and producing /w/ for /j/: skewer /skjuər/
7. Stopping, backing of /t/ and /d/, gliding: stream /stɹim/
8. Fronting velars and producing /w/ for /l/: glide /glaɪd/
9. Labialization of /θ/ and gliding: free /fɹi/
10. Assimilatory gliding of /ɹ/ when following a labial: spritz /spɹitz/
11. Assimilatory gliding of /l/ when following a labial: splash /splæʃ/
12. Stopping of /f/ and /v/ and gliding of /ɹ/: vroom /vɹum/
13. Stopping of /f/ and /v/ and gliding of /l/: fly /flaɪ/
14. Fronting velars and /w/ for /j/: skew /skju/
15. Alveolarization of palatals /ʃ/ and /ʒ/ gliding of /ɹ/: drum /dʒɹʌm/
16. Fronting velars and /j/ for /w/: quick /kwɪk/
17. Syllable deletion, initial consonant deletion, final consonant deletion: stretch /stɹɛʧ /
18. Limited consonant inventory, primarily consisting of vowels: swap /swɑp/
19. Assimilation errors of labialization of /s/ preceding bilabials: spray /spɹeɪ/
20. Gliding of /l/ and /ɹ/ only: scrape /skɹeɪp/, splat /splæt/ (pick 2)
21. Backing of /t/ and /d/ only: stream /stɹim/
22. Deaffrication only: drench /dɹɛnʧ /
23. Lateral list of /s/ only: scrape /skɹeɪp/, spray /spɹeɪ/, stretch /stɹɛʧ/ (pick 3 targets)
24. Frontal list of /s/ only: skewer /skjuər/, stream /stɹim/, splash /splæʃ/(pick 3 targets)
25. Rounding of /ɹ/ only: strike /stɹaɪk/, spring /spɹɪŋ/, scream/skɹim/ (pick 3 targets)

processes and sound error combinations? Assume the child can produce consonants accurately with maximum prompting unless indicated in parenthesis.

I have provided an example of a treatment target verb I would select. Could you provide another verb to deliver a preferred object or action to a child? Because speech is a continuous motor activity, these verbs will be targeted in the context of sentence(s). For example, "Can you *scrape* it to me please?" Complete ▶ Table 3.6 for practice in selecting efficacious treatment targets.

3.9 Chapter Summary

We walked through every step in selecting treatment targets that produce optimal gains quickly for children with speech sound disorders. Refer to Kelly's Corner Video 3.9 for a review of the stair step progression in selecting targets that produce optimal gains. Each maxim is presented with empirical support and therapeutic reasoning so that you can understand and explain why a therapy target was selected.

We also discussed the importance of producing words accurately in carrier sentences containing the treatment target to prevent negative practice.

In the next chapter we will make exceptions to this rule when we have considered pivotally important secondary goals. These goals could be increasing the length and complexity of language expression, and/or improving attention for preschoolers who present with concurrent expressive language delay and/or attentional deficits.

We also make exceptions in accuracy for children who present with severe speech impairment. In both scenarios, we reward successive approximations, productions that are closer to accurate over time. These improvements can be made as language length, complexity, attention, and speech clarity improve through differential reinforcement.

References

[1] American Speech-Language-Hearing Association. 2018 Schools survey. Survey summary report: numbers and types of responses, SLPs. Published in 2018. Available from www.asha.org

[2] Brumbaugh KM, Smit AB. Treating children ages 3–6 who have speech sound disorder: a survey. Lang Speech Hear Serv Sch. 2013; 44(3):306–319

[3] Sugden E, Baker E, Munro N, Williams AL, Trivette CM. Service delivery and intervention intensity for phonology-based speech sound disorders. Int J Lang Commun Disord. 2018; 53 (4):718–734

[4] Law J, Garrett Z, Nye C. The efficacy of treatment for children with developmental speech and language delay/disorder: a meta-analysis. J Speech Lang Hear Res. 2004; 47(4):924–943

[5] Gierut JA, Morrisette ML, Hughes MT, Rowland S. Phonological treatment efficacy and developmental norms. Lang Speech Hear Serv Sch. 1996; 27(3):215–230

[6] Gierut JA. Complexity in phonological treatment: clinical factors. Lang Speech Hear Serv Sch. 2001; 32(4):229–241

[7] Taps J. An innovative educational approach for addressing articulation differences. Perspectives on School-Based Issues. 2006; 7(4):7–11

[8] Elise B, Lynn WA. Complexity approaches to intervention. In: McCauley RJ, Williams AL, McLeod S, eds. Interventions for Speech Sound Disorders in Children. Baltimore: Paul H. Brookes Pub.; 2010

[9] Storkel HL. Implementing evidence-based practice: selecting treatment words to boost phonological learning. Lang Speech Hear Serv Sch. 2018; 49(3):482–496

[10] Greenberg JH. Universals of Human Language. Stanford, CA: Stanford University Press; 1988

[11] Gierut JA. Phonological complexity and language learnability. Am J Speech Lang Pathol. 2007; 16(1):6–17

[12] Miccio AW, Elbert M, Forrest K. The relationship between stimulability and phonological acquisition in children with normally developing and disordered phonologies. Am J Speech Lang Pathol. 1999; 8(4):347–363

[13] McLeod S, Masso S. Screening Children's Speech: The Impact of Imitated Elicitation and Word Position. Lang Speech Hear Serv Sch. 2019; 50(1):71–82

[14] Rosenbek JC, Lemme ML, Ahern MB, Harris EH, Wertz RT. A treatment for apraxia of speech in adults. J Speech Hear Disord. 1973; 38(4):462–472

[15] Gierut JA, Morrisette ML, Ziemer SM. Nonwords and generalization in children with phonological disorders. Am J Speech Lang Pathol. 2010; 19(2):167–177

[16] Cummings A, Hallgrimson J, Robinson S. Speech Intervention Outcomes Associated With Word Lexicality and Intervention Intensity. Lang Speech Hear Serv Sch. 2019; 50(1):83–98

3

4 Selecting Linguistic Contexts for Treatment Targets

Speech sounds can be analyzed into fundamental units called phonemes; these move around like protozoa in a drop of water, and, like protozoa, join together and split up.

—L. Sprague de Camp

Context matters. Effectiveness of your therapy target will largely be impacted by two factors. First, the phonetic context, the surrounding sounds of the treatment target, counts. Your phonetic context will impact how efficiently correct production can be established in the initial stages and generalized in the final stages of therapy.

Second, the syntactic context, the sentence structure that carries the treatment target(s), matters. The syntactic context impacts how effectively treatment targets are established and generalized. Whether the treatment targets are placed in simple sentences, expanded sentences, compound sentences, complex sentences, or paragraphs of connected speech can impact speech gains as well as language and attentional gains.

Repetition in producing more complex syntactically-rich linguistic contexts with multiple conjunctions results in complex language forms spontaneously developing. They also inherently require greater attention to task to complete longer utterances. This increase in utterance length can result in benefits in both sustained attention to a task and joint attention with others.

4.1 The Phonetic Context in the Establishment and Generalization Phases

4.1.1 Establishment Phase

Coarticulation, the influence of sounds before and after a sound, can result in sound errors. For instance, a child may produce "swing" as "fwing" due to regressive assimilation in which the bilabial /w/ impacts /s/ production.

Coarticulation can also provide support in establishing the correct production of a treatment target. For example, a child who typically mildly rounds [ɹw] can produce /ɹ/ in "green" (/gɹin/) due to both regressive and progressive assimilation in lip retraction required to produce neighboring /g/ and /i/ sounds.

Perhaps the oddest example of using a phonetic context to establish correct production of a treatment target was when we selected the word "ugly" (/ʌgli/) to suppress the phonological process of fronting velar sounds /k, g, ŋ/. Fronting was the only phonological process for the child to suppress.

After attempting numerous treatment target words that provided neighboring contexts to retract the tongue, the 3-year-old could only suppress fronting in the treatment target word "ugly" with a maximum level of prompting. At the initial stage, attempts were made to put "ugly" in the sentence "It's not ugly." That, however, proved to be too much of a mouthful to start. Therefore, following the initial therapy session, the parent was informed that the child should say "ugly" to request desired objects and actions in the natural environment.

The parent was initially taken aback when informed her daughter would be rewarded for producing an insulting adjective. The child's mother was reassured that this target was short term. In the next session, her treatment target became "It is not ugly." By the third session, she was able to request with "Can you scrape it to me please because I am a cool girl?" Without using "ugly" as a stepping stone, it's doubtful progress would have been so swift.

Why was "ugly" the only word to establish correct production of /g/ in suppressing fronting? For correct production to occur both regressive and progressive assimilation were necessary. The retraction of the tongue (from the frontal alveolar ridge at rest) to produce the central vowel /ʌ/ resulted in progressive assimilation in which the following /g/ sound was easier to produce. The alveopalatal /l/ sound resulted in regressive assimilation in which the alveopalatal placement of /l/, which neighbors the velum, also made the /g/ easier to produce.

Multiple treatment targets can positively impact one another in the treatment phase. For example, a child who produces a laterally lisped /s/ and a rounded /ɹ/, and a fronted /k/ can benefit from the treatment target "scrape" because of both progressive and regressive assimilation. The retracted lips in the production of /k/ makes both /s/ regressively and /ɹ/ progressively easier to produce. Additionally, the alveopalatal posterior location of /ɹ/, which neighbors the velum, results in /k/ being more easily produced through regressive assimilation. Assimilation is easily thought of as a sound's influence being "progress(ive)" forwards or "regress(ive)" backwards to impact neighboring sounds. In the

Putting Research into Practice: Selecting Establishment and Generalization Treatment Targets

Below, for five phonological processes, I provide an example of a 3-element establishment treatment target word that would aid in establishing correct production. Also, a 3-element generalization treatment target word is provided that would challenge correct production to occur through progressive and regressive assimilation. Can you come up with both an establishment and generalization treatment target for each phonological process?

Phonological Process	3-Element Establishment Target	3-Element Generalization Target
Backing of /t/, /d/	street /stɹit/	strike /stɹaɪk/
Fronting of velars /k/, /g/, /ŋ/	scrub /skɹʌb/	screen /skɹin/
Stopping of /s/, /z/	slice /slaɪs/	string /stɹɪŋ/
Gliding of /l/, / ɹ /	scrape /skɹeɪp/	spray /spɹeɪ/
Labialization of /s/ blends	squash /skwɑʃ/	spruce /spɹus/

video (Video 4.1), you'll see a clip of Luca saying "scrape" to improve /k/, /s/, and /ɹ / simultaneously in production of sentences "Can you scrape it to me please? I am a cool guy because I have sparkle teeth." It is the first day of therapy so a maximum level of prompting is provided. Luca, as you'll see in the video, has not yet learned the hand cues.

4.1.2 Generalization Phase

Unlike the establishment phase in which it is important to select neighboring sounds that will aid in the accurate production of targeted sounds, the generalization stage selects challenging neighboring sounds. At the generalization stage, select a 3-element consonant cluster that challenges the child to do acrobatics in the mouth. Select neighboring sounds that will regressively and progressively challenge accurate production.

For instance, for a child who has a lateralized (slushy) production of [s¹] and a rounded [ɹʷ], have the child say "spray" at the generalization phase. The /p/ would have a lip rounding impact, which would make suppression of both lateralized /s/ (in which airflow escapes due to a lack of labial and maxillary retraction) and rounded /ɹ/ more difficult.

Please refer to videos of Vance and Sampson in the generalization phase. Notice how differently the mouth moves to produce both /s/ and /ɹ / when producing each treatment target word. For Vance, the /s/ is impacted by the neighboring /p/ sound in the word "sparkle" through *regressive assimilation*. Whereas, the /ɹ / would be impacted by *progressive assimilation* in the "free" due the influence of the labiodental /f/ sound on /ɹ/ production. See Video 4.2.

For Sampson, "Drop" /dʒɹɑp/ is a challenging generalization word due to both the progressive assimilatory influence and the regressive assimilatory influence of /p/. Rounding of lips in both neighboring sounds will challenge his difficulty in correcting a rounded /ɹ/. See Video 4.3.

4.2 Selecting the Syntactic Context for a Treatment Target: Simple Sentence to Paragraphs

The syntactic context in which treatment targets are practiced is of critical importance. As speech is a continuous motor activity, I recommend addressing treatment targets in a sentence to paragraph level. Ideally, the child could produce every sound accurately within that sentence or paragraph. If the child presents with only speech impairment and no accompanying linguistic or attentional deficits, work to ensure that every sound in the child's carrier phrase, sentence, or paragraph is accurately produced to avoid negative practice.

There are four instances, however, where I recommend working with the treatment target in a

4

paragraph instead of a sentence context. First, when the child presents with a concurrent language impairment. Second, when the child presents with attentional issues. Third, when the child presents with structural phonological processes such as syllable and consonant deletion, which suggests a greater likelihood for concurrent language impairment.[1] Fourth, when the child presents with limitations in joint attention, which we will discuss in detail in Chapter 7, *Treating Motor Speech Disorders in Preschoolers with Autism Spectrum Disorder and Preschoolers with Neurological Differences.*

4.2.1 Advantages in Selecting a Longer and More Complex Syntactic Context in Working with a Child with Concurrent Language and Attentional Deficits

A 2004 meta-analysis by Law and colleagues indicates that speech language pathologists do not only effectively treat speech sound disorders, but also significantly improve expressive language, particularly in utterance length and complexity.[2] To achieve this, with children with limited verbal output regardless of etiology (Autism Spectrum Disorder, brain damage, cerebral palsy, Down's syndrome, specific language impairment), incorporate the treatment target as a complex sentence or paragraph.

Use maximum support to ignite expressive language improvement while treating the speech target. Some errors are acceptable in a shared focus on improving both speech and utterance length and complexity.

In the next clip, you will see Stella, a 4-year-old girl with an educational eligibility of ASD who presents with concurrent speech, language, and attentional deficits. In comprehensively treating the child, her therapist MaryLyn chose complex sentences: "Can you scrape it to me please? I am a cool girl because I have sparkle teeth," as Stella's request target.

You will notice in the video (Video 4.4), Stella becomes distracted numerous times but MaryLyn masterfully ignores those distractions and attends to the request sentences. Stella's attention joins MaryLyn's.

Although we have not yet tested the impact of increased language length and complexity on attention, we have observed qualitative improvements in attention to task, joint attention, and language expression in our clinical work.

4.3 Working with a Child with Structural Phonological Processes

Our research indicates that placing the treatment target in the context of sentences, complex sentences, or paragraphs results in greater gains than producing the consonant cluster word at a single word level to mand. For example, saying "Can you scrape it to me please?" results in greater gains in polysyllabic word production on standardized testing than having the child simply produce the word "scrape."

As described in Chapter 3, polysyllabic words can be treated indirectly by selecting 2- or 3-element consonant clusters. As a group, all 82 children whose baseline and post data were analyzed made gains in polysyllabic (three to four syllable) word production. These gains occurred despite none of the children having polysyllabic words selected as a treatment target or in their carrier sentence(s).

Because children with structural phonological processes are more likely to have concurrent language impairment and, therefore, at higher risk for literacy deficits, I recommend using a paragraph with temporal conjunctions such as *first, then,* and *lastly* to encourage early narrative development.

A paragraph using conjunctions *first, then,* and *lastly* provides a schema, which is simply an outline that organizes ideas logically. Repeating this paragraph multiple times results in automaticity of learning. Automaticity is the ability to do something without thinking about it because it is an overlearned behavior. Having this automaticity not only makes sequencing of ideas easier, but also frees the child to focus on the content of a subject in both comprehending and forming stories.

Please refer to Video 4.5 of Cameron learning his request paragraph at the establishment phase with a maximum level of verbal, gestural, and visual prompts provided.

At the generalization phase, Cameron has memorized the paragraph and is working on producing multiple variations of the /ɹ/ sound due to influence of varying phonetic contexts. In Video 4.6, you'll see that Cameron is requesting with increased independence as Torey's verbal model is faded out.

Creative Challenge

Create a request treatment target paragraph, complete with bolded print and pictures that incorporates first, then, lastly, and because. Uniquely create this treatment target for a 48-month-old girl who loves animals.

Have the paragraph include three treatment targets that suppress all of her phonological processes. Her phonological processes are stopping fricatives, fronting velars, cluster reduction, and gliding of /l/ and /ɹ/. She can suppress these phonological processes with a maximum level of prompting.

Note: To ensure that you have permission to use pictures for educational purposes from a Google Image search, scroll down to "Tools"→ "Usage Rights" → "Creative Commons licenses."

4.3.1 Advantages in Selecting a Simple Sentence as the Context for a Treatment Target

There are three possible advantages to embedding your treatment target into a simple linguistic context over a complex one.

Advantage 1: Quicker Transfer of the Locus of Control from the Adult to the Child

In selecting a simple sentence as the context for a treatment target, the child can more quickly assume the active role of teacher in the intervention process.

In Video 4.7, you'll see Chad, a 48-month-old child with mild articulation impairment and strong attention and language skills. He presents with the phonological processes of fronting velars, errors in devoicing /z/ at the conversational level, and producing /w/ for both /j/ and /l/. His intern selected the treatment target sentence, "Can you glide it to me please?" /kæn ju glaɪd ɪt tu mi pliz?/.

Please refer Video 4.7 and Video 4.8 for a glimpse of how scaffolding works in therapy. Video 4.7 will demonstrate a maximum level of prompting with slow, echoed speech. Chad and therapist Christina are working in his zone of proximal development. This zone is what a child can do with a more capable person's assistance.[3] He is heavily scaffolded. The locus of control is largely external in that he is dependent on the graduate intern to produce sounds correctly.

Watching Video 4.8, you'll see Chad assume an internal locus of control in which he is no longer dependent on the graduate student to improve his speech. He becomes his own teacher in teaching himself to speak correctly. The intern will dynamically provide cues only as necessary to ensure the maintenance of an 80% accuracy level to prevent reinforcement of errored speech, while fostering independence.

Chad had only three treatment target words, *can, glide,* and *please,* to learn in a single sentence. Had the intern Christina chosen more treatment targets and sentences to learn, do you think Chad would be as independent in self-cueing after only three sessions?

Christina chose a 2-element blend ("glide") instead of a 3-element blend ("scrape"). Do you think he would have also made greater gains if a 3-element blend was selected, such as "Can you scrape it to me please?" /kæn ju skreɪp ɪt tu mi pliz?/. This decision was made based on the intern's individual reasoning at that time. We had not yet completed research analysis indicating 3-element blends to ignite significantly greater gains than 2-element blends.

After completing five 45-minute therapy sessions using his carrier phrase "Can you glide it to me please?" across activities at a high level of density, Chad's number of single-word standardized testing errors had only decreased from 26 to 25, a minute 4% improvement in speech sound production.

Based on our experience, it is not uncommon for children who present with phonological processes of fronting and gliding at 3 to 4 years to demonstrate persistence with these errors until lingual strength develops with chronological age, which is typically between 4 and 5 years.

To start, Chad produced /t/ and /d/ for /k/ and /g/. After five sessions, he produced a glottal stop /ʔ/ as an approximation for /k/ and /g/. His glide was also less pronounced, with his previous full substitution of /w/ for /l/ and /j/ had become a mildly rounded production that could be detected in a single word testing situation but was hardly noticeable in conversational speech.

Standardized testing often will not capture these important qualitative gains. Yet these successive approximation improvements make a difference in overall speech clarity. For Chad, spontaneous speech in his perceived Percent Consonants Correct (PCC) went from 75% to 90% after only five therapy sessions.

Advantage 2: Increased Salience of an Error Sound with a Simple Sentence

Sometimes preschoolers have only a single distortion or substitution error in perhaps producing a lisped /s/ or glided /ɹ/. If not treated early, these errors can habituate and persist into adulthood due to their high frequency in the English language.

Additionally, recent research indicates that misarticulation of /s/ and /ɹ/ is largely correlated with misperception of /s/ and /ɹ/ in development of phonemic awareness skills.[4]

These are frequently occurring sounds and are therefore a concern for the child's phonemic awareness in literacy development. For this, /s/ and /ɹ/ should be given top priority as treatment

targets within the context of consonant clusters for maximum gains to occur.

These treatment targets would be most effectively improved upon in the context of consonant clusters in that they are more advanced and later developing than singleton sounds.

In selecting targets for single sounds, we have found that we can make improvements in distorted sounds, such as a rounded /ɹ/ more quickly by selecting 3-element cluster targets instead of 2-element cluster targets.

For instance, for a distorted sound such as /ɹ/, we may have a child say the complex sentence, "Can you scrape it, spray it, or drop it to me please because I have angry dog teeth?" /kæn ju skɹeɪp, spɹeɪ, ɔr/dʒɹɑp ɪt tu mi fɔɹ fɹi plizbɪˈkɔz aɪ hæv ˈæŋgɹi dɔg tiθ?/.

To appreciate the variations of /ɹ/, say this treatment target slowly in the mirror. Visually note the distinct change in position of your lips and cheeks while producing the /ɹ/ when saying each of the four treatment targets aloud. Also, feel in your mouth the unique placement of your tongue in each word while producing /ɹ/ to further appreciate the variability based on phonetic context.

Earlier we reviewed the advantages of selecting a simple treatment target to treat a phonological process to establish accurate production and to establish independence more quickly. In this scenario, we presented multiple treatment target exemplars containing /ɹ/ in a single sentence for generalization to occur.

Creative Challenge

Create a request complex sentence treatment target, complete with bolded print and pictures that incorporates three treatment target words to treat all phonological processes listed below. Uniquely create this complex sentence treatment target for a 48-month-old boy who loves vehicles, which include planes, boats, trains, and cars. His phonological processes are cluster reduction, deaffrication, and gliding of /l/ and /ɹ/. He can suppress all of these phonological processes with a maximum level of prompting.

Putting Research into Practice: Selecting a Syntactic Context from Sentences to Paragraphs

In the following scenarios, would you choose a simple sentence, complex sentence, or paragraph for treatment targets? Would you require an 80% minimal accuracy of all sounds presented or make exceptions for successive approximations in efforts to improve expressive language and attention?

Explain as you would to a colleague or superior your rationale for utterance length and required accuracy level for speech. Also, explain your reasoning for utterance length and accuracy level in lay terms as you would to a caregiver. Select utterance length and accuracy level for a preschool age child (3–5 years) who presents with:

1. Attentional deficits and articulation impairment
2. Concurrent language and articulation impairment
3. Structural phonological processes persisting for consonant and syllable deletion
4. Strong language skills and distortions of /ɹ/
5. Accuracy in structured therapy tasks of /s/; however, he or she frontally lisps /s/ in spontaneous speech
6. Limited joint attention and numerous immature phonological processes
7. Limited phonetic inventory, consisting of oral stops and centralized vowels

Advantage 3: Decreased Length of Request Utterances Allow for Increased Time for Repetitions

We use repetition of targets to establish automaticity of correct production of sounds. In this instance, increased accurate repetition of /ɹ/ across different phonetic contexts creates accurate speech production of /ɹ/ with "angry dog teeth." As saying a complex sentence takes less time than saying a paragraph, treatment targets can be produced more often. We know that with increased repetition myelin forms around the neuronal cells resulting in cells firing more efficiently and automatically, hence promoting generalization of new learning.

4.4 Chapter Summary

Context matters. Refer to Kelly's Corner Video 4.9 for an illustration of how linguistic context for the treatment target can globally improve outcomes for children with communication impairments.

In effectively differentiating instruction and comprehensively meeting the needs of children, rules change in both selecting phonetic and syntactic context.

At the establishment phase, select neighboring sounds to support accurate production. At the generalization stage, select sounds that will challenge accurate production.

These challenging sounds require acrobatics in the mouth for accurate production to occur. We call them our "tongue-twisting neighbors."

Rules additionally change based on the syntactic context of your treatment target. Will the child produce the targets in a simple sentence or within a paragraph? When the child presents with limitations in utterance length, complexity, and attention, go big.

Provide maximum support in having these children produce the longest and most syntactically complex utterances possible. Go to the paragraph level as soon as possible to ignite improvement globally in speech, language, literacy, and attentional skills.

When children with concurrent language or attentional impairments are speaking in paragraphs, some later developing sounds, such as /θ/ may be misarticulated. However, in this scenario consider the risk to reward ratio. The rewards of improving language expression and attention likely outweigh the risk of reinforcing inaccurate speech through negative practice.

At the preschool level, however, make every effort to suppress lisped /s/ and glided /ɹ/. These errors can persist through adulthood, so avoid reinforcing them. Provide a maximum level of cueing and use neighboring sounds to aid in accuracy through progressive and regressive assimilation.

Lastly, for children with strong language expression and a few distorted sounds at the generalization level, aim for saliency by selecting many variations of the sound. Present the sound with challenging neighboring sounds within the context of a sentence, while maintaining an 80% accuracy rate to prevent negative practice.

References

[1] Macrae T, Tyler AA. Speech abilities in preschool children with speech sound disorder with and without co-occurring language impairment. Lang Speech Hear Serv Sch. 2014; 45 (4):302–313

[2] Law J, Garrett Z, Nye C. The efficacy of treatment for children with developmental speech and language delay/disorder: a meta-analysis. J Speech Lang Hear Res. 2004; 47(4):924–943

[3] Vygotsky LS, Cole M. Mind in Society: The Development of Higher Psychological Processes. Cambridge, MA: Harvard University Press; 1981

[4] Hearnshaw S, Baker E, Munro N. The speech perception skills of children with and without speech sound disorder. J Commun Disord. 2018; 71:61–71

4

5 Developing Educationally Rich Activities

When you have teachers saying, "I don't have enough time for hands-on activities," we need to rethink the way we do education.

—Mae Jemison

If a newly certified speech-language pathologist asked me for the best piece of advice to improve therapy, I'd say, "Clean house!" Specifically, discard all of the two-dimensional drill work, including articulation decks, flashcards, worksheets, articulation bingo, print outs, and articulation maze games.

Children deserve better than drill and kill. Using these traditional, two-dimensional materials can result in decreased participation and engagement, thereby negatively impacting gains.

5.1 Treat the Whole Child

I blush in thinking of my own experience as a beginning speech-language pathologist in which I focused my efforts primarily on the mouth. My rationale was that my time was limited. For this, I needed to narrow my efforts to speech and language skills to have any sort of impact. If it were only that easy.

After 6 years as a speech-language pathologist, I had the opportunity to visit one of my very first students. She was a preverbal child who I could proudly state learned to talk in preschool. At the time, she was in the fifth grade. I couldn't wait to see how well she was doing.

Unfortunately, she wasn't doing well. When she saw me in her fifth-grade classroom, she repetitively yelled, "Speech with Miss Kelly!" She violently rocked, curled up in a fetal position, despite being seated in a metal, student chair.

In the physical world, she was with her peers and teacher in a classroom. In the emotional one, however, she was locked in the smallest of cells. Perhaps being in a straitjacket would best describe her confinement.

This was a defining moment. I had to rethink what the purpose of therapy was and whether I was actually impacting the child's ability to communicate with others and their environments in my meticulous "evidence-based practice." I resolved that I would do whatever it takes so that preschoolers whom I was treating at that time wouldn't be in this isolated state 6 years later.

The comprehensive treatment activities that I share today are the product of over a decade at the drawing board. This involved attending to successes and failures while consulting colleagues and researching across disciplines in charting unfamiliar territory. These activities will continue to improve over time as our knowledge base continually increases.

I missed the boat 17 years ago. I wasn't treating the child. I was treating body parts. At the preschool level, you have an amazing opportunity to open the world to the child by comprehensively treating them. Developmentally rich and engaging activities will produce optimal gains when neuroplasticity is at a high level.

A combination of the child overcoming neurological and environmental obstacles equates to learning. The therapist's role is to create challenging activities worth the struggle.

Challenge creates change. We cannot do children's push-ups for them. Think of yourself as simply a creator of a maze that is challenging, engaging, and educationally rich for the child to complete. Your job is to create a maze that is at the child's "challenge point" in which the child can independently complete the activity at an 80% accuracy rate.

An accuracy rate of over 80% is too easy. An accuracy rate below 80% is too challenging and risks habituation of error behaviors. After creating the maze, your job is to step back. Children are brilliant. They will learn most efficiently through trial and error.

5.2 Create Educationally Rich Activities across Developmental Domains

Provide engaging and educationally rich activities that comprehensively treat preschoolers. These activities will serve as a meaningful context in which children can request materials that will be strategically placed in reach of the adult, but not the child's.

This chapter presents educationally rich activities across the domains of art, engineering, math, movement, and science. Lastly, we present therapy activities that incorporate behaviors targeted to increase neuronal activity in the cerebellum, the ultimate control center of the brain.

Early literacy activities are additionally recommended because children with speech and language impairments are at elevated risk for literacy difficulties at school age. We cover early literacy intervention activities in Chapter 9.

5.3 Ensure That Activities Are Age Appropriate for All Children

In working with preschoolers with special needs, one challenge is to provide age-appropriate activities for every child regardless of the child's impairment or the child's developmental level.

We've found it to be challenging but important to take the extra time to consider individual needs so that all children can experience age-appropriate activities at an optimal level of independence. Most activities can be adapted to include an engaging individualized, cause-effect task-oriented component such as letters, numbers, shapes, vehicles, animals, and dinosaurs

5.4 Assign an Occupation

Notice how each child is assigned an occupation in the video clips presented throughout this book. This decision is not made flippantly for entertainment purposes. Rather, giving the child an occupation provides a realistic need for the child to complete the task-oriented activity to achieve important goals. An occupation also invites the child into the world of imaginary play.

5.5 Use Three-Dimensional Objects for Learning

Speech-language pathologists often print out papers, laminate, and velcro them, and start believing that they've created three-dimensional objects. That's unfortunate. Children learn from all of their senses, not just their eyes. Whenever possible, use real objects that engage multiple senses.

In this chapter we look at activities across multiple learning domains to comprehensively treat preschoolers. When viewing each digital clip, reference the activity checklist, *Evaluating Activities Scale* (▶ Table 5.1).

Evaluating these sessions will enable you to not only learn from the clips but also improve upon them. Apply this checklist to assist you in creating activities that are engaging, educationally rich, developmentally appropriate, and accessible to a diverse population of preschoolers.

In this chapter we look at activities across multiple learning domains to holistically treat preschoolers. When viewing each digital clip, reference the activity checklist, Evaluating Activities Scale (▶ Table 5.1). Evaluating these sessions will enable you to not only learn from the clips but also improve upon them. This checklist can also be helpful in evolving your activity development. Apply this checklist to assist you in creating activities that are engaging, educationally rich, and accessible to a diverse population of preschoolers.

5.6 Art

Research indicates that children with speech and language impairments are at greater risk for fine motor difficulties.[1,2,3] Art activities provide an enjoyable opportunity to manipulate materials while improving fine motor skills. Additionally, having multiple materials offers numerous opportunities for the child to request using the treatment targets.

With art activities, ensure that they are open-ended in nature. Open-ended activities are activities the child creates as he or she chooses. There is no right way or product that the child is asked to produce.

Conversely, art activities, in which the child is expected to create a predetermined product, are referred to as closed-ended activities and are not recommended. An example of a closed-ended mask making activity is the child being instructed to cut out face parts on a bolded line and glue them on designated areas. See ▶ Fig. 5.1 and ▶ Fig. 5.2 for examples of closed-ended versus open-ended mask making activities.

Video 5.1 and Video 5.2 show children requesting desired objects within art activities from Miss Taylor.

Putting Research into Practice: Creating Open-Ended Art Activities

See ▶ Table 5.2 for common preschool themes presented. What materials would you have the child mand? What motor actions would be required? Could this activity be adapted for children with different motor or developmental skill levels? Are there enough opportunities (i.e., pieces to request) for practice?

Table 5.1 Evaluating activities scale

	Strongly Disagree	Disagree	Neutral	Agree	Strongly Agree
Video Number:_____					
Please indicate your level of agreement to the following statements in reference to the video clip presented.					
1) Activity was reinforcing (i.e., fun and engaging).	1	2	3	4	5
2) Developmentally appropriate for age 3–5 years.	1	2	3	4	5
3) Incorporated 3-dimensional materials	1	2	3	4	5
4) Materials were strategically placed to motivate the child but not distract (e.g., in the child's view but out of the child's reach to elicit mands).	1	2	3	4	5
5) There were sufficient pieces for the child to mand the target numerous times.	1	2	3	4	5
6) Turns to engage in the activity could be quickly enough completed to ensure numerous treatment target mands.	1	2	3	4	5
7) The activity presented a sensory or cause-effect component that all preschool age children could actively participate in, regardless of developmental limitations?	1	2	3	4	5
8) Activity was 'hands-on' in which the child was able to independently manipulate materials.	1	2	3	4	5
9) Activity had a clear beginning, middle, end sequence.	1	2	3	4	5
10) Incorporated Tier 2 vocabulary meaningfully, as applicable, to encourage academic discourse development.	1	2	3	4	5

Strengths:

Weaknesses:

Suggestions for Improvement:

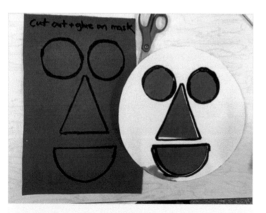

Fig. 5.1 Photo of a closed-ended mask making activity.

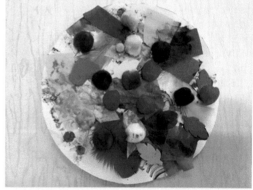

Fig. 5.2 Photo of an open-ended activity: child decided it was a mask.

Table 5.2 Creating open-ended art activities

Complex Consonant Cluster Request Sentence or Paragraph:_____			
Theme	Open-Ended Art Project	Materials to Mand	Child's Fine/Gross Motor Actions
Community Helpers			
Feelings			
On the Farm			
Sports			
Transportation			

Table 5.3 Creating open-ended engineering activities

Complex Consonant Cluster Request Sentence or Paragraph:				
Theme	Open-Ended Project	Materials to Mand	Child's Motor Actions	Spatial/Mathematical Concepts
All About Me				
Insects				
Rainbow Colors				
Five Senses				
Recycling				

5.7 Engineering

Improving spatial skills at the preschool level results in improved math skills at elementary age.[4] The word "engineering" may be daunting but I encourage you to think of activities that involve building, making, or simply tinkering with toys at the preschool level. As with emergent literacy in which you allow the child to take the lead while providing support as needed, treat emergent engineering in the same manner. Your enthusiasm and comfort in the child taking the lead to make open-ended creations will encourage the child to engineer with greater frequency, duration, and independence.

Common engineering materials that encourage spatial skill development in preschoolers include blocks, foam shapes, bricks, legos, wooden logs, magnetic blocks, gears, pegs, marble shoots, magnetic tiles, ramps, train tracks, play dough, clay, and tinker toys. These activities provide plenty of opportunities (or pieces) for children to request using their treatment targets. A good engineering activity would also have a cause-effect, task-oriented component that ensures that all children can participate regardless of developmental differences.

Please refer to Video 5.3, Video 5.4, Video 5.5, Video 5.6, and Video 5.7. In each video, note how the children have opportunities to improve visual-spatial thinking skills in the context of manding with their treatment targets.

Putting Research into Practice: Creating Engineering Activities

See ▶ Table 5.3 for the common preschool themes presented. What materials would you have the child request? What would the child be required to do? What spatial and mathematical concepts could you underscore? Could this activity be adapted for children of diverse developmental levels? Are there enough opportunities to request using the child's treatment target?

5.8 Math

Some research indicates that children with speech and language impairments are at greater risk for

Table 5.4 Incorporating math

Activity	How would you incorporate math?	How would you incorporate a fine/gross motor component?
Complex Consonant Cluster Request Sentence or Paragraph:		
Making Slime		
Car Wash		
Veterinarian		
Shaving Cream		
Ice Cream Shop		

mathematical difficulties at elementary age.[5] Math at the preschool age involves simple rote counting, quantitative counting, learning quantitative concepts (e.g., more, less, most, least), shapes, measuring, sequencing (e.g., first, second,...), and beginning number recognition. Math can easily be incorporated into any activity.

In Video 5.8, Video 5.9, and Video 5.10, math is meaningfully incorporated into speech-language therapy activities. In all situations, preschoolers are not expected to have mastered counting or number recognition. Their therapists are operating within their zone of proximal development, which is their level of capability with scaffolding, or with the assistance of another, to ensure success.[6]

At the therapeutic level, we are interested in the child's optimal level of functioning for maximum change to transpire with the limited therapy time we have available. Notice how fine and gross motor skills are concurrently addressed within the following videos.

Putting Research into Practice: Incorporating Math

See ▶ Table 5.4. For the engaging preschool activities presented, how would you add a math component that may include rote counting, counting quantities, quantitative vocabulary, shapes, sequencing, number recognition, measuring, and graphing? To increase meaningful fine motor opportunities, children can check off graphs with check marks, circles, X's, or tally marks when collecting data. How could you add a gross motor component as well?

5.9 Movement

Movement activities serve multiple purposes. First, they provide for generalization of concepts previously practiced in a more structured setting. Second, they provide for gross motor experiences, which are of unique value to children with communication impairments who are at greater risk for motor delays.[7] Third, they increase attention, cortisol, and dopamine levels to increase engagement and accelerate learning. Fourth, they provide meaningful, multistep experiences for narrative development. Fifth, they improve executive function skills in the child having to solve a problem, form a plan, execute the plan, and take a task to completion.

With movement activities, provide a clear schema of a beginning, middle, and end for the child to follow. This structure of a consistent routine provides organization for children who have self-regulation and organizational difficulties. Additionally, this multistep structure serves as a great linguistic opportunity in which children can request by connecting multiple steps into complex sentences that are conjoined by conjunctions, such as first, then, and lastly.

In Video 5.11, you'll see Alyssa working with a sensory seeking, highly distractible child with Autism Spectrum Disorder. She works at a quick pace and initiates a consistent routine with a clear beginning, middle, and end to maintain the child's attention and active participation while lessening distractions.

For further examples of motor movement activities that require complex motor movements, please see Video 5.12, Video 5.13, Video 5.14, Video 5.15, Video 5.16, Video 5.17, and Video 5.18.

Table 5.5 Incorporating movement

Theme	Activity	Beginning	Middle	End	Cause/Effect Component
Complex Consonant Cluster Request Sentence or Paragraph					
Beach					
Camping					
Carnival					
Safari					

Putting Research into Practice: Creating Movement Activities

See ▶ Table 5.5. Create a movement activity for each of the summer vacation themes with beginning, middle, and end steps to encourage complex language development. Also, include a task-oriented, cause-effect goal to achieve that signals completion of a task and also serves as a naturally occurring reward.

5.10 Science

Science activities are naturally present with exposure to rich academic discourse. Academic discourse is language that is used specifically in academic settings. Early, repeated, meaningful exposure to academic discourse within fun, hands-on activities empowers children with language impairments when they are faced with academic discourse in elementary school.

For science activities with preschoolers, we specifically focus on incorporating Tier 2 vocabulary. Tier 2 vocabulary involves words that are descriptive and cross academic subjects. Tier 2 words frequently occur in academic contexts but not routinely in everyday conversational speech.

Developing this vocabulary early on can empower children with greater comprehension and expression of academic content at elementary age. Some common words to use in describing the scientific process includes hypothesis, prediction, experiment, data, graph, analyze, and conclusion.

Tier 2 vocabulary could also be descriptive words such as transparent, opaque, dense, empty, heavy, light, expanded, contracted, lengthening, shortening, inflating, and deflating. When introducing Tier 2 vocabulary, simply define the words with callouts. Callouts are one or two words long simple explanations.

See Video 5.19, Video 5.20, Video 5.21, Video 5.22, and Video 5.23 for examples of children actively engaging in the scientific process. The scientific method is practiced within each activity. The steps are as follows: (1) ask a question; (2) predict or hypothesize; (3) experiment or test; and (4) graph data and analyze results. Notice how callouts are provided throughout for the child to learn these steps within his or her zone of proximal development.

Putting Research into Practice: Incorporating the Scientific Method and Tier 2 Vocabulary in Science Activities

See ▶ Table 5.6. Examples of common preschool science topics are presented. Write Tier 2 vocabulary and simple explanation callouts for each stage of the scientific process. What Tier 2 descriptive vocabulary words could be introduced with callouts?

5.11 Targeting the Cerebellum in Therapy

It has recently been discovered that the cerebellum plays a much larger role than originally thought. Previously, the cerebellum was considered largely responsible for not much more than motor movements, with neuronal activity primarily occurring in the anterior lobes of the cerebellum.

Table 5.6 Incorporating Tier 2 vocabulary in science

Complex Consonant Cluster Request Sentence/Paragraph:						
Activity	Tier 2	Question	Hypothesis	Experiment	Chart Data	Tier 2 Vocabulary
Feely Box	Callout					
Primary Colors	Callout					
Hot vs. Cold	Callout					
Rain Sticks	Callout					
Sweet vs. Sour	Callout					

However, recent advances due to improved brain imaging indicate the cerebellum to be the ultimate control center in the refinement of language, emotions, cognition, visual-spatial processing, and executive functioning. Neuronal activity of these higher level processes primarily occurs in the posterior lobes of the cerebellum.[8]

The cerebellum, located just behind the brain stem, can be considered the brain's powerhouse in that it is estimated to contain approximately 75% of the neuronal cells in the brain yet only occupies about 10% of its total weight. Also, the cerebellum attaches to nearly every area of the brain with approximately 250 million mossy fibers.[9]

The pervasive influence of the cerebellum on a child's ability to function is evident in children with cerebellar damage. Salman and Tsai's 2016 review indicates that approximately half of children who present with cerebellar damage demonstrate autism-like symptomology of poor eye contact, repetitive hand flapping, delayed speech and language, flat affect, global motor impairments, and impaired play skills.

This number of children with cerebellar damage presenting with these autism-like symptoms skyrockets to 80 to 100% when damage is located in the vermis cerebellar area of the brain. The vermis cerebellar is the midline that connects the left and right cerebellums.[10]

Could intervention that targets complex behaviors largely dictated by the powerhouse cerebellum result in optimal neuronal change? Could we exact optimal neuronal change through focused stimulation by effectively treating multiple behaviors controlled by the cerebellum concurrently? Would children with disorders associated with functional and structural differences in the cerebellum greatly benefit from this type of targeted intervention?

Populations at higher risk for cerebellar differences include children with attention deficit disorder,[11] autism spectrum disorder,[12] developmental coordination disorder,[13] cognitive impairment,[14] dyslexia,[15] language impairments,[16] speech motor disorders,[10] fine and gross motor disorders,[17] and very preterm infants.[18]

5.12 How to Behaviorally Target the Anterior and Posterior Portions of the Cerebellum

To target the anterior portion of the cerebellum, we can incorporate gross motor skills through meaningful task-oriented intervention activities that provide the necessary support for each child to operate at a challenging level.

For example, we can incorporate gross motor intervention by having children complete tasks of increased complexity. Incorporate fine motor intervention by having children engage in emergent writing activities such as graphing their data with tally marks. Improve oral motor coordination by having children request using complex consonant clusters.

By simultaneously focusing our efforts on a diversity of complex motor behaviors, our goal is to increase the amount of neuronal activity and complexity of connections in the cerebellum.

Why do we care so much about gross and fine motor movements? We are after all speech-language pathologists. In the anterior portion of the cerebellum, brain activity responsible for lingual movements is sandwiched between the most anterior portion, responsible for finger movements, and the posterior portion responsible for gross motor movements. To facilitate speech development, we want to increase neuronal activity in this area of the brain.

Table 5.7 Behaviorally Targeting the cerebellum: Provide examples from Video 5.21

Complex Consonant Cluster Request Sentence or Paragraph: Can you scrape it, spray it, or drop it because I have angry dog teeth?		
Anterior Cerebellum	Domain	How did the therapist target the following developmental domains in Video 5.21?
	Gross Motor	
	Fine Motor	
	Speech Motor	
Posterior Cerebellum	Emotion	
	Cognition	
	Language	
	Executive Function	
	Visual Spatial Processing	

To target the posterior portion of the cerebellum, we can incorporate activities that include focusing on learning a process to improve the higher level skill of executive function. We can do so by teaching the child the following steps: (1) "Problem" identification; (2) "Plan" development; (3) "Action" performance; and (4) "Check" for completion. Notice multi-modal gestures used in Video 5.6, Video 5.10, Video 5.13, Video 5.18, Video 5.21, and Video 5.23 that illustrate teaching executive function skills. The gestures are to (1) identify a "problem" with forefingers criss-crossed, tapping each other; (2) develop a "plan" with a football goal post created by thumbs and forefingers; (4) perform an "action" with alternate rowing of the forearms; and (5) self-monitor completion of a task with a "check mark" made by the thumb and forefinger.

To further treat the posterior portion of the cerebellum, we can increase accuracy of emotion identification.[19] These skills can be improved upon by improving motor imitation to increase mirror neuron activation for empathy development. We can also emphasize emotion through exaggerated facial, gestural, and vocal expressions within engaging activities.

To further target the posterior portion of the cerebellum in improving language skills, we can incorporate language of increased length and complexity. We can also incorporate Tier 2 vocabulary with callouts.

We can also target higher level literacy skills and multistep narration using first, then, and lastly.

Development of phonological awareness skills will also directly ignite neuronal development in the cerebellum.

Additionally, to improve executive function, we can provide guided practice using the scientific process. This helps develop higher-level, critical thinking skills, decision-making, problem-solving skills, and cognitive flexibility in that outcomes change depending on variables tested in experiments.

Explore three-dimensional materials and their characteristics using Tier 2 vocabulary through multi-sensory experiences enables new concepts and vocabulary to be learned more deeply.

See ▶ Table 5.7. Once again refer Video 5.21, Marine biologist Jillian examining sea animals. Provide an example of how Torey directly targeted behaviors related to the anterior and posterior lobes of the cerebellum.

Putting Research into Practice: Targeting the Anterior and Posterior Cerebellum

See ▶ Table 5.8. Create your own movement activity for preschoolers that targets the anterior and posterior portions of the cerebellum. Complete each aspect of the activity that will behaviorally target the cerebellum to increase its widespread neuronal activity.

Table 5.8 Create your own movement activity to behaviorally target the cerebellum

Complex Consonant Cluster Request Sentence or Paragraph:_____

Anterior Cerebellum	Domain	How will you target the following developmental domains?
	Gross Motor	
	Fine Motor	
	Speech Motor	
Posterior Cerebellum	Emotion	
	Cognition	
	Language	
	Executive Function	
	Visual Spatial Processing	

5.13 Chapter Summary

See Kelly's Corner Video 5.24 for an illustration of how we couple academic concepts with multimodal cueing to deepen the learning experience. This chapter delved into how to incorporate rich activities across developmental domains to comprehensively treat the child with a speech sound disorder. Our activities were quite dense in introducing academic discourse, the scientific method, and a process to improve executive function skills.

As a result, less time was often available for the child to request using speech-language treatment targets. With every educationally rich activity presented, density in terms of number of accurately produced requests containing treatment targets in a session is critically important in treating speech sound disorders to maintain the integrity of the intervention.[20]

In developing educationally rich activities, we leave this chapter on a new82frontier, applying behavioral interventions to target the cerebellum. In doing so, our goal is to produce optimal change in the brain when neuroplasticity is at a high level.

As our understanding of the connection between behaviors and neuronal activity improve with advances in science, particularly in the realm of functional magnetic resonance imaging (MRI) research, we can create therapy that more efficiently produces optimal change across developmental domains.

With these advances, we are on the cusp of a major evolution in how we comprehensively treat children to produce an impactful change early on for improved long-term outcomes.

References

[1] Bishop DV. Motor immaturity and specific speech and language impairment: evidence for a common genetic basis. Am J Med Genet. 2002; 114(1):56–63

[2] Iverson JM, Braddock BA. Gesture and motor skill in relation to language in children with language impairment. J Speech Lang Hear Res. 2011; 54(1):72–86

[3] Sanjeevan T, Rosenbaum DA, Miller C, Hell JGV, Weiss DJ, Mainela-Arnold E. Motor issues in specific language impairment: a window into the underlying impairment. Curr Dev Disord Rep. 2015; 2(3):228–236

[4] Verdine BN, Golinkoff RM, Hirsh-Pasek K, Newcombe NS, IV. Results-links between spatial assembly, later spatial skills, and concurrent and later mathematical skills. Monogr Soc Res Child Dev. 2017; 82(1):71–80

[5] Harrison LJ, Mcleod S, Berthelsen D, Walker S. Literacy, numeracy, and learning in school-aged children identified as having speech and language impairment in early childhood. Int J Speech Lang Pathol. 2009; 11(5):392–403

[6] Vygotskij LS, Cole M. Mind in Society: The Development of Higher Psychological Processes. Cambridge, MA: Harvard University Press; 1981

[7] Rechetnikov RP, Maitra K. Motor impairments in children associated with impairments of speech or language: a meta-analytic review of research literature. Am J Occup Ther. 2009; 63(3):255–263

[8] Schmahmann JD. The cerebellum and cognition. Neurosci Lett. 2019; 688:62–75

[9] Poretti A, Huisman TA. The pediatric cerebellum. Neuroimaging Clin N Am. 2016; 26(3):xiii–xiv

[10] Salman MS, Tsai P. The role of the pediatric cerebellum in motor functions, cognition, and behavior: a clinical perspective. Neuroimaging Clin N Am. 2016; 26(3):317–329

[11] Sjöwall D, Thorell LB. A critical appraisal of the role of neuropsychological deficits in preschool ADHD. Child Neuropsychol. 2019; 25(1):60–80

[12] Schmahmann JD, Guell X, Stoodley CJ, Halko MA. The theory and neuroscience of cerebellar cognition. Annu Rev Neurosci. 2019; 42(1):337–364

[13] Blank R, Barnett AL, Cairney J, et al. International clinical practice recommendations on the definition, diagnosis, assessment, intervention, and psychosocial aspects of developmental coordination disorder. Dev Med Child Neurol. 2019; 61(3):242–285

[14] He L, Parikh NA. Aberrant executive and frontoparietal functional connectivity in very preterm infants with diffuse white matter abnormalities. Pediatr Neurol. 2015; 53(4):330–337

[15] Borchers LR, Bruckert L, Dodson CK, et al. Microstructural properties of white matter pathways in relation to subsequent reading abilities in children: a longitudinal analysis. Brain Struct Funct. 2019; 224(2):891–905

[16] Yang HC, Gray S. Executive function in preschoolers with primary language impairment. J Speech Lang Hear Res. 2017; 60 (2):379–392

[17] McClelland M, Cameron CE. Developing together: the role of executive function and motor skills in children's early academic lives. Early Child Res Q. 2019; 46:142–151

[18] Herzmann CS, Snyder AZ, Kenley JK, Rogers CE, Shimony JS, Smyser CD. Cerebellar functional connectivity in term- and very preterm-born infants. Cereb Cortex. 2019; 29(3):1174–1184

[19] Adamaszek M, D'Agata F, Ferrucci R, et al. Consensus paper: cerebellum and emotion. Cerebellum. 2017; 16(2):552–576

[20] Edeal DM, Gildersleeve-Neumann CE. The importance of production frequency in therapy for childhood apraxia of speech. Am J Speech Lang Pathol. 2011; 20(2):95–110

5

6 Dynamically Prompting and Errorlessly Fading Multimodal Cues

The space between you and me is longer than forever and I will show them that forever is not so far away.

— Misty Copeland

What makes a speech-language pathologist different from the average lay person in improving speech of preschoolers with speech sound disorders? A primary difference is that the lay person does not have a toolbox of multi-modal cues to establish correct production. A child says, "Tan I have it? (/tæn aɪ hæv ɪt?/)" A lay person would say, "No, say 'can' (/kæn/)." The child again says, "Tan I have it? (/tæn aɪ hæv ɪt?/)" End of story.

Not only can we establish correct production of "can" but, more importantly, we can ignite robust cognitive and linguistic neurological connections. We can further increase neuronal connections by having the child say complex consonant cluster speech targets within utterances of increased length and complexity.

Instead of having the child simply say, "Can I have it?" we might have the child initially request with "Can you scrape it to me please?" Then, after correct production is established, we can increase the complexity to "First, can you scrape it out please? Then, can you spray it at me? Lastly, can you drop it on because I have angry dog teeth." (Refer to Appendix E.)

We are successful because of our elaborate tool box of cues that empower children to perform at their highest level in producing sounds and increasing expressive language length and complexity. Perhaps more importantly, we know of the neurological impact that more complex linguistic structures have on increasing brain activity.

Recent neurological evidence indicates that increased linguistic complexity not only improves speech intelligibility but can even rewire and reorganize neural networks in the brain.[1]

Over the past 10 years I've had the great fortune to work with talented graduate students to research and improve preschool age interventions for optimal gains. Collectively, we've developed over a hundred gestural cues. These invaluable cues have been effectively used to treat speech sound disorders, improve expressive language, comprehension, phonological awareness, narrative skills, numeracy skills, academic language, and reinforce prosocial behaviors.

These gestural cues are also effective in learning higher level processes of elements of a story, the scientific method, and executive function. Developing a strong foundation for these higher level thinking skills is of great value throughout an individual's lifetime.

Every graduate student has brought a unique brilliance to our intervention table. Over the years, I've taken detailed notes and improved my practice by incorporating the creativity and particular skills of each one.

This book is an opportunity to share effective and creative prompts that were collectively developed over the past decade. Also covered are scaffolding practices that have consistently resulted in both substantial gains in standardized single word testing and Percent Consonants Correct (PCC) in conversational speech.

In our summer speech intervention program, over a 5-year span, preschoolers with diverse etiologies and severity of speech impairment consistently showed substantive improvements after only four or five 45-minute therapy sessions. These improvements were replicated each year.[2,3,4,5]

6.1 Zone of Proximal Development

The zone of proximal development is the level a child is able to achieve with a more capable peer's or adult's assistance. To effectively implement the prompts in therapy, we'll review evidence-based practices which are implemented when introducing and fading multi-modal cueing. Visualize a scaffolded skyscraper in the construction phase. Your goal is to be that temporary scaffold that builds the child up to perform at an optimal level of performance for maximum growth to occur.[6]

6.2 Incorporating Principles of Nonspeech Motor Learning

Maas and colleagues have suggested incorporating efficacy research on the principles of (nonspeech) motor learning in treating motor speech disorders.[7]

Motor learning principles indicate that optimal learning occurs at a challenge-point. Guadagnoli and Lee, the authors of challenge-point theory, define challenge-point as when an individual learner's skill level is matched with a level of task difficulty that results in the learner performing at an optimal level.[8]

This theory emphasizes the interplay between the child's current skill level and a challenging task for an optimal performance. This theory is consistent with Vygotsky's theory of the zone of proximal development.

Both theories underscore that an interplay with more capable individuals (i.e., zone of proximal development) and with more advanced motor tasks (i.e., challenge-point) result in the occurrence of an optimal level of learning.

In using the construction of a skyscraper analogy, visualize this learning that involves the more advanced partner (i.e., the temporary scaffolds) and the challenge point target (e.g., 160 floors—the world's current tallest building) as a reference for therapy. In the initial stages, give a maximum level of support to operate at a challenge point. Fade support over time.[7]

6.3 Neurological Scaffolding

How does neurological scaffolding play out in the brain? As therapy progresses, scaffolds (others' temporary supports) are gradually faded as the child's neurological connections are built into place. These connections are strengthened due to frequent production of complex neurological behaviors—in this case, complex consonant clusters.

These newly built neurological connections are neural networks. A neural network is a group of neurons (nerve cells) interconnected by synapses (impulses that carry information to travel over spaces) to perform a function.

For instance, if a neural network is strengthened to produce 3-element consonant clusters (such as /spɹ/), simpler 2-element consonant clusters (e.g.,/sp/) and singleton consonants (/ɹ/) would naturally develop. This is due to the development of complex neural mechanisms through repeated production of 3-element consonant clusters. This results in the spontaneous development of simpler neural networks that produce simpler motor patterns.[1,4,9]

The take-home message is that our goal in therapy is to light up the brain. This occurs because the child is producing the most complex linguistic targets, thereby enabling optimal neuronal change to occur at younger ages when neuroplasticity is at a high level.

The neuroscientific research available from child and adult populations indicates that by selecting complex linguistic targets, simpler semantic,[10] syntactical,[11] morphological,[12] and phonological targets[13] will spontaneously develop. In treating each aspect of communication, rewiring and reorganizing children's brains is accomplished by teaching complex targets through dynamic multimodal cueing.[14,15]

6.4 Maxim #1: Provide Maximum Level of Support with Highest Level Targets to Ignite Optimal Change

Go big. Aim for the most complex 3-element consonant cluster if you are treating a speech sound disorder. If there is a concurrent language impairment, produce this complex speech target in a syntactic-linguistic context of increased length and complexity. You need to provide a maximum level of scaffolding for the child to accurately produce complex targets in the initial stages of therapy.

Following standardized articulation assessment, check for consonant clusters that the child can accurately produce with a maximum level of prompting using the *Supplemental Consonant Cluster Screener* from Chapter 3. What does a maximum level of prompting mean? The prompting hierarchy presented here is based on the work of Rosenbek and colleagues in treating adults with apraxia[16] and of Strand and colleagues in treating children with childhood apraxia of speech.[17,18,19]

It is adapted to treat a diverse population of preschoolers with speech sound disorders, using a most-to-least hierarchy that incorporates dynamic tactile and temporal cueing while maintaining an 80% minimal accuracy baseline throughout.

Tactile cueing refers to physical touch cues that aid the child in achieving accuracy in sound placement, manner, and voicing. These tactile cues can be self-administered by the child in being actively engaged. They can also be administered by an adult. In this case the child is more passively engaged.

Temporal cueing refers to spatial cues illustrated by fingers, hands, and arm movements in space to clearly aid the child in achieving accuracy in sound placement, manner, and voicing.

In the following text, refer to a highly effective six-step maximum to minimal prompting hierarchy that we have implemented and researched over a 5-year span in treating children of various etiologies and levels of severity.

In each case, this prompting hierarchy has ignited substantial gains for preschoolers with diverse underlying disorders and levels of severity over a short time period.

Refer ▸ Table 6.1 when viewing digital clips. The hierarchy of cueing may change depending on the child. For some children a visual model may be a maximum level of cueing and a verbal model may be of little to no assistance. For other children, a verbal model may be helpful while visual models are meaningless. Differentially adjust most-to least hierarchies based on a most-to-least helpful prompt sequence for each individual child.

6.5 Six-Step Process in Dynamically Prompting and Fading Multimodal Cues

Step 1: Speak in unison.

Speak in slow, choral speech with the child, prolonging consonants and vowels. Use accompanying tactile, temporal, visual, and verbal cues as necessary. Avoid pauses that exceed 2 seconds between sounds because speech is an automatic and continuous motor movement.

Increase rate slowly or continually while maintaining 80% accuracy. Quicken the speech rate when producing easier sounds and slow the rate by stretching out complex clusters to ensure accuracy in producing each sound. See Video 6.1.

Step 2: Focus on the child imitating your temporal or tactile cueing, while fading your verbal model. Encourage the child to mimic your hand movements as well as your speech to develop an internal locus of control. In this way the child assumes the role of the teacher in both temporal and tactile cueing.

Use exaggerated temporal cueing with your hands to make the manner, placement, and voicing salient. If you are using tactile cueing, have the child mirror you by touching his or her own face as you visually model.

Respect that some children have poor motor imitation skills and may never nonverbally imitate you. This does not mean that they are not attentively learning. Still, give an honest effort in developing this critically important skill of motor imitation. We've found that children who don't motorically imitate in therapy often demonstrate a lack of nonverbal participation in group settings.

Also, during the generalization stages, many children tend to focus 100% of their efforts on oral motor movements. Therefore, they will spontaneously phase out imitating temporal and tactile cues to fully attend to their mouth movements in producing complex consonant clusters. See Video 6.2.

Step 3: Provide intermittent verbal and nonverbal cues only when necessary.

Have the child say the words as independently as possible with you modeling temporal and tactile cues only when necessary. Dynamically provide intermittent cueing in which you insert verbal and nonverbal cues with harder to produce clusters and sounds. Pull back all cues with sounds the child can independently produce. Maintain 80% accuracy by dynamically removing and inserting support based on the child's moment-to-moment performance. See Video 6.3.

Step 4: Cue to prevent persistent errors.

When the child is independently saying the treatment target in a sentence or paragraph, fold your fingers together as the child is the teacher now and is assuming an internal locus of control.

Prevent persistent errors and suppress immature phonological processes by providing support for only these remaining error sounds. To prevent negative practice specifically insert choral speech, temporal cueing, tactile modeling, or a verbal call out (e.g., "snake in the cage") before the child produces a persistent error sound. See Video 6.4.

Step 5: Remind the child of the speech rule prior to the child's manding.

Remind the child of the speech rule before the child produces the treatment target request. For example, "Are you going to remember 'angry dog teeth ($/ɹ/$)'? I'm going to be on the lookout for scary, angry dog teeth ($/ɹ/$)." Each time you see the angry dog teeth pretend that you are afraid and pull back, biting your nails in fear.

After the request, prompt the child to also state the speech rule, asking, "What did you remember to do?" You could also provide a completion prompt: "You had _____."

Step 6: The child self-evaluates.

Have the child be the teacher in evaluating a puppet's speech, a peer's speech, your speech, or his/her own speech. You can hold up a thumb sideways and ask specific judgment of a speech behavior: "Did you stick your tongue out like a rude boy ($/θ/,/ð/$)?"

Remember to provide support so the child can be correct in judgment minimally 80% of the time. Perhaps the thumb can be held at a slight angle as a cue when the child seems unsure. (This strategy

Table 6.1 Evaluating prompting and fading multimodal cues

Video Number:_____

Please indicate your level of agreement to the following statements in reference to the literacy digital clip presented.	Strongly Disagree	Disagree	Neutral	Agree	Strongly Agree
1) Therapist has child's attention.	1	2	3	4	5
2) Child is nonverbally imitating cues.	1	2	3	4	5
3) Direct verbal modelling is faded as much as possible, while maintaining 80% accuracy.	1	2	3	4	5
4) Speech is presented as a continuous motor movement with pauses between sounds not exceeding 2 seconds within words.	1	2	3	4	5
5) Level of cueing ensures a minimal 80% accuracy level.	1	2	3	4	5
6) Pace is appropriate based on child's skill level to ensure 80% accuracy level. (Too slow=child is inefficiently challenged. Too fast=less than 80% accurate.)	1	2	3	4	5
7) Cues are presented to prevent errors ensuring a minimal 80% accuracy level.	1	2	3	4	5
8) Call outs clearly instruct desired behavior or incompatible rule to a speech error and are used repeatedly to instill the concept.	1	2	3	4	5
9) Therapist exaggerates temporal gestural cues to ensure saliency of desired speech motor movement.	1	2	3	4	5
10) Cueing is downplayed on easier sounds/words and emphasized on complex sounds/clusters.	1	2	3	4	5
11) Child is encouraged to actively participate by stating the speech motor rule.	1	2	3	4	5
12) At generalization stage, child is encouraged to self-evaluate after producing the target.	1	2	3	4	5
13) Therapist responds enthusiastically to correct production of complex sounds/clusters.	1	2	3	4	5
14) Therapist provides objective and specifically feedback regarding the child's production.	1	2	3	4	5
15) Therapist provides objective encouragement for the child assuming an internal locus of control (i.e., role as teacher).	1	2	3	4	5

Strengths:

Weaknesses:

Suggestions for Improvement:

6

can be easily implemented into a whole group speech perception activity with children actively participating with their judging thumbs.) See Video 6.6.

Research has suggested that principles of motor learning may be applied in providing two types of objective feedback to a speech motor target: *Knowledge of Performance* (KP) and *Knowledge of Results (KR)*. KP refers to providing specific feedback regarding the motor movement, such as "you kept an angry dog smile /ɹ/." Refer Video 6.1, Video 6.2, Video 6.3, Video 6.4, Video 6.5 for KP feedback.[7]

Conversely, KR refers to providing feedback regarding accuracy versus inaccuracy after the motor movement is completed (Video 6.6). At the preschool age level, opt to focus attention on KP, in which objective feedback regarding the desired motor movement is provided at a 1:1 behavior to reinforcement ratio. This is in consideration of continuous reinforcement being indicated at preschool age over an intermittent schedule for improved outcomes.[20] Additionally, with increased complexity of the motor act of producing 3-element clusters, increased feedback in learning more complex motor patterns will be required.[7,21]

At the generalization level, a child can begin to focus on KR, which is judgment of accurate versus inaccurate performance immediately after producing treatment targets. Developing independence in self-monitoring through a focus on KR can further assist the child in developing an internal locus of control in self-evaluating his or her own speech.

6.6 Maxim #2: Go Errorless by Placing 99.99% Effort in Prevention of the Error

Often a child will produce a sound incorrectly and then produce the sound correctly. The child is then rewarded with desired materials provided or actions administered within an engaging activity. The problem with reinforcement of this accuracy level is that the child was correct 50% of the time and incorrect 50% of the time with a reward following. The incorrect form is as likely to be rewarded as the correct production. To prevent randomly rewarding incorrect speech:

1. Front-load by stating the rule with accompanying gestures prior to requesting with the treatment target. For instance, give a completion prompt, "The snake stays in___ (child: 'the cage')" prior to attempting to produce an /s/ that is typically frontally lisped as a /θ/.
2. Prevent an error sound if you see it coming. If you see the child with rounded lips about to produce /w/ for /l/, you may call out (e.g., "teeth, teeth, teeth–big smile!" for a labially retracted /l/).
3. Strategically prompt by planning to pull back prompting when it is unnecessary and preemptively deciding which challenging sounds to cue before and during production.

See Video 6.7 of Elon with Taylor. Note how prompting is dynamically faded and inserted prior to production of more difficult consonant clusters. Verbal call outs are also used for errorless production to occur.

6.7 Maxim #3: Develop Cues That Are Incompatible with the Error

Developing incompatible cues that prevent the error sound from being produced is a highly effective strategy in establishing correct sound production. For instance, if the child maintains an open mouth posture, the child simply cannot front velars in producing /k/, /g/ as /t/, /d/. Refer ▶ Table 6.2 and ▶ Table 6.3, which list common phonological processes and distortions followed by incompatible strategies to prevent these errors from occurring.

As mentioned in Chapter 3, do not waste therapy time intervening on simpler phonological processes of consonant or syllable deletion because consonant cluster treatment targets effectively suppress these earlier syllable structure phonological processes spontaneously.[2,3,4,5]

Parents may ask for a way to cue correct production of multisyllabic words. You can advise that caregivers clap syllables as spoken to improve phonological awareness skills.[22] However, emphasis on later developing phonological processes of cluster reduction and cluster simplification results in greater efficiency in ameliorating both sound and syllable deletion. See Video 6.8.

Putting Research into Practice: Hands-On Practice in Cueing Consonant Clusters

Refer to the *Consonant Cluster Stimulability Screener* in Chapter 3. Provide a maximum level of cueing for every item on the screener in a mirror or with a partner using choral speech. Emphasize the consonant clusters and later developing sounds. Provide explicit verbal "call outs" as well to ensure accurate production. If you have a partner, have the partner present with common phonological processes and distortions for you to prevent. Keep in mind that speech is an automatic, continuous motor activity. Therefore, pauses between sounds should not extend beyond 2 seconds.

6.8 Maxim #4: Fade Verbal Modeling as Soon as Possible while Maintaining 80% Accuracy

Children can easily become dependent on the verbal model provided in choral speech. They often stop talking when our verbal model in choral speech is removed. Pointing to the child helps cue a transfer of responsibility for speaking to to the child. sentences independently in the child assuming the teacher's role.

Notice in Video 6.9 Alyssa is fading out the verbal model with Jacob on words that he is able to produce independently. She is prompting dynamically, providing supports for blends and sounds that remain challenging for him. At the same time,

Table 6.2 Phonological processes and incompatible strategies

	Incompatible Strategy: Have the child....
Backing of /t/ and /d/	produce /s/ or /z/ and stop the airflow
Fronting of /k/, /g/, /ŋ/	place a finger horizontally across the mouth like a horse-bit to ensure it remains open
Stopping	hold the sound longer and release it in a neutral vowel position /ʌ/ to ensure continuation of airflow
Deaffrication	have the child hold cheeks in for "choo-choo" sound or turn the key with fists rotating for "engine revving" /dʒ/ sound loudly
Cluster Reduction	produce every sound in the cluster sound *slowly* in echoed speech
Final Consonant Deletion*	hold finger in the air like popping a bubble–pop it when it's produced (leave finger in air until the final sound is produced)
Weak Syllable Deletion*	clap hands together with production of each syllable

*Note: Final consonant deletion and weak syllable are not recommended as treatment targets in that more complex consonant cluster targets directly suppress these phonological processes and result in greater gains. Parents, however, often request cues to work on these simpler phonological processes within the natural environment.

Table 6.3 Distortion errors and incompatible strategies

Distortions	Incompatible Strategies
Gliding of /l/ and /ɹ/	smile big to prevent rounding of lipsand make "angry dog teeth" for /ɹ/
Lisping of /s/ frontally	teeth together, "keeping the snake in the cage"
Lisping of /s/ laterally	smile big to prevent air escaping laterally
Misarticulation of /θ, ð/	stick tongue out like a rude child and blow
Labializations of /f/ and /v/	say alphabet letter "F" (/ɛf/) before /f/ and "eh" (/ɛ/) before /v/ to curl the lower lip over the bottom teeth
Rounding of lips with /j/	say alphabet letter "E" (/i/) before /j/ to achieve lip retraction
Retracting lips with /w/	Say "oo" /u/ before /w/ to achieve lip protrusion

6

When to Use Tactile Cueing and When to Use Temporal Cueing?

Temporal cueing is the preferred cueing method if sounds can be produced accurately. This is because temporal cues can be easily faded and are less intrusive to the speed and automaticity of speech movements than tactile cues.

Tactile cueing is effective in establishing labial phonemes /p, b, m/ when the child has poor proprioception, which is the sense of knowing where his or her own body parts are in space. When the child touches his or her own lips, the child can be sure they are closed. Additionally, some children have poor proprioception of their tongue and have difficulty protruding it to produce the /θ/ and /ð/ sound. For this, I have instructed children to touch their tongue with their forefinger (when clean) to establish production and self-awareness of the rude boy /θ/ and /ð/ sounds.

For children with poor motor coordination, glides /w/ and /j/ can be challenging. Both /w/ and /j/ involve lip protrusion and retractions as the airflow literally glides over the tongue. To produce the /w/, have the child start with the rounded tense vowel /u/ and quickly retract the lips into a smile.

Opposite to /w/, the /j/ begins with lips retracted in producing the tense labially retracted, like the vowel /i/, and ends with lips protracted forward.

With both sounds, the child can use a forefinger and thumb on the corners of the lips to provide proprioceptive feedback and assist in both retracting and protracting the lips.

Children with poor maxillary strength often present with chubby cheeks, downturned corners of the lips, and mouth breathing at rest. Due to these weaknesses, protrusion of lips to produce the palatal /ʃ/ and /ʒ/ sounds, as well as the alveopalatal affricates /tʃ/ and /dʒ/, is often difficult.

We've found that children pinching their cheeks together with the thumb on one cheek and fingers on the other cheek and pulling forward to effectively cue palatal sounds.

A tactile technique that we have not found successful is children tucking their lip under their top teeth with their forefinger for the labial dentals /f/ and /v/. (See ▶ Table 6.4 for effective /f/ and /v/ strategies.)

For the remaining English phonemes, which are produced inner-orally, we have also found tactile cues to be ineffective. For these sounds, we've found temporal cues to be more effective.

---

she is fading support for simple singleton sounds and easier clusters.

6.9 Maxim #5: Create Catchy Slogans or Songs for Children to Learn Speech Rules

Though probably tone deaf, I have learned to create songs for every phonological process and common speech distortion. My colleagues and "therapy roommates" are not my biggest fans but my preschoolers love singing our speech rule songs and dancing with accompanying gestures. Use a tune from a classic children's song or perhaps a catchy chorus from a popular song on the radio. Children will more quickly and memorably learn the speech rule because of the engaging manner in which it is presented. See Video 6.10.

Putting Research into Practice

For each phonological process and common distortion listed below, create with a slogan for how to produce the sound to be sung in a classic children's song. Complete ▶ Table 6.4 for practice.

6.10 Maxim #6: Encourage Independence Every Step of the Way

Children love hearing, "You're the teacher now!" Whenever a verbal model is faded, make sure to acknowledge that the child is in charge. This may be a powerful motivator because communication is

Table 6.4 Making speech rules meaningful through slogans and tunes

Name of Process	Definition	Example	Refrain of Song: Tune
Fronting	A palatal or velar sound becomes an alveolar sound.	Cow: /kaʊ/ → /taʊ/	
Stopping	A stop replaces a fricative.	Four: /fɔr/ → /bɔr/	
Gliding	A liquid becomes a glide.	Red: /ɹɛd/ → /wɛd/	
S-blend Simplification	/s/ in a consonant cluster is deleted.	Spoon: /spun/ → /pun/	
L-Blend Simplification	/l/ in a consonant cluster is deleted.	Fly: /flaɪ/ → / faɪ/	
R-Blend Simplification	/ɹ/ in a consonant cluster is deleted.	Broom: /bɹum/ → /bum/	
Deaffrication	An affricate becomes a palatal fricative	Jar: /dʒɑr/ → /ʒɑr/	

power and children with communication impairments often are deprived of control of their own bodies, control of others, and control over their environments.

When the child is able to say the paragraph independently and accurately, he or she will often instruct you to not help with your hands. They are not only teaching you now, but also themselves. This behavior demonstrates development of an internal locus of control.

6.11 Maxim #7: Emphasize Accuracy Over Speed

Do not worry about the child's rate of speech. A child will increase the rate of speech for natural rewards to be delivered more quickly. Err on the side of speaking too slowly, which gives children time to self-monitor while engaging in accurate practice.

Differentiate practice for each individual child. There are children with attentional deficits that require quicker speech and cueing to maintain attention. The price for speed may be decreased accuracy.

Over time, attempt to slow the pace with these children to increase both accuracy and attention.

Children will also naturally develop a quicker speaking rate as their request target sentence or paragraph becomes more automatic. Use a mixed pace method in carrying a normal speed with easier sounds and words. Conversely, slow down with complex consonant clusters and later developing sounds.

Be cautious of going too slowly, which makes speech a series of disjointed effortful motor movements. This is completely unlike speech. For instance, in producing the 3-element blend /skɹ/ in "scrape," the therapist has left the automatic realm of speech in instructing the child to make three disparate motor movements by saying, "Make the snake sound /s/. Put the tongue in the back of your mouth /k/. Make an angry dog sound /ɹ/."

Schmidt and Wrisberg argue that speech is an example of a behavior dictated by an open-loop 89control center in which the behavior will occur before the speaker can change it based on sensory feedback.23 Open-loop control systems are movements that are completed without reference to the environment. If a wrong movement is planned, a wrong movement will be executed.

This contrasts with closed-loop control systems, in which movements are purposeful, slow, and effortful. Closed-loop control movements are constantly modified based on feedback from the environment. Schmidt and Wrisberg argue that closed-loop control movements are too purposeful and slow to account for the automatic, fast movements of speech.

Conversely, consider any human motor act in depth and you'll find it difficult to categorize it as being governed by either a closed-loop motor system or an open-loop motor system behavior.

In speech therapy, the motor movements of speech could be controlled by both an intentional closed-loop system and an automatic open-loop system. In the initial stages of therapy, producing accurate complex sound clusters are learned through a slowed, purposeful closed-loop system that incorporates multi-modal feedback every step of the way.

With repeated accurate practice, however, speech is produced under an open-loop system in which neuronal automaticity has developed over time. As

6

Determining if Human Behaviors Are Controlled by Open-Loop or Closed-Loop Motor Systems

To illustrate open-loop control systems versus closed-loop control systems, picture a baseball pitcher throwing a pitch to a batter. The minute the pitcher begins the wind up, he or she is engaged in an open-loop control system in which he or she is simply moving too fast to change the motor movement based on sensory feedback. The batter, however, is engaged in a closed-loop activity in which he or she uses the environmental feedback of the ball height and distance from the plate to decide whether or not to swing the bat.

Could closed-loop versus open-loop control systems really be that simple? No. Human behavior is just too complex to place in these binary categories. For instance, suppose the batter starts to swing, it would mean open-loop control system is immediately in place. However, what if the batter suddenly pulls back, deciding the pitch is out of reach, in which case is the closed-loop control system newly in place? It is up to a discerning umpire to decide whether the activity was an open-loop swing (i.e., strike) or a closed-loop, checked swing (i.e., ball) that doesn't cross midline.

Unlike human behavior, mechanical behavior can be easily categorized. Mechanical objects can be either controlled by open-loop motor systems, such as a timed toaster or closed-loop motor systems, such as a thermostat that continually adjusts in response to room's temperature.

the child develops automaticity in speech accuracy, the child's speech will fluidly move from a closed-loop motor system to an open-loop system.

This ability to fluidly and creatively move in and out of these complex motor systems is a uniquely human behavior that even the most advanced artificial intelligence cannot currently replicate. Similarly, it is in this art of creatively stepping forward and backward in response to one another that both the therapist and the client will reach optimal levels of potential.

6.12 Chapter Summary

In this chapter, we examined the dynamic dance of pushing in and pulling back support based on a child's moment-to-moment performance. The goal from the onset of therapy is always to transfer the locus of control from the therapist to the child. The child is, from the initial stages, encouraged to take responsibility for speech by assuming the teacher role as early in the intervention process as possible.

In therapy, be present. Your total dedication to the child in every response and cue in each moment will reap dividends in the future. Personally, I focus on the quality of the interaction in providing a graduated level of prompting so that each and every response maintains an 80% accuracy level. See Kelly's Corner Video 6.11 for a discussion of the importance of adhering to the 80% accuracy rule.

For all of my clients with speech sound disorders, I administer a single-word standardized test approximately every 8 weeks. Meta-analytic research indicates this to be generally a sufficient time frame for gains to accrue.[24]

References

[1] Kiran S, Thompson CK. Neuroplasticity of language networks in aphasia: advances, updates, and future challenges. Front Neurol. 2019; 10:295

[2] Vess K, Hansen L, Mae-Smith M, Ridella M, Steinberg E. Evidence-based intervention strategies to effectively treat preschoolers with speech sound disorders. Poster session presented at Annual American Speech, Language and Hearing Association; November, 2015. Denver, CO

[3] Vess K, Burgess R, Corless E, Discenna T. Selecting complex consonant cluster targets: are certain sound combinations more efficacious than others? Poster session presented at Annual American Speech, Language and Hearing Association; November, 2016. Philadelphia, PA

[4] Vess K, Coppiellie J, Ingraham B, Reidt M. Targeting /ɹ/ consonant clusters: does generalization occur across phonetic contexts? Poster session presented at Annual American Speech, Language and Hearing Association; November, 2017. Los Angeles, CA

[5] Vess K, Liovas M, Mocny A, Vuletic D. Applying the complexity approach to effectively treat severe speech impairment in preschoolers with ASD. Poster session presented at Annual American Speech, Language and Hearing Association; November, 2018. Boston, MA

[6] Vygotsky LS, Cole M. Mind in Society: The Development of Higher Psychological Processes. Cambridge, MA: Harvard University Press; 1978

[7] Maas E, Robin DA, Austermann Hula SN, et al. Principles of motor learning in treatment of motor speech disorders. Am J Speech Lang Pathol. 2008; 17(3):277–298

[8] Guadagnoli MA, Lee TD. Challenge point: a framework for conceptualizing the effects of various practice conditions in motor learning. J Mot Behav. 2004; 36(2):212–224

[9] Gierut JA, Champion AH. Syllable onsets II: three-element clusters in phonological treatment. J Speech Lang Hear Res. 2001; 44(4):886–904

[10] Kiran S. Complexity in the treatment of naming deficits. Am J Speech Lang Pathol. 2007; 16(1):18–29

[11] Thompson CK, Shapiro LP, Kiran S, Sobecks J. The role of syntactic complexity in treatment of sentence deficits in agrammatic aphasia: the complexity account of treatment efficacy (CATE). J Speech Lang Hear Res. 2003; 46(3):591–607

[12] Van Horne AJO, Fey M, Curran M. Do the hard things first: a randomized controlled trial testing the effects of exemplar selection on generalization following therapy for grammatical morphology. J Speech Lang Hear Res. 2017; 60(9):2569–2588

[13] Storkel HL. Implementing evidence-based practice: selecting treatment words to boost phonological learning. Lang Speech Hear Serv Sch. 2018; 49(3):482–496

[14] Dick AS, Raja Beharelle A, Solodkin A, Small SL. Interhemispheric functional connectivity following prenatal or perinatal brain injury predicts receptive language outcome. J Neurosci. 2013; 33(13):5612–5625

[15] Ghotra SK, Johnson JA, Qiu W, Newton A, Rasmussen C, Yager JY. Age at stroke onset influences the clinical outcome and health-related quality of life in pediatric ischemic stroke survivors. Dev Med Child Neurol. 2015; 57(11):1027–1034

[16] Rosenbek JC, Lemme ML, Ahern MB, Harris EH, Wertz RT. A treatment for apraxia of speech in adults. J Speech Hear Disord. 1973; 38(4):462–472

[17] Strand EA, Stoeckel R, Baas B. Treatment of severe childhood apraxia of speech: a treatment efficacy study. J Med Speech-Lang Pathol. 2006; 14(4):297–307

[18] Strand EA. Application of principles of motor learning to the treatment of severe speech sound disorders: especially CAS. Invited presentation at Annual American Speech, Language and Hearing Association; November, 2013. Chicago, IL

[19] Strand EA. Diagnosis and management of CAS: dynamic temporal and tactile cueing. Video presentation hosted by University of Texas at Dallas, Callier Center, sponsored by Once Upon A Time Foundation. Published 2017. Website: https://www.utdallas.edu/calliercenter/events/CAS/. Accessed October 14, 2018

[20] Kazdin AE. Behavior Modification in Applied Settings. Belmont, CA: Wadsworth/Thomson Learning; 2013

[21] Swinnen SP, Lee TD, Verschueren S, Serrien DJ, Bogaerds H. Interlimb coordination: learning and transfer under different feedback conditions. Hum Mov Sci. 1997; 16(6):749–785

[22] Vess K, Hunter S. Integrated ASD literacy peer groups: the impact on literacy skills of typically developing preschoolers. Poster presented at Annual American Speech, Language and Hearing Association Convention; November, 2014; Orlando, FL

[23] Schmidt RA, Wrisberg CA. Motor Learning and Performance: A Problem-Based Learning Approach. 3rd ed. Champaign, IL: Human Kinetic; 2008

[24] Law J, Garrett Z, Nye C. The efficacy of treatment for children with developmental speech and language delay/disorder: a meta-analysis. J Speech Lang Hear Res. 2004; 47(4):924–943

6

7 Treating Motor Speech Disorders in Preschoolers with Autism Spectrum Disorder and Preschoolers with Neurological Differences

There is always, always…the Third Door. It's the entrance where you have to jump out of line, run down the alley, bang on the door a hundred times, crack open the window, sneak through the kitchen— there's always a way.

—Alex Banayan

7.1 Background

For almost two decades, I've specialized in treating and researching intervention for preschoolers with autism spectrum disorder (ASD). I feel instantly connected and devoted to this population. In every child, I see a treasure. Treasures take work. It takes knowledge, vision, creativity, talent, patience, drive, and gallons of elbow grease. This effort makes every step along the way rewarding. As much as you give to these children, they give back exponentially more. Working with this exceptional population will make you an extraordinary therapist.

Every year, I can attest that I have become a more effective therapist. This is evident by impressive increases in growth in data and observational gain each year. As you will see in this chapter, these intervention gains have been widespread in terms of speech, language, and social communication for preschoolers with ASD.

These children often have to take an entirely different path than their neurotypical peers in order to blossom. For these children, to find and enter the "Third Door" requires trying multiple creative methods.

Research indicates that the visual cortex for children with ASD is a relatively intact area of the brain. Perhaps children with ASD have even greater visual perception abilities than their neurotypical peers.[1] Therapists need to take advantage of this strength to help overcome neurological challenges to get to the "Third Door."[2,3]

7.2 Treat the Motor Speech Disorder in Preschoolers with ASD

Motor speech disorders result from functional or structural neurological differences that affect perception, speech motor planning, programming, control, and/or execution. A plethora of research indicates that children with ASD present with neurological differences in perception, motor functions, and oral motor coordination skills.

Because of this, we must first acknowledge the existence of a motor speech disorder before we can effectively treat it.[4] Fortunately, we don't need to reinvent the wheel to effectively treat motor speech disorders in children with ASD. We can effectively treat them with a best practice stew consisting of well-researched strategies.[5] Evidence based strategies that would serve as ingredients include milieu therapy,[6] Dynamic Tactile Temporal Cueing,[7] multimodal cueing,[8] core vocabulary,[9] and Lee Silverman voice treatment (LSVT)[10] to improve dysarthric speech.

Taking this research base into consideration, the best advice that I can give on working with preschoolers with ASD is to focus on treating the *motor speech disorder.* Our current research indicates that doing so can ignite gains globally in speech, expressive language, and even social communication. A cascading effect can occur across domains by selecting not only a complex speech target but also a complex linguistic context when treating the motor speech disorder.

Lastly, treatment of motor speech disorder strategies presented in this chapter can be adapted to treating children with childhood apraxia of speech, inconsistent speech sound disorder, or dysarthria. Dysarthria, which is speech affected by weakness, paralysis, or incoordination, can be associated with common conditions such as very pre-term prematurity, cerebral palsy, Chromosome 11q deletion, Down's syndrome, pediatric strokes, Lyme disease, and traumatic brain injury.

7.3 Neurological Differences Prevalent in People with ASD

How can we significantly and consistently improve our practice in treating children with ASD? In this chapter, we will reference neurological research pertaining to preschoolers with ASD in order to strategically provide practice that capitalizes on strengths while overcoming weaknesses.

Evaluate each digital clip of therapy using ▸ Table 7.1. Hone your efforts into the "Suggestion for Improvements" section when watching each digital clip of therapy to improve upon our work. As we gain a better understanding of neuronal challenges so will our therapy that directly addresses these differences.

7.4 Mirror Neuronal Deficits in Child with ASD

The mirror neuron system of the brain includes the inferior frontal cortex and inferior parietal lobule. It is largely responsible for speech and motor imitation. This area of the brain activates mirror neurons when observing others' behaviors.[2]

Typically, this activation of motor neurons occurs in both passive observation or when actively imitating others. Electroencephalography (EEG) research indicates that children with ASD have less mirror neuronal activation when observing others.[2]

Interestingly, neuronal activity of mirror neurons increases in children with autism when they are viewing either their own hand movements or actions of parents or siblings.[11]

This underscores the importance of children with ASD actively engaging in self-cueing their verbal expression with their hands to increase mirror neuronal activity when imitating motor actions. It additionally indicates the value of forming a strong therapeutic bond to increase mirror neuron activity.

Mirror neuron activity is also substantially increased when the observer additionally motorically imitates.[12] Prelinguistic motor imitation without objects is highly predictive of later language outcomes for children with ASD.[13] Conversely, a decreased degree of mirror neuron activity is correlated with decreased social functioning.[2]

See Video 7.1 of Stella, a child with ASD, who is imitating Ms. MaryLyn's temporal cues as she requests with a complex sentence. As discussed earlier, Stella is both viewing her hands and imitating Ms. MaryLyn's speech, fine, and gross motor movements, which dramatically increase mirror neuron activity.

Improved mirror neuronal activity not only increases children's ability to learn by example, but also develop empathy for others. When children see another person smiling or crying, the activation of motor neurons enable them to physically experience those feelings. Whereas, teaching or discussing feelings does not.

See Video 7.2 for another example. Ida, a child with ASD, is engaging in speech, and fine and gross motor imitation with Ms. Torey in both temporal cueing and imitating various animals' gaits to increase Ida's mirror neuronal activity.

7.5 Functional and Structural Differences in the Cerebellum

See Video 7.3 of Deenie. She does not have ASD. However, she was born very prematurely with a resultant underdeveloped cerebellum. When watching Video 7.3, note the similarities in symptomology that you would see in a child with severe ASD. She is preverbal with limited vocalizations. She demonstrates difficulty in initiating movement, coordinating movement, responsively navigating her environment, and completing movements. She additionally demonstrates a lack of eye contact, impaired play skills, and repetitive hand flapping. This autism-like symptomology underscores the pervasive impact of structural and functional damage to the cerebellum. (Reference sentence strip in ▸ Fig. 7.1.)

Often what happens in the body, happens in the mouth. Children demonstrating hypotonic muscular weakness in gross motor movement may hang their head forward or to the side with shoulders rounded forward and arms passively swinging.

There's a shuffle quality to their gait instead of a fluid, well-differentiated use of hip, knee, and ankle joints when walking. Their mouths, matching their limb movements, are often passively hanging ajar at rest and demonstrate excessive jaw movement (like a puppet talking) to compensate for poor oral motor coordination of the lip, tongue, and cheek musculature when producing sounds or speech.

Conversely, with motor coordination deficits, muscular weakness is not evident but motor coordination difficulties in the mouth and body often coexist. These children often demonstrate difficulty in initiating movement, responsively navigating environmental obstacles, completing tasks, and ceasing movement.

They often demonstrate proprioception difficulties evident by toe walking. In the mouth, these proprioceptive difficulties often present as difficulty with nonspeech intentional movements, such sticking the tongue out on demand.

7

Table 7.1 Evaluating treatment of speech motor disorders

Video Number:_____

Please indicate your level of agreement to the following statements in reference to the literacy digital clip presented.	Strongly Disagree	Disagree	Neutral	Agree	Strongly Agree
1) Child is actively engaged and enjoying learning.	1	2	3	4	5
2) Therapist proactively adapts activity to establish to maintain an individual child's interest (e.g., incorporating highly desired objects into a neutrally rewarding activity).	1	2	3	4	5
3) Therapist is maintaining a joyful learning experience in which the child "gets" to talk rather than "has to" talk with pressure to speak decreased.	1	2	3	4	5
4) Therapist is a reinforcer in enthusiastic responses, warmth, and conveying positive facial and vocal expression.	1	2	3	4	5
5) Therapist ensures that all directions and questions are responded to on a 1:1 ratio or prompts a response within 2–3 seconds (i.e., no blow-offs).	1	2	3	4	5
6) Therapist attains the child's attention prior to giving a direction or asking a question.	1	2	3	4	5
7) Therapists adjusts pace for a balance of accuracy in slowing down and speech in maintaining attention.	1	2	3	4	5
8) Therapist is at the child's eye level.	1	2	3	4	5
9) The child is producing the treatment at a high level of frequency.	1	2	3	4	5
10) Therapist has natural rewards placed within therapist's (not child's) each during manding for optimal attention to speech production.	1	2	3	4	5
11) Therapist is making sounds salient with slow, exaggerated movements using multiple modalities.	1	2	3	4	5
12) With muscular weakness, the therapist is speaking loudly and moving loudly with exaggerated limb movement (like a cheerleader).	1	2	3	4	5
13) Therapist is challenging the child to produce speech at maximum level of phonetic and linguistic complexity.	1	2	3	4	5
14) Therapist is able to assist the child in participating in developmentally appropriate activities with the child actively participating at a maximal "hands on level."	1	2	3	4	5

7

Table 7.1 (*Continued*) Evaluating treatment of speech motor disorders

Video Number:_____					
Please indicate your level of agreement to the following statements in reference to the literacy digital clip presented.	Strongly Disagree	Disagree	Neutral	Agree	Strongly Agree
15) Therapist is encouraging motor imitation with speech imitation.	1	2	3	4	5

Strengths:

Weaknesses:

Suggestions for Improvement:

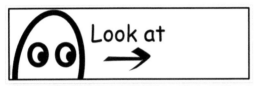

Fig. 7.1 "Look at" augmentative and alternative communication sentence strip.

Repetitive motor acts such as hand flapping and difficulty completing multistep gross and fine motor actions generally present with concomitant oral apraxia of speech.

Similarly, in the mouth you'll see struggle in initiating speech, continuous repetition of sounds and words, and difficulty with complexly coordinated sounds, clusters, and polysyllabic words. You'll also generally see greater difficulty with performing both motor movements and speech on demand than spontaneously.

This difficulty with on demand versus spontaneous movements is evident in both the body and the mouth. Parents often wonder how their child with ASD can climb cabinets to the top of the refrigerator like a superhero and open and operate a complex candy dispenser, located in a tightly closed jar.

However, this same child, when called upon, does not independently cross the room even with the lure of a highly rewarding object in view. Parents also wonder why the child won't join them in singing a song that the child repetitiously sings throughout the day. These are common examples of the discrepancy between on demand versus spontaneous movement.

Look closely at the children you work with who can verbally request wants and needs yet they are effectively locked in. Many of these children may be able to talk yet are unable to independently physically engage with others or their environments.

Conversely, you'll meet children with ASD who can nonverbally meet their wants and needs but continue to be preverbal. They underscore the need to comprehensively treat the child to fully interact with the world.

See Video 7.4, Video 7.5, and Video 7.6. In which we target the cerebellum through task-oriented activity based intervention. Complete the cerebellum lesson plan presented in Chapter 5 for each video.

This will provide valuable practice in identifying how to comprehensively treat children with ASD by targeting behaviors largely dictated by the cerebellum. This type of active learning will empower the viewer to create targeted interventions.

7.6 Treat the Cerebellum to Comprehensively Treat the Child

The latest research empowers us to treat speech and motor development comprehensively as they transactionally impact each other.[14] Choi and colleagues refer to the direct impact of motor development on communication as an example of a developmental cascade.[15]

Developmental cascades refer to the effects of interactions and transactions between developmental domains that result in widespread effects across systems.[15] Motor movements in the body directly impact linguistic development.

An example of a developmental cascade is research associating learning to walk with increasing the frequency and quality of parent-child interactions.[16]

When a child learns to walk, the child's hands are free to hold objects or freely point for the purpose of showing others. This is known as a deictic gesture. A deictic gesture is used for commenting purposes and is a type of gesture that is uniquely highly predictive of improved expressive vocabulary development.[17]

Semantic development occurs as the child is provided with labels and descriptions. Syntactic development increases as description of actions and locations increase with this newfound mobility to travel.

Phonologically, the number of sounds perceived increases with greater exposure to a variety of words. Pragmatically, increases in opportunities for joint attention occur with greater frequency, duration, and variety of communication partners.

The developmental cascade from learning to walk is even more widespread in cognitive development This occurs because the child is able to more fully experience the environment with adults and more capable peers within a zone of proximal development.

Social emotional gains occur as the child is able to manipulate toys using both hands at an increased level of complexity and independence in play.

Fine motor gains are made because the child is able to manipulate an increased number of objects, such as door knobs. The child's sensory system develops through increased exposure to novel stimuli.

Thus, when a child learns to walk, frequency of all of these new experiences create multiple new neuronal connections and myelin development as nerve cells fire more efficiently through repeated practice.

In extensively working with children with ASD, I've found many have never learned to walk. They are typically "being walked" by an adult. Many do not yet independently or functionally navigate their environment through initiation, coordination, responsive navigation of obstacles, completion of a task, and cessation of movement.

Nor do they respond to environmental stimuli along the way while independently traversing space. Therefore, the widespread impact of this crucially important developmental milestone may never be experienced.

Despite movement disorders being highly prevalent in an estimated 80% of children with ASD, they are no more likely to receive physical therapy services than children without movement disorders.[18,19,20] This needs to change.

7.7 The Body→Mouth Connection

I've directly observed over the years that often what happens in the body, happens in the mouth. Children who demonstrate imprecise, distorted, and inaudible, weak speech articulation often demonstrate these challenges in their gait as well. These children often walk with their heads hanging forward or to the side with arms passively swinging. This is due to a lack of well-coordinated, differentiated movement between joints and surrounding musculature. The observable stiff and shuffled gait quality largely stems from compensatory overuse of hip, knee, and ankle joints. Children demonstrating hypotonic muscular weakness in gross motor movement often do so in the mouth as well. They may hang their head to the side, arms passively swinging, and have a shuffle quality to their gait instead of a well-differentiated use of hip, knee, and ankle joints when walking. Their mouths, matching their limb movements, are often passively hanging ajar at rest.

Conversely, with motor coordination deficits, muscular weakness is not evident but motor coordination difficulties in the mouth and body often concur. These children often demonstrate difficulty in initiating movement, responsively navigating environmental obstacles, completing tasks, and ceasing movement. They often also demonstrate proprioception difficulties evident by toe walking. In the mouth, these proprioceptive difficulties often present as difficulty with nonspeech intentional movements, such sticking the tongue out on demand.

Repetitive motor acts such as hand flapping and difficulty completing multistep gross and fine motor actions generally present with concomitant oral apraxia of speech. Similarly, in the mouth you'll see struggle in initiating speech, continuous repetition of sounds and words, and difficulty with complexly coordinated sounds, clusters, and polysyllabic words. You'll also generally see greater difficulty with performing motor movements and speech on demand than spontaneously.

This difficulty with on demand versus spontaneous movements is evident in both the body and the mouth. Parents often wonder how their child with ASD can climb cabinets to the top of the refrigerator like a superhero and open and operate a complex candy dispenser, located in a tightly closed jar. However, this same child, when called upon, does not independently cross the room even with the lure of a highly rewarding object in view. Parents also wonder why the child won't join them in singing a song that the child repetitiously sings throughout the day. These are common examples of the discrepancy between on demand versus spontaneous behavior often seen in preschoolers with ASD who have motor coordination difficulties.

For some children there is also a mouth and body disconnect. These children with ASD can speak yet are completely locked in. You too may have observed these children who, rather than purposefully interacting with the environment, experience life largely through repetitive self-stimulatory behaviors. Look closely at the children you work with who can verbally request wants and needs yet they are effectively locked in. Many of these children may be able to talk yet are unable to independently physically engage with others or their environments.

Conversely, you'll meet children with ASD who can nonverbally meet their wants and needs but continue to be preverbal. They underscore the need to holistically treat the child to fully interact with the world. See Video 7.4, Video 7.5, and Video 7.6. Holistically treat the child by targeting the cerebellum. Complete the cerebellum lesson plan presented in Chapter 5 for each video. This will provide valuable practice in identifying how to holistically treat children with ASD by targeting behaviors largely controlled by the cerebellum. This type of active learning will empower the viewer to better create targeted interventions.

7.8 Incorporate Movement Activities into Therapy to Increase Verbal Output

In treating preverbal preschoolers with motor speech disorders, we have found it beneficial to incorporate movement activities. Our research on five preverbal preschoolers indicated all five showed an increase in pleasurable verbal output during movement activities over seated ones.

The younger the preverbal preschoolers were, the greater the impact of movement on verbal output.[21] This increase in communicative vocalizations is correlated with improved expressive language outcomes.[22] Watch Video 7.7.

Notice how Ms. Holly responds with a calm enthusiasm, acknowledging even the quietest of sounds, with "Nice talking!" Hear the increase in Davey's vocalizations from the second session in Video 7.7 to the fifth session in Video 7.8 and Video 7.9. Notice how Davey's vocalizations only occur concurrently with his finger tapping and hand movements.

Finger and hand movements are primarily processed in the cerebellum of the brain adjacent to tongue movements.[23] My occupational therapist colleagues, Dianne Stall and Joseph Evens, report that children often stick out their tongues when performing challenging fine motor tasks, such as beading, and drawing. They also often open and close their mouths when cutting. In both scenarios, hand movements mirror mouth movements.

7.9 Advance Neuronal Development by Increasing Complexity of Targets and the Linguistic Context

The latest neurological research underscores the pivotal role of linguistic complexity in maximizing brain development.[24] Recent research indicates that longer and more complex utterances are more beneficial to preschoolers with ASD.[25,26]

This may be in part due to auditory processing deficits and attention deficits prevalent in this population. Longer utterances could provide the child with more time to attend to and auditorily process verbal input. It could also provide a greater variety and number of words from which the child could comprehend.

In current practice, however, there is a mismatch. It has been recently reported that 82% of speech-language pathologists surveyed report using telegraphic speech in therapy.[27] Telegraphic speech is simplified, ungrammatically correct speech, often spoken to a child with the misguided notion that less speech would improve comprehension for children with ASD. In applying research to practice, let's all evolve from Neanderthals and say goodbye to caveman talk.

See Video 7.10. Liam produces dramatically simplified consonant clusters. We continue to focus on requesting at the paragraph level to increase Liam's attention, joint attention, joint engagement, and language expression. This is an example of making an individualized clinical decision to forgo the 80% speech accuracy rule in order to ignite gains across developmental domains.

7

7.10 Treating Children with ASD Who Are Preverbal and Minimally Verbal

Currently, it is estimated that 25–30% of children with ASD will remain minimally verbal despite years of intervention and a range of educational services.[28] We can do better. Typically, each school year, one of the seven children graduating our ASD preschool program to elementary school will be preverbal or minimally verbal. Minimally verbal refers to very limited use of speech for functional communication.[28]

Our program consists of two classrooms, each with seven moderately to severely impaired preschoolers with ASD who attend our half day, self contained TEACCH (Treatment and Education of Autistic and Communication related handicapped Children) based program. Our talented intervention team consists of one ASD teacher, two teaching assistants, an occupational therapist, and myself.

Based on parent report, approximately 50% of the children in our program additionally receive 15 to 20 hours of private Applied Behavioral Anal ysis therapy in a week. Approximately 30% additionally receive private speech services. Approximately 15% receive occupational therapy services privately.

Today, I can still vividly recall each student who graduated remaining preverbal or minimally verbal. Why? Because learning to talk is life-changing. The ability to speak predicts whether children will grow to develop friendships, work, or live independently.[29] For this reason, I am always researching my practice, learning new strategies, and giving it my all in every session.

In developing new empirically and theoretically based strategies, at times I fail and it is through these failures that I've made great strides. Specifically, the failures reveal the ineffective aspects of intervention which can be cut so that only effective strategies are implemented within our limited therapy time.

I envision a time in the near future when I can report 100% of preschoolers graduating fluently verbal every year. It is my belief that great promise lies in advances in neuroscience, which will continue to inform and evolve our practice.

In working with minimally verbal children, I've encountered children with a verbal output profile similar to symptomology of childhood apraxia of speech or inconsistent speech sound disorder.

Both are primarily motor coordination disorders, presenting with inconsistent production of words in the absence of muscular weakness or paralysis. I've also encountered children who demonstrate a verbal profile similar to dysarthric disorders caused by paralysis or muscular weakness.

Inconsistent speech sound disorder is similar to childhood apraxia of speech except that in children with this disorder, speech is clearer when imitated than spontaneously spoken. On the other hand, children with childhood apraxia of speech generally produce spontaneous speech more clearly than imitated. See Chapter 1 for a review of differential diagnosis of motor speech disorders.

I've also encountered children with motor speech disorders who presented with a blend of symptomatology common to dysarthria, childhood apraxia of speech, and inconsistent speech sound disorder. For these children, in particular, trial therapy will guide your direction as to whether to take a more responsive "follow the child's lead" approach, a direct elicitation of speech approach approach, or a hybrid of the two.

As a child's speech motor disorder improves, it can evolve into a phonological disorder, and perhaps an articulation impairment with some distorted sounds. Lastly a speech motor disorder can evolve into clear speech. Throughout, the protocol will remain the same, requesting with linguistically complex treatment targets across engaging and meaningful learning experiences with increased levels of independence.

Children with ASD are like anyone else. Under pressure, some will thrive, some will survive, and others will fold. In appreciation of the diversity of temperament, we'll cover a responsive and direct elicitation approach to treating children with ASD, childhood apraxia of speech, and dysarthria. First, we'll cover how to improve outcomes for children with sensitive temperaments.

7.11 Taking a Responsive Approach to Improve Communication Skills when Treating a Child with a Sensitive Temperament Who Is Minimally Verbal

You have probably met a child like Saheen. Saheen whispers when singing his favorite songs spontaneously throughout the day. Yet, he will quickly stop singing when you try to join him. He labels numbers, colors, letters, and shapes.

However, he doesn't use these labels communicatively to request, comment, or respond to questions. Looking at his body, you do not detect muscular weakness. His mouth is closed at rest and he has well-shaped cheeks.

His fine motor strength also appears normal in that he draws with appropriate firmness. For gross motor activity, Saheen often requires physical or hand over hand prompting to both initiate and cease movement. He walks on his toes in a curvy, rather than a straight, line, suggesting poor proprioception. Instead of a controlled gradualness in initiating and ceasing movement, he starts and stops with a jerky quality. He does not navigate around obstacles, such as other children or furniture. His walk indicates breakdowns in proprioception, motor planning, programming, and execution.

When pressure is put on Saheen to verbally imitate, read a Picture Exchange Communication System (PECS) sentence strip aloud, or verbally request in response to an expectant time delay prompt, he invariably screams.

Children like Saheen, who present with a profile consistent with childhood apraxia of speech, speak more clearly and fluidly spontaneously than when imitating. With imitated speech, breakdowns often occur.

Less pressure to speak produces greater and more consistent verbal output from Saheen. It seems as if the pressure to speak, in children like Saheen, switches on a fight or flight response, diminishing their ability to coordinate motor movements that underlie the complex task of speech.

Children with motor coordination difficulties can teach you about the challenges of producing complex sounds, which involve shifts of movement, by observing their attempts to produce them.

With short sounds, such as labial stops, it is not uncommon to see pursing of the lips but an inability to release the airflow. These children additionally demonstrate difficulty with complex phonemes in which articulators shift during production. These include diphthongs, glides, and labial-dentals /f/ and /v/ in which quick movement of articulators during production is required to produce them.

With diphthongs, children with coordination difficulties may produce each vowel separately with a pause inserted incorrectly. They may also demonstrate difficulty in producing glides (e.g., "want"→ /jant/ and "yes" → /wɛs/).

With consonant clusters, they may engage in epenthesis by often inserting a schwa /ə/ between consonants ("blue"→ /bə...lu/). Production of polysyllabic words can be inconsistent, perfect at times

and completely unintelligible at other times, particularly when on demand.

To assist in producing these complex shifting sounds, we want to make sounds and movement patterns salient by producing sounds slowly and using exaggerated multimodal cues in choral speech to capitalize on visual strengths (see Dynamic, Tactile, Temporal Cueing in Chapter 6). This technique has demonstrated efficacy in treating children with childhood apraxia of speech.[7]

You'll note in Video 7.11 that Ms. Christina is whispering, almost sneaking in, "What's that?" The goal in treating populations that present with a profile consistent with childhood apraxia of speech is to develop consistency. Christina is improving the consistency and functionality of Saheen's expressive output by gently fading in questions.

We are using a core vocabulary approach that has been effectively researched for inconsistent speech sound disorder by having the child use a core vocabulary on a consistent basis across settings and people.[30] We continue building consistency in expanding his core vocabulary of favorite things appropriate to the context (e.g., colors, letters, shapes).

Additionally, we are calmly celebrating spontaneous speech instead of demanding it. Saheen's favorite song is the "You are talking" song that we made up and he likes to spontaneously sing it.

Over the past year, Saheen's speech has increased in frequency and consistency. Demanding speech continues to only result in his dysregulated screaming. His speech is at his highest level of frequency and clarity when he is engaged in movement activities, such as walking, and the pressure to speak is removed.

7.12 Treating Children with a Sensitive Temperament Who Are Inconsistently Verbal

You may come to know a child like Ardo. Ardo has a sensitive temperament. Like Saheen, he screams when pressured to speak. Specifically, his screams are in response to directly being asked to verbally imitate and answer questions on demand. Like Saheen, Ardo speaks more when there is less pressure to talk.

Our goal is for Ardo to speak as much as possible to improve speech, expressive language, and joint attention. Demands to speak in the form of responding to questions or imitating may be slowly faded in over time within the context of his favorite activities as Ardo's speech develops in consistency. This pairs speech with enjoyable experiences.

See Video 7.12. Note how Ms. Katelyn creates a high level of engagement with Ardo by entering his world. She encourages turn-taking responses by responding to Ardo's actions as intentional communicative turns aimed at her. She also dramatically responds to his behaviors to elicit his emotional responses. Ms. Katelyn additionally indirectly elicits both verbal and motor imitations through repeatedly modeling actions and language in a sportscaster role for Ardo to spontaneously produce. Ms. Katelyn sneaks in verbal directions for Ardo to follow in the context of play.

Katelyn takes on a sportscaster role in providing an ongoing verbal commentary of Ardo's interests and actions on a play-by-play basis. A combination of these socially engaging techniques and verbally mapping the interests of children with ASD have been found to be globally predictive of improved engagement in play, expressive language, and social communication outcomes.[31]

7.13 Taking a Direct Elicitation of Speech Approach for Children with a Stable Temperament

The approach you take with a child should be highly individualized based on the child's temperament, communicative profile, and needs. While this chapter provides you with generalizations, your clinical expertise and intuition in differentially responding to each child should always guide your practice.

In Video 7.13 and Video 7.14, you'll see the therapists use a direct elicitation of speech approach with children verbally requesting natural rewards and activities.

Regardless of whether a responsive or direct elicitation approach is used to foster communication development, it's important to note that speech should always be a choice. It should never be demanded by a therapist or parent.

7.14 Treating Dysarthria Caused by Muscular Weakness or Paralysis

Dysarthria can present as weakness, paralysis, or poor motor coordination impacting speech. Earlier in this chapter we discussed treating poor motor coordination through the use of slowed, echoed speech with dynamic use of tactile and temporal cueing. We also covered responsive strategies in following the child's lead and sportscasting to increase the child's verbal output.

With muscular weakness or paralysis, the goal is to improve speech accuracy through differentially rewarding to successive approximations. In treating dysarthria, there are observational studies indicating support for increasing vocal loudness coupled with exaggerated limb movement to improve speech clarity.[10] Increasing airflow through loudness results in improved vocal fold contraction and articulatory contact. This creates clearer speech that can be attributed to the *Bernoulli Effect*.

What Is the Bernoulli Effect?

The Bernoulli Effect is a phenomenon when airflow moves faster, less pressure is placed on an object. and Therefore, that object will be drawn to it and away from the slower, more static, denser airflow. This is because the static airflow which applies more pressure on the object.

For instance, if you are riding your bike and a fast truck passes, the speed of the air will actually dangerously draw your bike towards the increased air speed from the truck and away from the curb where air is denser.

In the vocal folds, with increased airflow from the lungs, the air moves faster through the glottis, the opening in the vocal folds. As a result, folds are drawn together to the area of decreased pressure. Therefore, they close more strongly. As a result, increased airflow from the lungs builds up from is even further increased by the pressure of the previously, tightly closed folds and the process repeats itself.

Similar to an airplane taking off from a runway, increased airflow gliding over the tongue will also result in the tongue lifting up to the lighter level of air pressure. At the articulation level, the greater lift of the tongue makes stronger connections at places of articulation. This results in clearer speech.

Thus, the Bernoulli Effect can improve both vocal fold vibration and speech clarity in the face of muscular weakness or paralysis through increased airflow.

See Video 7.15. Harry presents with muscular weakness and partial vocal fold paralysis and imprecise articulation secondary to a pediatric stroke. Our goal is to increase vocal fold vibration and speech clarity through loudness. The increase in volume engages the Bernoulli Effect for improved vocal fold vibration and for the tongue to make stronger articulatory contacts. Ms. Katelyn is modeling both loud speech and big, exaggerated temporal cues from an increased physical distance in order to improve articulation and encourage voicing instead of whispered speech.

I've also found modeling loud speech with grandiose movements from a distance to be a highly effective technique in working with preschoolers with ASD who speak in whispered or inconsistently vocalized speech. This technique results in both a decrease in whispered speech and an increase in speech clarity. As shown in Video 7.15, I have children with stable temperaments use loud speech and large movements in unison in the context of requesting in a direct elicitation of speech approach.

Lastly, for children with speech sound disorders who have difficulty voicing consonants, I've found this technique of using a louder voice coupled with large limb movement to be effective. For instance, if the child says, "Sue" for "zoo" (/su/ → /zu/), I'll prompt with my fingers high in the air, exclaiming "Louder! Let's hear the loud bumble bee sounds," while producing loud buzzing /z/ sounds in unison with the child.

Here the Bernoulli Effect is in effect in with the increased airflow necessary for loudness resulting in vocal fold vibration.

7.15 Selecting Maximally Distinct Consonant Clusters for Children with a Very Limited Consonantal Inventory

In selecting a therapy target, never base your target on what a child can do independently, the severity of speech impairment, or the child's diagnostic label. Doing so is limiting to both the child's potential and yours.

Of interest to you should only be the child's highest level of performance with your skillful assistance. Go big. Aim for 3-element clusters with every child you encounter. If they can't produce 3-element clusters with a maximal level of support, go for 2-element clusters. Slow the speech, yet keep the flow continuous by pausing less than 2 seconds between each sound to maintain the automaticity of speech. Jump to 3- element clusters as soon as possible.

Use the same treatment target repeatedly. This develops consistency in motor planning, programming, and execution. Darren, a child with ASD, began the summer program primarily using the centralized vowel /ʌ / to request highly preferred items with "uh-uh." We selected "sweep it to me" (/swip ɪt tu mi/) as his treatment target because he could produce it with a maximum level of prompting. Refer to Video 7.16.

7.16 Combining a Responsive Approach with a Direct Elicitation Approach

Next, you'll see Ava who presents with dysarthria in the form of muscular weakness and poor motor coordination related to having Turner's syndrome. Turner's syndrome is caused by partial or complete deletion of an X chromosome.

Ava has a slightly sensitive temperament. When too much pressure is put on her to speak, she will shut down and be silent. See how she is actively involved in requesting with her treatment target when dancing (Video 7.17) and also when sitting on Ms. Holly's lap (Video 7.18). These contexts establish a positive affective domain in which pressure to perform is decreased for optimal speech improvements to occur.

See Video 7.18. As soon as Ava was able to imitate an /skw/ blend with accuracy, Ms. Holly chose to increase Ava's request sentence by adding a 3-element cluster "squeak" to her treatment target to increase the efficiency of therapy.

Why /sw/? For this child, /sw/ was the highest level of cluster that could be produced with a maximum level of cueing on the *Supplemental Consonant Cluster Screener*. Why did we choose an /s/ blend over a different initial consonant blend? The /s/ is more complex and therefore would have a cascading impact on more earlier developing sounds.

Also, /s/ is long in duration, allowing the child time to both perceive the sound and join in.

Why did we not choose /s+stop/ such as "'sneak' /snik/ it to me?" These are not maximally distinct sounds, which are sounds that significantly differ in both placement and manner to challenge oral motor coordination.

7

For instance, /sn/ would have been a fricative + stop cluster (both obstruents of airflow) in the same position in the mouth (alveolar). We want to select blends that perform acrobatics in the mouth. With /sw/, /s/ is an alveolar in placement and fricative in manner. Distinctly, /w/ is a labio velar in placement, and a glide in manner. This makes them an appropriate maximally distinct target in terms of both placement and manner. The blend /sl/ was not selected because Darren and Ava could not produce /l/, even with a maximum level of prompting.

Consistently, in working with children with limited phonetic inventories of centralized vowels and with both weakness and coordination difficulties, we've found using /sw/ blends results in optimal gains by quickly increasing the child's consonantal inventory and improving intelligibility.

Also note that it is important not to teach a child "more" or "yes" at the emerging speech stage. These words could provide access to *everything*, deeming specific vocabulary development to be unnecessary.

Be mindful and select unique targets for every child you work with based on the individual needs and the most complex target stimulable.

That said, /sw/ treatment targets at the simple sentence level have consistently produced impressive gains in working with preschoolers who have only a centralized vowel inventory at baseline to encourage optimal gains. The /skw/ sound is recommended over /sw/ if the child is able to produce it with a maximum level of cueing.

7.17 Paying Attention to the Details to Effectively Assess and Treat Speech Sound Disorders

Details matter. Throughout this book, we've covered details of our practice in working with diverse groups of preschoolers that truly make a difference.

Details that optimize intervention gains within limited time constraints include selecting complex treatment targets; providing a most-to-least 80% accuracy level using errorless prompting; multimodally cueing of communication and academic concepts; incorporating movement; fostering an internal locus of control; incorporating the child's interests; and, developing hands-on, engaging, 3-dimensional, educationally rich activities that comprehensively treat preschoolers with communication impairments.

Each of these details are active ingredients that expedite change. Together, they have a powerful, cumulative impact that produce life-long outcomes when neuroplasticity is at a high level.

7.18 Presence of Multiple Atypical Phonological Processes in Speech Testing May Indicate Neurological Differences

Concluding this chapter are atypical phonological processes that often surface during baseline testing of preschoolers with motor speech disorders or more pervasive developmental delays. With progress, I've generally found atypical phonological processes evolve into typical phonological processes and distortions over time.

My clinical experience suggests that the presence of multiple atypical phonological processes may indicate concurrent linguistic delays or neurological differences. This is because atypical processes tend to violate universals of speech sound development.

Generally, easier to produce sounds develop before later developing sounds. Speech errors, therefore, are typically substitutions of simpler sounds for more complex ones. You'll notice a pattern, however, with atypical processes in that later developing, more difficult to produce sounds often replace earlier developing ones.

In 2008, Preston thoroughly presented atypical phonological processes based on atypical syllable structure (▶ Table 7.2), atypical placement (▶ Table 7.3), and atypical manner (▶ Table 7.4). Referencing Preston's work are examples taken from our diverse group of 76 preschoolers with speech sound disorders who participated in our summer speech intervention program.

Examples are taken from their responses on either the Clinical Assessment of *Articulation and Phonology-2* (*CAAP-2*)[32] or the *Supplemental Consonant Cluster Screener* from Chapter 1.

Based on performance on these assessments, multiple atypical phonological processes were found to be largely present in populations with more pervasive impairments. Specifically, from my diverse sample of 76 preschoolers with speech impairments, the 31 children who presented with concurrent language impairment, ASD, childhood apraxia of speech, inconsistent speech sound disorder, or Down's syndrome presented with multiple atypical processes.

Conversely, few of the 42 children we studied with a sole diagnosis of speech impairment presented atypical phonological processes. For this,

Table 7.2 Putting research into practice: Preston's atypical syllable structure processes

Atypical Syllable Structure Processes	Definition	Example: correct → typical	correct → atypical (provide an example)
Atypical /s/ Cluster Reduction	Initial /s/ clusters: /s/ remains with a stop or nasal deleted	Snake: /sneɪk/→ /seɪk/	School: /skul /→
Atypical Liquid Cluster Reduction	Liquid clusters: /l/ or /ɹ/ liquids remain	Clown: /klaʊn/ → /laʊn/ Broom: /bɹum/ → /rum/	Fly: /flaɪ/ → Pretzel: /'pɹɛtzəl/→
Atypical Glide Cluster Reduction	Stop + glide clusters: /w/ or /j/ glide remains	Tweet: /twit/ → /wit/ Puke: /pjuk/ → /juk/	Queen: /kwin/ → Cute: /kjut/ →
Initial Consonant Deletion	Word-initial singleton consonants are deleted	Dog: /dɔg/→ /ɔg/	Pig: /pɪg/ →
Medial (Intervocalic) Consonant Deletion	Intervocalic consonants are deleted	Lemonade: /'lɛmə'neɪd/ → /'lɛmə'eɪd/	Treasure: /'tɹɛʒɚ/ →
Addition of Consonants, Vowels, or Syllables	Addition of consonants, vowels, or syllables (not between consonant clusters, which is epenthesis)	Sheep:/ʃip/ → /ʃlip/	Fish: /fɪʃ/ →
Migration	Consonant/syllable is moved to another part of the word	Thermometer: /θɚ'mamətɚ/ → /'mɑməθɚ/	Elephant: /'ɛləfənt/ →
Strong Syllable Deletion	Syllable/vowel with primary or secondary stress is deleted	Basketball: /'bæskət,bɔl/ → /'kʌ,bɔ/ (primary stressed deleted) Basketball: /'bæskət,bɔl/ → /'bæs,bɔ/ (secondary stressed deleted)	Computer: /kəm'pjutɚ/ →

Table 7.3 Putting research into practice: Preston's atypical placement processes

Atypical Placement Processes	Definition	Example: correct → typical	correct → atypical (provide an example)
Glottal Replacement	Glottal stop /ʔ/ replaces a consonant, except final /t/	Cage: /keɪdʒ/ → /ʔeɪdʒ/	Shoe:/ʃu/ →
Atypical Backing of Velars	A labial, dental, alveolar, or palatal is backed to a velar (not assimilation)	Tweet: /twit/ → /kwit/	Yo-yo: /joʊ-joʊ/ →
Palatalization	A non-palatal fricative or becomes a palatal fricative (not assimilation)	Zoo: /zu/ → /ʒu/	Seal: /sil/:
Atypical Labialization	Velar or palatal phoneme becomes labial (not assimilation)	king: /kɪŋ/ → /mɪŋ/	Gate: /geɪt/ →
Gliding Interchange of /w/ becoming /j/	Interchange between /j/ and /w/	Watch: /watʃ / → /jatʃ/	Water: /'wɔtər/ →
Liquid Interchange	Interchange between /ɹ/ and /l/	rake: /ɹeɪk/ → /leɪk/	Leaf: /lif/ →

Table 7.4 Putting research into practice: Preston's atypical manner processes

Atypical Sound Processes	Definition	Example: correct → typical	correct → atypical (provide an example)
Denasalization	Nasal phoneme becomes voiced stops at the same place of articulation (i.e., homorganic)	Clown: /klaʊn/ → /klaʊt/	Van: /væn/ →
Nasalization	Non-nasal phonemes become nasal at the same place of articulation (i.e., homorganic)	Bed: /bɛd/ → /mɛd/	Sheep: /ʃip/ →
Fricatives Replace Stops	Fricatives replace stops at the same place of articulation (i.e., homorganic)	Pig: /pɪg/ → /fɪg/	Gate: /geɪt/ →
Liquids Replace Glides	Glides become liquids	Watch: /wɑʧ/ → /ɹɑʧ/	Web: /wɛb/ →
Tetism	/f/ becomes /t/	Fish: /fɪʃ/ → /tɪʃ/	Leaf: /lif/ →
Atypical Gliding of Intervocalic Consonants	Intervocalic consonants (other than fricatives) are replaced by glides	Dinosaur: /'daɪnəˌsɔr/ → /'daɪwəˌsɔr/	Treasure: /'tɹɛʒər/ →
Atypical Stopping of Liquids or Glides	Glide or liquid becomes a stop at the same place of articulation	Leaf: /lif/ → /tif/	Yo-Yo: /joʊ-joʊ/ →

there is a heightened need for a more thorough language evaluation when multiple atypical phonological processes surface during speech testing.

Furthermore, presence of concurrent language impairment indicates greater risk for later literacy deficits.[33,34,35] Therefore, phonological awareness testing is proactively recommended as well. Additionally, focus on integrating literacy rich activities as contexts in treating speech disorders to increase intervention efficiency. Reference Chapter 9 for evidence-based strategies to improve phonological awareness skills.

For further practice in actively identifying atypical phonological processes, apply Preston's terminology and definitions in ► Table 7.2 and ► Table 7.3 by providing an example of each atypical production using the International Phonetic Alphabet (IPA).

Identifying these atypical processes can provide a better clue to a therapist as to where breakdowns are occurring so that these areas can be more prominently addressed in therapy through incompatible cues, expression, increased slowness, and increased volume.

7.19 Identifying Speech Errors Prevalent in Preschoolers with ASD

What are challenges unique to children with ASD in learning to talk? To find out, I compared seven preschoolers with ASD and severe speech impairment to seven preschoolers without ASD who had language impairment and severe speech impairment.

In attempts to identify the impact of the ASD disorder on speech production, participants were selected based on gender, age, and severity of speech impairment. Each group consisted of two girls and five boys. The age range of preschoolers in the speech and language impairment group was 39 to 72 months, with an average age of 55 months and an average score of 40 errors on the *CAAP-2*. The closely matched preschoolers in the ASD impairment group had an age range of 46 to 72 months, with an average age of 56 months and an average score of 41 errors on the *CAAP-2*.

7

Children in both groups presented with a severe level of speech impairment with scores at the 2%ile, 1%ile, impairment. All scores ranged from the less than 1 percentile to 2 percentile in comparison to their age-matched peers on the CAAP-2.

In item analysis of these 14 children's performance on the CAAP-2, two patterns emerged for children with ASD. First, they demonstrated difficulty in producing stop consonants, which are the shortest sounds in the English language (averaging 50 milliseconds in length). Second, they demonstrated greater difficulty in producing the "start" of words in which they were more likely to delete initial syllables in polysyllabic words and slightly more likely to delete initial consonants in CVC words.

7.20 Short Stop Consonants Are Difficult to Perceive and Therefore Difficult to Produce

The McGurk Effect is the impact of auditory and visual modalities operating as one in an audiovisual nature to perceive speech.[36] Preschoolers with ASD are frequently shown to present with deficits in auditory perception. Because of this, these children often lack the ability to concurrently use audio and visual perception to process speech.

Perhaps as a compensatory measure, children with ASD may even present with advanced visual perception skills when compared to the neurotypical population.[1] Children with ASD likely present with a mismatch in slower auditory processing and with faster visual processing.[1] This mismatch could be likened to children with ASD viewing life as a poorly dubbed foreign film that is visually fast forwarded with the sound slowed down.

In item analysis, I compared the production of the word "snake" (/sneɪk/) by preschoolers with ASD to that of the preschoolers with speech and language impairment. All of the children in the ASD group could produce the /s/ in "snake." However, only two of the seven preschoolers with ASD could produce the /n/ in "snake." Interestingly, the /n/ typically develops in English a full year before the letter /s/.[37]

On the other hand, the speech and language impairment group errored in a more typically developing manner. Six of the children could produce the /n/ in "snake." (The single child who could not produce /n/, could also not produce /s/.) Only three of the seven children with speech and

language impairment could accurately produce the later developing /s/ in "snake."

Because these differences were found in a limited number of participants, they could be attributed to chance. Yet this is important to note because these children with ASD are breaking the universals of sound development. Let's ask, "Why?" The earliest developing sounds in the English language are oral and nasal stops, which are also the shortest, averaging 50 milliseconds in length, such as the /n/ in "snake." Whereas, the later developing continuant airflow /s sound/, averages 130 milliseconds in length.

This is approximately three times longer than the /n/ in duration. With auditory processing deficits, it is possible that these short sounds could easily go undetected and therefore not produced.

Even Chomsky in his *Innate Theory of Language Development* acknowledges that perception is necessary for production: "External stimulation is necessary during formative times in maturation. This exposure should occur for the child to self-generate linguistic rules from his or her environment."[38]

Now, think about the plethora of oral and nasal stops that we typically focus on as "step one" when working with minimally verbal children with ASD. The commonly used words *ball, bubbles, pop, my turn, in, on, go, all done,* and *bye-bye* come to mind.

It may be beneficial to rethink our initial vocabulary by focusing on longer sounds, with continuant airflows, such as fricatives /s/, /z/, /ʃ/, and /ʒ/ and liquids /l/ and /r/.

Using these longer sounds within a Dynamic, Temporal, Tactile, Cueing methodology (covered in Chapter 6) could empower children with poor auditory perception and oral motor coordination to both better perceive and produce speech.

More consequential than our invaluable "stops, stops, more stops" core vocabulary for therapy time is the knowledge that an inability to audiorily perceive short oral stops would negatively impact a child's ability to produce them.

In the larger scheme of life, caregivers are universally addressed by stop consonants.[39] If an infant or a toddler could not perceive and therefore not produce oral or nasal stops, a caregiver's attention would not be verbally called. The resulting impact of a child's inability to call a caregiver's attention is immeasurable.

I would not have found this proverbial "snake in the grass" had I not been playing in the field or digging with my own hands. Mindfully working as a speech-language pathologist will result in developing keen intuition through numerous first-hand experiences.

Furthermore in collecting, entering, and analyzing your own data, you will discover the details to becoming a more effective therapist. (Refer to Chapter 10 for a simple, yet effective, methodology to research your practice.)

7.21 Putting Research into Practice: Decreasing Rate of Speech to Increase Both Perception and Production

In therapy, speech can be considerably slowed so that children are able to both perceive and produce auditory stimuli. Notice in Video 7.19 that Ms. Alyssa holds fricatives and lengthens stop consonants so that the child with ASD is able to join her.

Over the years, I've used this slowed speech technique effectively to teach many preverbal children with ASD to talk. The method is simple: holding sounds at length until the child joins in. Children seem to enjoy the sensory feedback of the vibrations from our choral speech. This technique allows the child with auditory processing deficits the time necessary to both perceive and produce the sound in slow, unison speech.

7.22 The Child with Auditory Processing Deficits May Be Slower to Orient, Therefore Missing the Start of Words

Through item analysis research of the 14 preschoolers aforementioned, I also found that children in the group with ASD were more likely to delete initial syllables and sounds. In both groups, four of the seven children deleted final consonants. A discrepancy in performance between the two groups was noted in initial syllable deletion.

Five of the seven preschoolers in the ASD group deleted the initial syllable of polysyllabic words. Whereas, only two of the seven preschoolers in the speech with language impairment group did. (Note: The test item "computer" was not used in the analysis because we've found "puter" for "computer" to be an error common to a majority of preschoolers we've tested.)

This is a small study of 14 preschoolers and therefore the discrepancy in performance may again be attributed to chance. However, it is in these small

studies that we detect "something in the water" for further investigation. If children with ASD were more in fact more likely to delete initial syllables, why?

Could we revisit Chomsky's stance on language development that speech production requires speech perception?

Not perceiving therefore producing beginnings of words could be attributed to difficulty in orienting attention, which has been indicated as a life-long challenge for individuals with ASD.[40]

Perhaps auditory processing and orienting attention difficulties take together can manifest as children with ASD deleting initial syllables of multisyllabic words.

Let's look at therapy that can provide support for both orienting attention and increasing auditory perception. In this next video, attention is attained through a motor imitation. This is performed prior to speaking for increased engagement.

See Video 7.20 in which Ms. MaryLyn is preparing Stella for initial sound production by having Stella join her in temporally cueing the sound prior to Stella producing it.

Stella imitating motor cues prior to beginning choral speech accomplishes four goals: (1) It orients Stella's attention; (2) emphasizes the initial sounds by temporally cueing tongue placement; (3) increases perception through slowed speech; and (4) cues correct production through slowed verbal and temporal cues.

7.23 Supplementing and Encouraging Speech Development with Augmentative and Alternative Communication

In the preverbal and minimally verbal stages, the immediate focus is for functional communication with augmentative and alternative communication incorporated immediately to optimize communication gains.[41]

With improvement, the course of therapy will evolve to include an emphasis on increased complexity of speech targets and linguistic contexts (e.g., clusters in the context of elaborate complex sentences within paragraph long formats). Selection of type of alternative and augmentative communication is an individualized decision based on the child and his or her family with a variety of options. In consideration of the constraints of one chapter, I will cover my personal adaptation of the popular low-tech Picture Exchange Communication System (PECS). The six stages of PECS are intended to progress from requesting to commenting through the use of communication symbols. A most-to-least hand-over hand prompting hierarchy is used in which prompting is provided with an adult shadowing the child. Hand-over-hand prompts are successively faded in the teaching stages while maintaining an 80% accuracy level.[42]

The child is to complete the six stages with a most to-least, beginning with a hand-over-hand prompting hierarchy. The six phases with graduated levels of independence are as follows:

Stage I: Exchange a single picture, photo, or object for an item.

Stage II: Move across a distance to exchange a picture with a communication partner.

Stage III: Discriminate between an array of two to five pictures.

Stage IV: Adhere a picture from an array to a sentence strip ("I want X").

Stage V: Answer "What do you want?" with a sentence strip.

Stage VI: Comment ("I see a _____.").

PECS is a widely used, research-based intervention for increasing functional communication skills of preschoolers with ASD. It has been found to increase social communication and speech production while decreasing problem behaviors.[43] Research has indicated that children with limitations in joint attention additionally benefit from the PECS in increased functional requesting skills over a more naturalistic responsive milieu teaching approach. In this study, the more responsive enhanced milieu teaching approach was indicated for children with stronger joint attention skills at baseline.[44]

Our very small study of six preverbal and minimally verbal preschoolers with ASD indicated that the PECS sentence strip is most effective for increasing verbal output for children who produce less than five word approximations or words in a 5-minute period. Common Core Boards were relatively more effective for children who produced more than one word per minute on average.[45]

Further research is indicated for clinical decision-making regarding selection of PECS versus a Common Core Board's impact on verbal output with preverbal and minimally verbal preschoolers.

Despite these evidence-based positive gains using PECS, it is important to note that meta-analytic research indicates gains in verbal speech development for children with ASD using PECS are not substantial. Clinicians and parents should be knowledgeable of these limited outcomes considering the immense impact of not learning to talk.[46]

Importantly, research indicates that the greatest amount of speech production occurs at the sentence strip level, Stage IV of PECS.[47] This requires the child to print reference words as read by an adult to the child. It is unknown if this correlation is due to these children being naturally more advanced and therefore able to reach a higher level of PECS stages.

Perhaps, the motor act of print referencing in finger tapping syllables or words stimulates increased oral motor neuronal activity, thereby encouraging speech. Both factors could influence this finding of Stage IV associated with greater speech production.

For this, I personally reorder the sequence of PECS. I begin at Stage IV and then go through each phase. There are multiple reasons that I begin with a sentence strip instead of a single picture to comprehensively treat the child:

1. I want the child to learn to verbally comment, which indicates greater outcomes than request ing.[48] Therefore, I use the carrier phrase "Look at ___" instead of using an "I want ___" (See ▶ Fig. 7.1).
   Additionally, in using the carrier phrase "Look at ____", I've systematically observed: Children are more likely to attain eye contact with the communication partner when 119 | 16.10.20 - 13:45 Treating Motor Speech Disorders in Preschoolers with Autism Spectrum Disorder an reading "look," which is what pragmatically appropriate speakers do when initiating interactions; and

2. Quicker learning of speech production with less practice is required in that the carrier phrase "Look at ____" does not require the complex coordination to produce the diph thongs ("I" /aɪ/) and glide ("want" /w/). I've found these sounds to be challenging for minimally verbal children with ASD in that they require complex articulatory shifts to produce them.

3. Speech is a continuous motor activity. It makes no sense to speak at a single word level, especially considering that children with ASD benefit from exposure to lengthier utterances.[26]

4. In holistically treating the child, I see fine motor benefits in initially using the PECS sentence strip over a single picture. This is because it requires children to engage in the multistep fine motor activity of pulling a picture from a velcro board, adhering it to a sentence strip, pulling the sentence strip, physically

exchanging the strip to a communicative partner, and pointing to multiple syllables as spoken. Research indicates that fine motor skills at 2 years of age are importantly correlated to expressive language outcomes at 3 years of age.[14]

5. The sentence strip and presentation of print capitalize on what neurological researchers indicate to be the strongest modality for children with ASD, visual perception.[1] Additionally, research indicates that preschoolers with ASD have alphabet knowledge comparable to their neurotypical peers.[49,50] I inform parents that their child may learn to read first and talk later. Reading will serve as an important avenue to learning to talk.

See Video 7.21 of Deenie. Deenie does not have ASD but has an underdeveloped cerebellum due to being born very prematurely. As a result, Deenie presents with ASD-like symptomology. As presented in Chapter 5, recent research indicates deficits associated with ASD can be attributed to Video 7.21 differences in the cerebellum.

This video demonstrates backward chaining in which hand-over hand prompting continues to be provided in the initial stages with fading of support in the final steps. Support will continue to be faded in a backward sequence with support faded on the final before the first steps. Notice that Deenie is independently tapping syllables as spoken, the last step in the sequence.

7.24 Putting Neuroscientific Research into Practice: Judicious Use of Limited Time to Ignite Dramatic Change

In treating preschoolers with ASD, using a combination of the complexity approach, multi-modal cueing, natural reward milieu strategies, and core vocabulary approach has resulted in remarkable gains on both standardized speech testing and Percent Consonant Correct (PCC) within connected speech samples.[5]

After only five therapy sessions over a 6-week period, three verbal preschoolers with ASD (the only ones with ASD participating in this intervention at that time) produced an average of 14 less errors on the CAAP-2 test,[5] indicating efficient generalization to untreated targets. They additionally produced an average 20% improvement in PCC in spontaneous, connected speech samples.

Preschoolers with diverse impairments participating in this intervention showed substantial improvements. However, the gains of these three preschoolers with ASD were the most impressive in terms of both speech testing performance and improvement in speech intelligibility within conversation as measured by PCC.

In both standardized test gains and PCC, the group of three preschoolers with ASD out performed preschoolers with speech and concurrent language impairment as well as preschoolers with only speech impairment who received the same intervention.

In objectively analyzing the data, it should be noted that the preschoolers with ASD presented with the most severe level of impairment at baseline. Therefore, regression toward the mean, in which extreme scores move toward average, may have played a role in inflating their gains. Digital clips of these three preschoolers are presented in this chapter under the pseudonyms of Darren, Cadge, and Stella for a glimpse of their intervention.

7.25 Efficiently Impact Multiple Domains Concurrently through Linguistic Complexity

These impressive gains were achieved after five 45-minute outpatient therapy sessions.[5] Could these types of gains occur with the limited therapy time and high caseload of a practicing speech language pathologist within the public school system?

Meet Kelly Vess. This is my life 9 months out of the year. Perhaps it sounds familiar. I have over 50 preschoolers on my caseload. Approximately 50% have speech only impairment, 20% have concurrent speech and language impairment, and 30% have ASD or another pervasive developmental disorder.

I additionally perform all incoming speech and language evaluations for preschool age children at my school. All students receive 30 to 60 minutes of therapy weekly. Research indicates 30 to 60 minutes of direct therapy time to be standard practice regardless of the child's disorder.[51]

Table 7.5 Gains made in a 6-month period for preschoolers with autism spectrum disorder (ASD) in comparison to normative data of neurotypical peers based on pre- and post 20 continuous utterance language sample

Avg Increase in Mean Length of Utterance following 6-Months ASD (N=9) (30 mos-66 mos)	Avg Increase in Mean Length of Utterance following 6-Months Neurotypical (30 mos-66 mos)	Avg Decrease in Number of Errors on CAAP-2 following 6-Months ASD (N=9) (30 mos-66 mos)	Avg Decrease in Number of Errors on CAAP-2 (X=100) following 6-Months Neurotypical (30 mos-66 mos)
Average increase of .52 in MLU following 6 months	Average .29 increase in MLU for each 6 month interval[a]	Average 19 less errors in 6-month period	Average 3 less errors in a 6-month period[b]
Average Percent Verbal Requests in Language Sample at Baseline (N=9)	Average Percent Verbal Requests in Language Sample Post-intervention 6-Months Later (N=9)	Average Percent Verbal Comments* in Language Sample at Baseline (N=9)	Average Percent Verbal Comments* in Language Sample Post-intervention 6-Months Later (N=9)
Requests: 54%	Requests: 21%	Comments: 44%	Comments: 79%

*Comments were defined as contextually-based language not used for the purpose of requesting.
Normative Neurotypical Peer Data Comparison: a) Rice ML, Smolik F, Perpich D, Thompson T, Rytting N, Blossom M. Mean length of utterance levels in 6-month intervals for children 3 to 9 Years with and without language impairments. Journal of Speech, Language, and Hearing Research. 2010;53(2):333–349. b) Secord W, Donohue JS. Clinical Assessment of Articulation and Phonology-2nd Ed (CAAP-2). Torrance, CA. WPS Publishing; 2013

I'm sharing this because I want you to know that even with severe time constraints and high workload demands, significant gains in working with preschoolers with ASD can be made through judicious use of therapy time.

Our current research study of nine verbal preschoolers with ASD over a 6-month period during the school year quantifiably indicates that we can substantially increase speech clarity, mean length of utterance (MLU), and social commenting. This is accomplished through production of a complex paragraph in the context of requesting.

Refer ▶ Table 7.5 which displays data gleaned from language samples of 20 continuous utterances for each child. Language samples were collected in the fall and 6 months later in the spring for the nine preschoolers in our study. Data displayed also indicates performance on the CAAP-2 in the fall and 6 months later in the spring.

Refer to the request paragraph in Appendix E. Note the 3-element consonant clusters and the overall length of the utterance. This results in an increase in joint attention, and increase in joint engagement required to complete the paragraph.

Also, notice the use of narrative conjunctive tier 2 vocabulary, first, then, lastly, and because. Finally, see how alphabet knowledge and pictorial demonstration of speech rules capitalize on the visual processing strengths of preschoolers with ASD.

There was a developmental cascade impact in gains. Within only a six-month time period, MLU,

speech clarity, and commenting increased substantially. How was that possible?

I would propose that the complexity of our treatment target in terms of phonology (3-element consonant clusters) and syntax (conjoined complex sentences) played a role in these measurable global improvements. How? Having the child produce the most complex targets at the greatest degree of length and complexity resulted in optimal speech, expressive language, and joint attention gains.

Joint attention can be defined as two individuals having coordinated attention to each other and to a third object or event. In this case, both the child and adult have coordinated attention to reciting and acting out the "angry dog teeth" request paragraph. The act of speaking with an adult echoing or gesturing, while conjointly referencing a paragraph, could be characterized as an extended act of joint attention with a high level of engagement.

Development of joint attention and a high level of engagement is of critical importance in early intervention for preschoolers with ASD.[52] Research indicates that improvement in joint attention results in a developmental cascade across domains with improvement in play, social initiations, positive affect, imitation, and spontaneous speech.[53]

The significant increase in commenting within spontaneous language sampled following a 6-month period may be partially attributed to an increase in joint attention. Perhaps, speech and motor imitation additionally served as active agents of change. Imitation promotes mirror neuron development and may have also contributed to the increase in social communication evident by commenting.

Brain research indicates that the complexity approach ignites neuronal activity with increased nerve impulses firing across multiple regions of the brain.[24] By requesting with the paragraph, you may also appreciate the visual-temporal and narrative storytelling with tier 2 vocabulary developing in automaticity with a high dose of repetition of first, then, lastly, and because.

Building an ability to tell a story with automaticity at the preschool level can be of pivotal importance to later social-emotional outcomes.[54,55] Being able to more easily articulate social frustrations, sensory dysfunction, or academic challenges can serve as a protective social-emotional functioning factor later on.

In this chapter, refer digital clips of preschoolers Ida and Liam requesting with a complex paragraph for a glimpse of the intervention approach used with these nine verbal preschoolers with ASD during the school year. These preschoolers with ASD made requests using this paragraph to induce optimal change in speech, language, joint attention, and social communication.

7.26 Respecting the Child's Current Capacity

After sharing these successes of effectively working with verbal preschoolers with ASD, I'll end this chapter on a somber note. I've worked with two preschoolers with ASD who were minimally verbal. With a maximum level of prompting they both spoke only when it was required to request the highest rewarding objects and actions. Upon returning from summer vacation, however, both had completely stopped talking.

In both cases, their well-meaning parents decided to take the "Nothing is free" approach to improve speech. One of the children whispered. The parent was hoping to encourage louder speech by not rewarding whispered speech, which unfortunately was the only speech the child appeared to be capable of producing at the time. This child most likely could not coordinate vocal fold vibration with articulation.

The other child with ASD who was minimally verbal fronted velars, substituting /t/ and /d/ for /k/ and /g/. His parents opted to not reward the "baby talk" in hopes of improving his speech. He most likely had not yet developed the oral motor strength to retract the tongue to produce velars. He too ceased talking.

Please share these stories with parents of children with ASD. Speech is a complex motor activity in which many instruments must fluidly work together. Like an orchestra, a lot of unforced, joyful practice will aid in unique sections seamlessly blending together with increased practice over time.

7.27 Chapter Summary

For the past 30 years, meta-analytic research indicates that we have largely not improved outcomes for preverbal and minimally children with ASD. The rate today mirrors that of 30 years ago with an estimated 25–30% of children with ASD not developing functional speech in their lives.

In Kelly's Corner, Video 7.22, I discuss the importance of treating the speech motor disorder and concurrent motor impairment for many children with ASD. In this chapter, please reference digital clips of Davey, a child who was preverbal and producing minimal vocalizations. He additionally presented with sensory and motor impairment challenges.

Today, a year later, Davey fluidy and joyfully vocalizes throughout the day using word approximations. Every day, his spontaneous speech becomes clearer through his constant self-generated practice. His speech is calmly, yet joyfully appreciated as not a requirement, rather the gift that it is. Speech is never something pressured or forced to do. Davey is showing us a better way for children with ASD to learn to talk.

This is an exciting time in intervention for children with ASD. The neuroscience will give them a voice in which they will be better treated with neuro-divergent approaches that capitalize on strengths, with focused attention to neurological challenges inherent to these children.

We know from the research that the "one size fits all" approach is not working for these children who present with a multi-faceted, complex disorder.

These non-science based approaches uniformly fail. When they do, it is often attributed to the child having a cognitive impairment. The impairment does not lie in the child rather the intervention. Neuroscience gives these children a voice. We need to listen.

References

[1] Derrick D, Bicevskis K, Gick B. Visual-tactile speech perception and the autism quotient. Front Commun. 2019; 3

[2] Neuhaus E, Beauchaine TP, Bernier R. Neurobiological correlates of social functioning in autism. Clin Psychol Rev. 2010; 30(6):733–748

[3] Zhang J, Meng Y, He J, et al. McGurk effect by individuals with autism spectrum disorder and typically developing controls: a systematic review and meta-analysis. J Autism Dev Disord. 2019; 49(1):34–43

[4] Peeva MG, Tourville JA, Agam Y, Holland B, Manoach DS, Guenther FH. White matter impairment in the speech network of individuals with autism spectrum disorder. Neuroimage Clin. 2013; 3:234–241

[5] Vess K, Liovas M, Mocny A, Vuletic D. Applying the complexity approach to effectively treat severe speech impairment in preschoolers with ASD. Poster presented at: Annual American Speech, Language and Hearing Association Convention; November, 2018; Boston, MA

[6] Kaiser AP, Scherer NJ, Frey JR, Roberts MY. The effects of enhanced milieu teaching with phonological emphasis on the speech and language skills of young children with cleft palate: a pilot study. Am J Speech Lang Pathol. 2017; 26 (3):806–818

[7] Murray E, McCabe P, Ballard KJ. A systematic review of treatment outcomes for children with childhood apraxia of speech. Am J Speech Lang Pathol. 2014; 23(3):486–504

[8] Dale PS, Hayden DA. Treating speech subsystems in childhood apraxia of speech with tactual input: the PROMPT approach. Am J Speech Lang Pathol. 2013; 22(4):644–661

[9] Crosbie S, Holm A, Dodd B. Intervention for children with severe speech disorder: a comparison of two approaches. Int J Lang Commun Disord. 2005; 40(4):467–491

[10] Finch E, Rumbach AF, Park S. Speech pathology management of non-progressive dysarthria: a systematic review of the literature. Disabil Rehabil. 2020; 42(3):296–306

[11] Oberman LM, Ramachandran VS. The simulating social mind: the role of the mirror neuron system and simulation in the social and communicative deficits of autism spectrum disorders. Psychol Bull. 2007; 133(2):310–327

[12] Oberman LM, Ramachandran VS. Preliminary evidence for deficits in multisensory integration in autism spectrum disorders: the mirror neuron hypothesis. Soc Neurosci. 2008; 3 (3–4):348–355

[13] McDuffie A, Yoder P, Stone W. Prelinguistic predictors of vocabulary in young children with autism spectrum disorders. J Speech Lang Hear Res. 2005; 48(5):1080–1097

[14] Choi B, Leech KA, Tager-Flusberg H, Nelson CA. Development of fine motor skills is associated with expressive language outcomes in infants at high and low risk for autism spectrum disorder. J Neurodev Disord. 2018; 10(1):14

[15] Masten AS, Cicchetti D. Developmental cascades. Dev Psychopathol. 2010; 22(3):491–495

[16] Karasik LB, Tamis-Lemonda CS, Adolph KE. Crawling and walking infants elicit different verbal responses from mothers. Dev Sci. 2014; 17(3):388–395

[17] Özçalışkan Ş, Adamson LB, Dimitrova N. Early deictic but not other gestures predict later vocabulary in both typical development and autism. Autism. 2016; 20(6):754–763

[18] Fournier KA, Hass CJ, Naik SK, Lodha N, Cauraugh JH. Motor coordination in autism spectrum disorders: a synthesis and meta-analysis. J Autism Dev Disord. 2010; 40(10):1227–1240

[19] Green D, Charman T, Pickles A, et al. Impairment in movement skills of children with autistic spectrum disorders. Dev Med Child Neurol. 2009; 51(4):311–316

[20] Ming X, Brimacombe M, Wagner GC. Prevalence of motor impairment in autism spectrum disorders. Brain Dev. 2007; 29(9):565–570

[21] Vess K, Abou-Arabi M. Increasing verbal output of prelinguistic preschoolers with autism spectrum disorder through movement. Poster presented at: Annual American Speech, Language and Hearing Association Convention; November, 2018; Boston, MA

[22] McDaniel J, D'Ambrose Slaboch K, Yoder P. A meta-analysis of the association between vocalizations and expressive language in children with autism spectrum disorder. Res Dev Disabil. 2018; 72:202–213

[23] Buckner RL. The cerebellum and cognitive function: 25 years of insight from anatomy and neuroimaging. Neuron. 2013; 80(3):807–815

[24] Kiran S, Thompson CK. Neuroplasticity of language networks in aphasia: advances, updates, and future challenges. Front Neurol. 2019; 10:295

[25] Crandall MC, McDaniel J, Watson LR, Yoder PJ. The relation between early parent verb input and later expressive verb vocabulary in children with autism spectrum disorder. J Speech Lang Hear Res. 2019; 62(6):1787–1797

[26] Sandbank M, Yoder P. The association between parental mean length of utterance and language outcomes in children with disabilities: a correlational meta-analysis. Am J Speech Lang Pathol. 2016; 25(2):240–251

[27] Venker CE, Yasick M, McDaniel J. Using telegraphic input with children with language delays: a survey of speech-language pathologists' practices and perspectives. Am J Speech Lang Pathol. 2019; 28(2):676–696

[28] Tager-Flusberg H, Kasari C. Minimally verbal school-aged children with autism spectrum disorder: the neglected end of the spectrum. Autism Res. 2013; 6(6):468–478

[29] Biller MF, Johnson CJ. Social–cognitive and speech sound production abilities of minimally verbal children with autism spectrum disorders. Am J Speech Lang Pathol. 2019; 28(2):377–393

[30] McIntosh B, Dodd B. Evaluation of core vocabulary intervention for treatment of inconsistent phonological disorder: three treatment case studies. Child Lang Teach Ther. 2008; 24(3):307–327

[31] Bottema-Beutel K, Yoder PJ, Hochman JM, Watson LR. The role of supported joint engagement and parent utterances in language and social communication development in children with autism spectrum disorder. J Autism Dev Disord. 2014; 44(9):2162–2174

[32] Secord W, Donohue JS. Clinical Assessment of Articulation and Phonology-2nd Ed (CAAP-2). Torrance, CA. WPS Publishing; 2013

[33] Preston JL, Hull M, Edwards ML. Preschool speech error patterns predict articulation and phonological awareness outcomes in children with histories of speech sound disorders. Am J Speech Lang Pathol. 2013; 22(2):173–184

[34] Hayiou-Thomas ME, Carroll JM, Leavett R, Hulme C, Snowling MJ. When does speech sound disorder matter for literacy? The role of disordered speech errors, co-occurring language impairment and family risk of dyslexia. J Child Psychol Psychiatry. 2017; 58(2):197–205

[35] Masso S, Baker E, McLeod S, Wang C. Polysyllable speech accuracy and predictors of later literacy development in preschool children with speech sound disorders. J Speech Lang Hear Res. 2017; 60(7):1877–1890

7

[36] McGurk H, MacDonald J. Hearing lips and seeing voices. Nature. 1976; 264(5588):746–748

[37] McLeod S, Crowe K. Children's consonant acquisition in 27 languages: a cross-linguistic review. Am J Speech Lang Pathol. 2018; 27(4):1546–1571

[38] Chomsky N. Aspects of the Theory of Syntax. Cambridge, MA: The MIT Press; 2015

[39] Nichols J. Linguistic Diversity in Space and Time. Chicago: The University of Chicago Press; 2017

[40] Patten E, Watson LR. Interventions targeting attention in young children with autism. Am J Speech Lang Pathol. 2011; 20(1):60–69

[41] Kasari C, Kaiser A, Goods K, et al. Communication interventions for minimally verbal children with autism: a sequential multiple assignment randomized trial. J Am Acad Child Adolesc Psychiatry. 2014; 53(6):635–646

[42] Frost L, Bondy A. PECS Training Manual. Newark, DE: Pyramid Educational Consultants; 2002

[43] Hart SL, Banda DR. Picture Exchange Communication System with individuals with developmental disabilities: a meta-analysis of single subject studies. Remedial Spec Educ. 2010; 31(6):476–488

[44] Yoder P, Stone WL. A randomized comparison of the effect of two prelinguistic communication interventions on the acquisition of spoken communication in preschoolers with ASD. J Speech Lang Hear Res. 2006; 49(4):698–711

[45] Devine K, Vess K. Comparing efficacy of Picture Exchange Communication System (PECS) versus Common Core Communication Board (CCCB) on speech development for preschoolers with ASD. Poster presented at: Annual American Speech, Language and Hearing Association Convention; November, 2017; San Diego, CA

[46] Schlosser RW, Wendt O. Effects of augmentative and alternative communication intervention on speech production in children with autism: a systematic review. Am J Speech Lang Pathol. 2008; 17(3):212–230

[47] Flippin M, Reszka S, Watson LR. Effectiveness of the Picture Exchange Communication System (PECS) on communication and speech for children with autism spectrum disorders: a meta-analysis. Am J Speech Lang Pathol. 2010; 19(2):178–195

[48] Shumway S, Wetherby AM. Communicative acts of children with autism spectrum disorders in the second year of life. J Speech Lang Hear Res. 2009; 52(5):1139–1156

[49] Lanter E, Watson LR, Erickson KA, Freeman D. Emergent literacy in children with autism: an exploration of developmental and contextual dynamic processes. Lang Speech Hear Serv Sch. 2012; 43(3):308–324

[50] Dynia JM, Brock ME, Logan JAR, Justice LM, Kaderavek JN. Comparing children with ASD and their peers' growth in print knowledge. J Autism Dev Disord. 2016; 46(7):2490–2500

[51] Brumbaugh KM, Smit AB. Treating children ages 3–6 who have speech sound disorder: a survey. Lang Speech Hear Serv Sch. 2013; 44(3):306–319

[52] Bottema-Beutel K. Associations between joint attention and language in autism spectrum disorder and typical development: a systematic review and meta-regression analysis. Autism Res. 2016; 9(10):1021–1035

[53] Whalen C, Schreibman L, Ingersoll B. The collateral effects of joint attention training on social initiations, positive affect, imitation, and spontaneous speech for young children with autism. J Autism Dev Disord. 2006; 36(5):655–664

[54] Basil C, Reyes S. Acquisition of literacy skills by children with severe disability. Child Lang Teach Ther. 2003; 19(1):27–48

[55] Lyons R, Roulstone S. Well-being and resilience in children with speech and language disorders. J Speech Lang Hear Res. 2018; 61(2):324–344

7

8 Generalization Coming from Within

Begin with the end in mind.

—Stephen Covey

When I first wrote an outline for this book, I titled this chapter "Generalization across People and Settings" with a plan to share with you what a *therapist* can do to make generalization happen. The problem is that the therapist doesn't make generalization happen. The *child* does. For this, I changed the title to "Generalization Coming from Within."

After much research, I've found that generalization is an internal process that can't be controlled externally. It is ultimately the child, not the adult, who is responsible for generalization to occur through the following: (1) The child assuming an internal locus of control. and (2) The internal workings of the child's brain through a process known as *myelination* strengthens new neuronal pathways through repetition of accurate speech.

8.1 Generalization through Child Assuming an Internal Locus of Control

People often think of generalization as the final step in the therapy process. It is actually the first step. When you first meet the child, develop a relationship in which the child, not the therapist, is in charge of the learning experience. This is the most important life-changing impact speech-language pathologists can have on children.

The overarching goal is to help each child develop an *internal locus of control*. An *internal locus of control* is a belief that outcomes can be influenced by *internal factors* that the child can control, such as perseverance and hard work. Conversely, *external factors*, which are factors beyond the child's control, such as environment, inherited traits, or even neurological differences, produce very realistic challenges. However, for a child with a well-developed internal locus of control, external factors do *not* necessarily dictate outcomes.

For children with communicative impairments, *self-efficacy*, a belief in an individual's ability to create desired results, matters.[1] As a speech-language pathologist, you do not have a magic wand. You may not be able to completely ameliorate neurological damage. You cannot replace poverty, unsafe environments, broken schools, and broken homes with golden, yellow brick roads.

The children we work with will likely have to work exponentially harder than their neurotypical peers due to neurological differences. For this, they must know that they themselves can create success through effort and by independently and actively functioning as their own teacher.

To help the child develop an *internal locus of control*, establish from day one a relationship in which the *child* is his or her own teacher. Your role will be to provide a level of support that empowers the child to engage in linguistic behaviors that are currently outside of the child's reach by working within the child's *zone of proximal development*.[2]

The *zone of proximal development* is what the child can accomplish with a more capable individual's support. Through engaging in these more complex linguistic behaviors, optimal neurological change will transpire at an age when neuronal plasticity is at a greater level.[3]

8.2 The Initial Assessment: Establishing an Internal Locus of Control

The child taking the teacher's role, and you assuming the role as the child's assistant, begins the first day you meet the child for an initial assessment. You begin by only providing feedback that promotes a growth mindset.[4] A growth mindset is one that specifically acknowledges effort, actions, and perseverance. It does not prejudge or label the child as having fixed attributes, such as being labelled as "smart" or "good."

During testing, provide specific objective feedback regarding effort, attention to task, active participation, compliance, and self-regulation. The corresponding Video 8.1 demonstrates how prosocial communication rules presented in Chapter 2 are routinely reviewed and practiced in a small group setting with verbal presentation coupled with movements. Additionally, these rules are routinely taught and reviewed in classroom settings of approximately 20 preschoolers with speech and language impairments in which *all* children are expected to chorally and gesturally participate.

At the beginning of standardized speech testing explicitly acknowledge the child as the teacher, "You get to be the teacher and to tell me what each of these pictures are." After completing the standardized single-word assessment, administer the

Supplemental Consonant Cluster Screener in which the child is again explicitly instructed to say the words with you clearly like a teacher when provided a maximum level of cueing.

There are two steps in administering the *Supplemental Consonant Cluster Screener*. First, have the child imitate all words. Next, re-administer words that the child incorrectly imitated with a maximum level of prompting and without picture reference (which could elicit errors due to inaccurate prior learning of the word).

Recent research indicates that words containing initial position consonant clusters are produced similarly by children, whether spontaneously produced or directly imitated.[5] This research is clinically relevant in consideration of 45-minute evaluation time constraints typically imposed by insurance companies.

Single-word speech assessments can be completed in one-third of the time with children imitating words instead of spontaneously producing them.[5] Testing information can be coupled with a 5- to 10-minute speech sample for Percent Consonant Correct for a reliable, naturalistic snapshot of the child's current speech.[6] Therefore, correctly imitated consonant cluster target words would *not* be selected as treatment targets as it can reasonably be assumed that they are correctly produced spontaneously.

The exception to this rule is in assessing preschoolers with autism spectrum disorder (ASD). Our research indicates that imitated speech with this population tends to be more accurately produced than spontaneously elicited speech.[7] Our findings that preschoolers with ASD perform better when imitating may be partially due to the influence of echolalia. Echolalia is the exact repetition of

---

Is a Preschool Age Child with Severe Speech Impairment Able to Produce 3-Element Consonant Clusters?

Yes. We studied 27 preschoolers with severe speech impairment and assigned 9 preschoolers to one of three groups based on educational eligibility label: (1) speech impairment only; (2) speech and language impairment; and (3) speech and ASD. These preschoolers were compared across closely matched groups based on baseline Standard Score (SS) on the *Clinical Assessment of Articulation and Phonology-2* (X = 100, SD = 15) and age.

There were nine preschoolers with severe speech impairment alone (average SS = 62; average age = 45 months), nine preschoolers with both severe speech impairment and language impairment (average SS = 59; average age = 50 months), and nine preschoolers with both severe speech impairment and ASD (average SS = 62; average age = 49 months). They were closely matched in terms of baseline single-word SS test performance and age to indicate impact of disorder on ability to produce 3-element consonant clusters with maximum prompting.

We found an overwhelming majority of the 27 children could produce at least one 3-element cluster with a maximum level of cueing, regardless of disorder. Importantly, *all* 27 children in this study could produce minimally a 2-element s-blend complex cluster.[8] We've selected s-blend targets to be the most efficacious two-blend cluster.

In this study, each child was provided a maximum level of dynamic, tactile, temporal cueing with an allowance of two attempts to produce the consonant clusters accurately on the *Supplemental Consonant Cluster Screener* from Chapter 1.

We found that all nine of the preschoolers with severe speech impairment, seven of the nine preschoolers with severe speech impairment and language impairment, and eight of the nine preschoolers with severe speech impairment and ASD could accurately imitate at least one 3-element consonant clusters at baseline with maximum cueing.[9]

Be confident in what the child is capable of with your assistance. A majority of the preschoolers in this study were receiving cues from speech-language pathology graduate students with minimal clinical experience, not from me—an experienced therapist.

Both our research and systematic observation have consistently indicated that even preschoolers with severe speech impairment and concurrent language impairment or pervasive developmental delays can produce 3-element consonant clusters with a maximum level of cueing. Never discriminate in determining what a child is capable of based on severity of impairment or disorder. Not only is it unfair to the child but it undermines your pivotal role as an agent of change.

another's verbal output instead of the child independently generating sounds, words, or sentences.

Treatment targets that would be selected are consonant clusters that the child is able to produce with a maximum level of prompting provided. These clusters are in the realm of the child's *zone of proximal development*. Of importance is discovering the most complex 3-element consonant cluster that the child can produce with your assistance that treats both the child's phonological processes and distortions.

Only if the child is unable to produce a 3-element consonant cluster with maximum cueing, would the most complex 2-element consonant cluster be selected to directly treat the child's most complex phonological processes or distortions.

8.3 Informing the Parents of the "Child as Teacher" Intervention Plan

At this point we've completed the assessment and selected a therapy target. Now we're going to explain the reasons behind the therapy decisions made to support generalization. These are questions that we want to answer in the initial stage of intervention.

In reviewing the child's individualized treatment plan, take time to flesh out the logic behind strategies so that the parent can be an educated partner in the therapy process and actively involved in generalization every step of the way. Below are explanations of evidence-based strategies for therapists to review with parents during the intervention plan stages.

8.4 Putting Research into Practice: Explaining Evidence-Based Practices to Parents

1. *Why Select 3-Element Consonant Clusters as a Starting Point?*

Explain the efficiency of working on more advanced treatment targets due to the cascading impact on untreated, less complex, earlier developing sounds. This impact is unidirectional. We've completed six intervention studies over six years with preschoolers of diverse etiologies and severity levels. There has *never* surfaced an upward impact in which earlier developing treatment targets impacted later developing sounds. There is, however, consistent evidence showing that more complex treatment targets impact earlier developing ones.[8,9,10,11,12]

2. *Why Select 3-Element Consonant Clusters Embedded in Complex Syntax, Such as an Elaborate Sentence, Complex Sentence, or Paragraph-Level Linguistic Context to Start Therapy?*

Unfortunately, speech-language pathologists report therapy time to be limited regardless of the child's severity level, which is typically a cumulative time of 30 to 60 minutes at a frequency of one to two times per week.[13] In fact, there is a gap between our practice and the evidence base we reference. The research we reference in treating speech sound disorders is largely based on a greater frequency of two to three 30- to 60-minute sessions, resulting in the cumulative therapy time of 60 to 180 minutes per week.[14] More therapy equals greater gains.[15,16] For this, we have to use our limited time judiciously.

We can improve *efficiency* of therapy by focusing efforts on what we can change by not only improving speech clarity, but also increasing sentence length and complexity.[17,18] Additionally, it is beneficial to have the child print for reference a syntactically complex linguistic treatment target card as words are spoken. Doing so can positively impact early literacy skills in both print-referencing and in building automaticity of orally conjoining ideas to foster narrative skill development.[19,20]

3. *How Should the Parent Use the Child's Treatment Request at Home?*

I advise parents to put the treatment target paragraph on the fridge and to have it as part of the everyday routine, like brushing teeth. The child should make at least one request daily. Frequency of practice is important in improving speech.[21]

4. *Why Use the Treatment Target as a Request?*

Research indicates that if children receive natural rewards for producing the treatment target, learning will occur quicker and will be more resistant to regression.[22]

5. *Why Are We Using the Same Treatment Target for the Entire Course of Therapy?*

We want children to develop an internal locus of control in which they are not dependent on an adult teaching them new words and phrases. Use of the same target allows them to focus on *how* they are talking, not *what* they are saying.

We want children to focus on the correct motor speech behaviors so that they can self-instruct,

8

self-monitor, and self-generalize. Additionally, research indicates that repeated use of the same target results in consistency in neuronal pathway development of motor planning, programming, and execution. This results in improved outcomes in both speech accuracy and consistency.[23]

6. *Will Use of the Same Treatment Target for the Entire Course of Therapy Result in Generalization to Other Words and Untreated Sounds?*

Yes. Research indicates that use of the same treatment target exemplar results in generalization to untreated targets.[8,9,10,11,12,24,25,26]

7. *Do We Need to Practice Consonant Clusters in the Middle and at the End of Words as Well?*

No. Consonant clusters in the initial position of words are later developing.[27] Our research has supported the premise that working on the cluster in the initial word position would have a cascading impact to other positions.[11]

8. *Where Are the Flashcards, Worksheets, and Apps (Which Are Basically Electronic Worksheets) That Our Private Therapist Gives Our Child?*

Meaningless activities lead to mindless practice. Preschoolers should be engaged in *mindfulness* in their learning through play, which is being aware, perceptive, and attentive.[28] This behavior will foster generalization as the child assumes both active participation in *constructively learning*, in which the child constructs knowledge and meaning through experiences in further developing an internal locus of control.[29]

Conversely, an example of *mindless practice* would be having the child passively producing a word correctly a prescribed number of times in drill format when shown a flashcard. Another would be labeling 20 exemplar pictures of a treatment target sound, 10 times each, on a worksheet. These activities will likely foster habituation of inaccurate production of sounds through mindless repetition. Mindless practice will not result in generalization. Mindful practice will.

Additionally, preschoolers should experience learning three-dimensionally for optimal neurological growth with multiple senses engaged in novel experiences that result in increased neuronal activity. With flashcards, worksheets, and screens, primarily visual senses are engaged.

We know that preschoolers learn from actively manipulating three-dimensional objects, which engage multiple senses, in the context of play. For this reason, our therapy activities and home practice "presents" are always hands-on, fun, and open-ended to foster creative, active learners.[30]

9. *Why Do We Provide Objective Feedback Instead of Praise?*

We want to teach the child to objectively self-evaluate. We can do this by providing objective feedback at a higher rate with younger, preschool age populations.[31] Also, the use of praise, such as "good job," can deter the child from taking risks. After all, an error would mean a "bad job."[32] We want to develop risk takers. It is by operating outside of comfort zones that neurological change will occur.

Children are also encouraged to judge whether they followed a speech rule by holding their thumbs up or down. For example, with a frontal lisp distortion of /s/, I would ask, "Did you keep the snake in the cage?" The child puts a thumbs up to affirm or thumbs down to deny. (You can add a little drama and excitement here by waiting a few seconds to affirm or deny their judgment with your own thumb—drum roll please.)

10. *Where and with Whom Should Children Practice Their Treatment Target?*

Generally, everywhere and with everyone to request desired objects and access to desirable activities. Remind caregivers to ensure that the child is provided with enough support for *accurate* practice to occur at a minimal 80% accuracy level across settings and people. The greater the number of accurate productions, the greater the speech gains.[33,34,35]

8.5 Beginning Therapy: Learning the Treatment Target

Many graduate students start with as little prompting as necessary in a commitment to providing naturalistic therapy and preventing prompt dependency. Do the opposite. At stage one of therapy, when plasticity levels are greatest, provide maximum level of prompting so the child can perform at the highest level possible. For therapeutic purposes, we're not interested in what the child is individually capable of doing. We're only interested in what the child is capable of with assistance in the *zone of proximal development*.

From day one of therapy, establish the most complex consonant cluster treatment target possible. Do this based on results from the single-word standardized single-word speech testing, connect speech sample, and the *Supplemental Consonant Cluster Screener.*

The most complex consonant cluster treatment target could be presented in a sentence, complex sentence, or paragraph. With introduction of the treatment target on the first day of therapy, the child is given a treatment target card (refer to **Appendix E**). Even if the child is not producing the target perfectly, the child can begin by memorizing the carrier sentences to request. As a result, the child will be able to focus efforts on speech accuracy at an earlier time.

8.6 Developing Neurological Automaticity to Achieve Generalization

People often think of generalization as something that can be fostered through application of highly repetitive activities, like homework worksheets in which you produce the sound in isolation, syllable, and word to sentence level, produce the sound in a number of different words, say the sound in every position within words, say the sound in words with one to multiple syllables, say the word and its minimal pair, and say the sound in poorly written, tongue-twister "stories." Parents may even be encouraged to bring these ridiculous flashcards and worksheets on vacation.

If you're doing these things, stop. You risk the child developing a dislike for learning and reading. Any situation that requires unrelated extrinsic rewards, such as stamps, stickers, tokens, or magnetic chips, is a testament to the fact that these activities are not intrinsically rewarding. Preschool age is a highly impressionable time in which children learn that learning and reading are either joyful experiences or taxing.[36] Our goal is to develop, not squash, a life-long love of learning and reading.

Within educationally rich activities, in which the child is actively engaged, provide and pull support to ensure a minimal 80% accuracy level with these challenging targets. Just as accurate practice results in creation and strengthening of accurate speech motor neurological pathways, inaccurate neurological pathways can also be created and strengthened through repetition.[37]

As a therapist, be present in this transactional learning experience. This dance in which scaffolds are removed and inserted dynamically in the *zone of proximal development* based on the child's response will keep you on your toes. The child is performing new, more advanced behaviors both incorrectly and correctly, as you are being constantly challenged to creatively respond.

You'll especially grow exponentially when working with neurologically diverse populations as you'll often have to step further out of your comfort zone, building new neuronal pathways yourself in response to both understanding and responding to unique behaviors. Please see Video 8.2 to observe this transactional experience. Refer ▶ Table 8.1 to evaluate generalization promoting responses specifically discussed in this chapter.

Practicing these new and advanced behaviors will directly result in the child forming new, more complex neurological pathways. Development of complex neural pathways will naturally create simpler pathways without valuable therapy time spent on attention to simpler sounds and linguistic concepts. These simpler sounds and concepts will naturally develop as a by-product of more complex neuropathway construction. The repeated practice of 3-element clusters presented in complex linguistic contexts.[3,38] See Video 8.3 for an example of therapy aimed to expedite gains through use of a complex speech and language treatment target.

8.7 Generalization through Myelination

See ▶ Fig. 8.1 to visualize how *nerve impulses*, the transfer of electrical or chemical activity, occur across nerve cells. When engaging in a new activity, neurons will connect to other neurons through *axons*, which serve as conduction cables. The electrical impulses cross tiny gaps, known as a *synapses*, while transferring to other neurons until they reach their destination.

This process of generalization is internally controlled in the child's brain. With repeated activity, white, fatty myelin sheaths are formed around the child's axons. This process is known as *myelination*. Increased *myelination*, which directly occurs as a result of increased practice, results in nerve impulses firing with increased strength and speed.

Typically, 300 to 400 nerve impulses occur every second in the brain. Maximally, 1,000 nerve impulses can occur in a second.[39] I encourage you to look at development of myelination as the primary objective in generalization. The myelination resulting in automaticity during firing of nerve impulses occurs from frequent, meaningful,

8

Table 8.1 Evaluating generalization strategies

Video Number:_____

Please indicate your level of agreement to the following statements in reference to generalization strategies in each digital clip presented.	Strongly Disagree	Disagree	Neutral	Agree	Strongly Agree
1) Child is actively engaged and enjoying learning.	1	2	3	4	5
2) Child is encouraged to actively participate by verbally and/or nonverbally stating the speech motor rule.	1	2	3	4	5
3) Direct verbal modelling is faded as much as possible, while maintaining an 80% accuracy level.	1	2	3	4	5
4) Child's prosocial communication behaviors of paying attention, answering every question, following every direction, keeping hands to self, and working super hard are objectively encouraged.	1	2	3	4	5
5) Therapist provides objective and specific feedback regarding the child's speech rules in engaging and creative ways.	1	2	3	4	5
6) Cueing is downplayed on easier sounds and words to make cueing of challenging sounds and words more salient.	1	2	3	4	5
7) Child is objectively recognized for increased independence. For example: "Wow, you're the teacher now. I didn't even help you."	1	2	3	4	5
8) Therapist attempts to spontaneously elicit a mastered target within an activity (e.g., What color do you want? Child answers, "blue" for a child who glides /l/.)	1	2	3	4	5
9) The child is producing the treatment target accurately at a high level of frequency to encourage myelination development.	1	2	3	4	5
10) At the generalization stage, child is encouraged to self-evaluate whether a speech rule was followed (e.g., thumbs up vs. thumbs down) after producing the target.	1	2	3	4	5

Strengths:

Weaknesses:

Suggestions for Improvement:

8

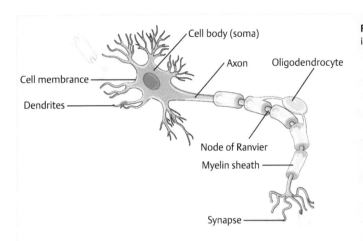

Fig. 8.1 Conduction of a nerve impulse across neurons.

accurate practice within naturally rewarding, educationally rich activities.

See Video 8.4 of Cadge, a child with ASD. Note the high dose of repetition of his treatment target that encourages myelination development.

How Does the All-Important Myelin Grow and Deteriorate?

How does *myelin* form around axons in newly learned behaviors? With repetition of a newly learned behavior, scientists believe two glial (i.e., non-neuronal) cells are primarily responsible for creating myelin sheaths. First, a glial cell known as an astrocyte monitors axons for activity. When an astrocyte detects repeated activity on an axon, it stimulates another glial cell, the oligodendrocyte, to produce myelin around that particular axon. As the myelin continues to form around the axon, automaticity occurs resulting in generalization of the accurate newly learned behavior.

Myelin matters. At young ages, children develop myelin at an incredible pace as they newly acquire information about the world around them and themselves. With age, myelin production declines. In fact, recent research suggests that cognitive decline in aging is largely linked to a deterioration of myelin, which directly results in a decrease in connections between neurons.[40,41]

8.8 Teaching Caregivers Prompting Strategies: Live and Through Video

There are two methods of teaching cues to adults who spend a lot of time with the child, such as parents, grandparents, and caregivers. First, we can directly model cues following therapy sessions. At the end of sessions, I have a "present" for the child, which is a hands-on home practice activity that was earned for following prosocial rules presented in Chapter 2. I directly model dynamic, tactile, temporal cueing with the child's treatment request in front of the parent for the child to finally receive the "present" after therapy.

Recent research indicates that a majority of preschool age children are from dual income homes in the United States.[42] Therefore, you may have limited direct interaction with either parent during both the evaluation and therapy process because of the necessity of both to work.

In this situation, sharing YouTube digital clips of therapy that illustrate effective cues can be invaluable. The benefit of emailing or texting a YouTube clip is that it does not require memory from the parent or you for storing or requiring data usage to view clip. An emerging body of research indicates that there is great potential in parents of preschoolers being effectively educated through video presentation to overcome this commonplace, realistic barrier of a lack of face time with their child's therapist due to conflicting work schedules.[43,44,45]

8

8.9 Assigning a Treatment Target

In **Appendix E**, you'll see treatment targets of increasing levels of linguistic complexity used from the beginning to the later stages of therapy. At the generalization stage, you'll notice treatment cards that contain multiple complex treatment targets in a single sentence for preschoolers who continue to distort /ɹ/ and /s/, which can be persistent error sounds into adulthood if not effectively treated early due to habituation.

Generally, we want preschoolers to practice the most linguistically rich paragraph and say all of the sounds correctly with and without cueing. Multiple targets are put in a single sentence at the generalization level when the goal is for the child to truly master production of /ɹ/ and /s/ by making varied productions of /ɹ/ and /s/ due to the surrounding phonetic context of scrape (/skɹeɪp/), spray (/spɹeɪ/), and drop (/dɹɑp/). See Video 8.5 and Video 8.6 for examples of children using the complex paragraph during the establishment phase and a complex sentence during the generalization stage.

As mentioned in Chapters 4 and 7, if the child has concurrent language and/or attentional issues, I select the treatment target in the longest and most complex utterance possible with a maximum level of prompting to ignite concurrent improvement in attention and language expression. With these populations, I accept successive approximations of speech sounds, realizing that language development is as important as speech development and a concurrent focus will require less stringency in speech accuracy. In Video 8.7, you'll note inaccurate speech with an emphasis on increasing language length, complexity, and attention to task.

Treatment targets, like those seen in **Appendix E**, are laminated on recycled file folders for durability to remain in the home throughout the course of therapy. The card is sent to the child's home in the first session with a hands-on activity provided weekly to be used in conjunction with the treatment target.

With the parent, the child can practice the target by saying the treatment target at least once a day to request a desired object or activity in the natural environment. The parent is advised to place the card in an area of high traffic, such as the refrigerator, and incorporate it into a daily routine such as dinner time.

8.10 Middle Stages of Therapy: The Child Has Learned the Treatment Target but "Don't Drop the Baby!"

At this stage, parents know that we keep the treatment target the same so that children are focused on *how* they are speaking and not *what* they are saying. The child has memorized the treatment target at this point so the therapist is silent and allows the child to be the teacher on all words that the child is able to say correctly. The therapist may explicitly state, "What? You are the teacher now!"

With sounds that remain difficult, seamlessly fade in a prompt, which could be a maximum level of prompting, a temporal level of prompting, a tactile cue, or a verbal call-out as a reminder of a speech rule to prevent misarticulation depending on the individual child's level of need.

During this stage, I remind graduate students and parents, "Don't drop the baby!" Always maintain a minimum of 80% accuracy level with prompting dynamically faded and provided based on the child's performance to prevent the habituation of incorrect motor speech patterns.

At this stage you may note a persistent phonological process or distortion that you'll want to make salient to suppress. Make a catchy slogan or song with accompanying gestures that you'll have the child mimic. Say this slogan or song both before and after the child requests as both a preventative prompt and objective feedback. In Video 8.8, note how Xander is stating his rule "slowly and smoothly" for fluent speech. Always aim for the child to say the rule and perform the accompanying gestures with as much independence as possible. Children will particularly love scaring you with their "angry dog teeth."

8.11 The Final Stage of Therapy

The child is clearly the teacher at this point. The child is saying his or her treatment target independently and accurately. The child has developed an internal locus of control, and is automatically producing more earlier developing untreated single sounds, affricates, and simpler 2-element cluster blends correctly that weren't directly targeted.

The impact of selecting a 3-element consonant cluster is that sounds will develop more quickly, but maintain a developmental order in progress.

Respecting the Path of Progress for Children with Attentional Issues

With children with attentional issues, I've found that that progress in standardized testing and generalization outside of the structured therapy environment can be slow. This can be due to a lack of attention to the task and a lack of self-monitoring. Be patient with these children. Generalization will occur. It'll just take more time.

Stay the course, making sure that *accurate* practice is occurring and naturally reinforced. Remember that with repetition of the newly learned accurate motor behavior, the myelin sheath is strengthening. This results in automaticity of accurate speech motor patterns developing. Use of highly preferred natural rewards in response to speech accuracy will additionally expedite gains, specifically for populations with attentional issues.[51]

In the past 18 years I've found that it is not uncommon for children with attentional difficulties to demonstrate minimal progress for an entire calendar year and then, without any change in the course of therapy, demonstrate extraordinary gains and improvement in standard testing scores in a short time frame. Children at the 1% percentile, indicating an extremely severe level of impairment at baseline, advance to the 50th percentile, indicating no impairment, as they finally "get it" a year later. I jokingly will refer to these moments as our speech "exorcisms." I look at the child and think to myself, *I knew you were in there the whole time.*

I share these experiences with you because I believe you will encounter children with attentional deficits who will make a slower rate of progress in the initial and medial stages of therapy but will make substantial progress later. It is important that you're able to explain this growth trajectory to parents so they don't lose faith in the therapeutic process. Know that you are right in staying the course. Accurate practice is resulting in myelination that can't be visibly seen by the human eye.

Table 8.2 Implicational universals for phonological development: a stair step progression

3-Elements Clusters (require presence of 2-element clusters)
2-Element Clusters (require presence of affricates)
Affricates (require presence of fricatives)
Fricatives (require presence of stops)
Stops (aspirated voiceless stops generally require voiced stops)

As stated in previous chapters, earlier developing sounds generally develop before later. In our research I've found the following: post-vocalic /l/ and /ɹ / will develop before prevocalic /l/ and /ɹ /, and singleton sounds will develop before affricates. Affricates will develop before 2-element clusters, simpler 2-element clusters (e.g., stop blends) will develop before more complex ones (e.g., fricative blends), and lastly, 2-element clusters will develop before 3-element clusters.

In the same manner, earlier developing phonological processes will be suppressed before later ones. Over a 6-year period of researching how complex consonant clusters as treatment targets impact untreated sounds, we observed this developmental trajectory to occur consistently.[8,9,10,11,12]

Refer ▶ Table 8.2, *Implicational Universals for Phonological Development: A Stair Step Progression*. This universal progression was referenced earlier in the book in selecting complex treatment targets. Here you will reference this stair step progress by simply explaining to parents how generalization is occurring across untreated sounds.

In summary, working on 3-element consonant clusters does not change the universals of sound development. Simpler sounds and phonological processes will develop later regardless of the treatment target selected.[46,47] However, in our current research in working with preschoolers with ASD, we have observed exceptions to this developmental progression of sounds. We attribute this nondevelopmental trajectory, of both speech development and response to therapy, to neurological differences inherent to this population.[48,49,50] See Chapter 7 for further detail.

In the final stages of therapy, the child's behavior clearly reflects an internal locus of control. It is as if a light switch goes on in the head. A sort of extraterrestrial look often emerges as the child independently applies speech rules to novel words and phrases within conversation. At this level the child independently produces targets accurately across people and settings.

It is always a thrill when a child who previously frontally lisps /s/, fronts /k/, and glides /l/, out of the blue, cocks the head to the side and spontaneously addresses me by my name, "Miss Kelly," correctly and with mindful deliberation. At that point, the child realizes that he or she truly is the teacher. That is what a well-developed internal locus of control looks like in preschoolers, which is the ultimate goal of therapy.

8.12 Exiting Therapy

See Video 8.9 for an example of children taking on the teacher's role. In holistically treating the child, always proactively emphasize the prosocial behaviors of being attentive, working hard, following directions, answering questions, and demonstrating self-regulation by keeping hands to self. Emphasize these behaviors from the beginning of therapy to dismissal.

Lastly, they are "talking like a teacher" as they have truly taken on the role as teacher. See Kelly's Corner Video 8.10 in which I discuss the importance of frequency in practice to ensure both maintenance and generalization after exiting therapy. I encourage the child to say the paragraph as part of the daily routine to encourage both maintenance and generalization after exiting therapy.

8.13 Chapter Summary

This chapter underscores the value of frequency in practice for a newly established behavior to generalize. The latest neurological research clearly supports the notion that *neurons that fire together, wire together*. Repetition results in both correct and incorrect complex speech behaviors being habituated. Because of this, diligence is required in adhering to a minimum 80% accuracy rule.

How to ensure that correct repetition occurs with our limited therapy time? The answer lies in connecting treatment targets to routines that reliably occur on a daily basis in the child's natural environment. First, consult caregivers to select daily routines for treatment target practice. Second, provide a visual in that location to serve as a reminder. (See **Appendix E** for ready-for-use visuals.)

Lastly, review whether or not the child is practicing treatment targets on a daily basis. If not, try a different routine or changing the treatment target. Perhaps a less hectic time of day, or pairing the treatment target with a more rewarding experience would increase the likelihood of practice.

Also, creating an easier treatment target could encourage everyday practice to take place.

References

[1] Jerome AC, Fujiki M, Brinton B, James SL. Self-esteem in children with specific language impairment. J Speech Lang Hear Res. 2002; 45(4):700–714

[2] Vygotsky LS. Mind in Society: The Development of Higher Psychological Processes. Cambridge, MA: Harvard University Press; 1978

[3] Kiran S, Thompson CK. Neuroplasticity of language networks in aphasia: advances, updates, and future challenges. Front Neurol. 2019; 10:295

[4] Dweck CS. Mindset: How You Can Fulfil Your Potential. London: Robinson; 2012

[5] McLeod S, Masso S. Screening children's speech: the impact of imitated elicitation and word position. Lang Speech Hear Serv Sch. 2019; 50(1):71–82

[6] Shriberg LD, Austin D, Lewis BA, McSweeny JL, Wilson DL. The percentage of consonants correct (PCC) metric: extensions and reliability data. J Speech Lang Hear Res. 1997; 40(4):708–722

[7] Vess K, Szczembara R. Testing speech of preschoolers with autism spectrum disorder: impact of imitated versus spontaneous productions. Poster presented at: Annual American Speech, Language and Hearing Association Convention; November, 2019; Ft. Lauderdale, FL

[8] Vess K, Burgess R, Corless E, Discenna T. Selecting complex consonant clusters: are certain sound combinations more efficacious than others? Poster presented at: Annual American Speech, Language and Hearing Association Convention; November, 2016; Philadelphia, PA

[9] Vess K, Abou-Arabi M. Stimulability in production of consonant clusters: comparing preschoolers with ASD, language impairment, articulation impairment. Poster presented at: Annual American Speech, Language and Hearing Association Convention; November, 2018; Boston, MA

[10] Vess K, Hansen L, Smith MM, Ridella M, Steinberg E. Evidence-based strategies to effectively treat preschoolers with speech sound disorders. Poster presented at: Annual American Speech, Language and Hearing Association Convention; November, 2015; Denver, CO

[11] Vess K, Coppiellie J, Ingraham B, Reidt M. Targeting /ɹ/ consonant clusters: does generalization occur across phonetic contexts? Poster presented at: Annual American Speech, Language and Hearing Association Convention; November, 2017; San Diego, CA

[12] Vess K, Liovas M, Mocny A, Vuletic D. Applying the complexity approach to effectively treat severe speech impairment in preschoolers with ASD. Poster presented at: Annual American Speech, Language and Hearing Association Convention; November, 2018; Boston, MA

[13] Brumbaugh KM, Smit AB. Treating children ages 3–6 who have speech sound disorder: a survey. Lang Speech Hear Serv Sch. 2013; 44(3):306–319

[14] Sugden E, Baker E, Munro N, Williams AL, Trivette CM. Service delivery and intervention intensity for phonology-based speech sound disorders. Int J Lang Commun Disord. 2018; 53(4):718–734

[15] Jacoby GP, Lee L, Kummer AW, Levin L, Creaghead NA. The number of individual treatment units necessary to facilitate functional communication improvements in the speech and language of young children. Am J Speech Lang Pathol. 2002; 11(4):370–380

8

[16] Cummings A, Hallgrimson J, Robinson S. Speech intervention outcomes associated with word lexicality and intervention intensity. Lang Speech Hear Serv Sch. 2019;50(1):83–98

[17] Law J, Garrett Z, Nye C. The efficacy of treatment for children with developmental speech and language delay/disorder: a meta-analysis. J Speech Lang Hear Res. 2004; 47(4):924–943

[18] Kamhi AG. Treatment decisions for children with speech-sound disorders. Lang Speech Hear Serv Sch. 2006; 37 (4):271–279

[19] Justice LM, Kaderavek JN, Fan X, Sofka A, Hunt A. Accelerating preschoolers' early literacy development through classroom-based teacher-child storybook reading and explicit print referencing. Lang Speech Hear Serv Sch. 2009; 40(1):67–85

[20] Griffin TM, Hemphill L, Camp L, Wolf DP. Oral discourse in the preschool years and later literacy skills. First Lang. 2004; 24(2):123–147

[21] Allen MM. Intervention efficacy and intensity for children with speech sound disorder. J Speech Lang Hear Res. 2013; 56(3):865–877

[22] Gamba J, Goyos C, Petursdottir AI. The functional independence of mands and tacts: has it been demonstrated empirically? Anal Verbal Behav. 2014; 31(1):10–38

[23] Iuzzini J, Forrest K. Evaluation of a combined treatment approach for childhood apraxia of speech. Clin Linguist Phon. 2010; 24(4–5):335–345

[24] Gierut JA, Morrisette ML, Ziemer SM. Nonwords and generalization in children with phonological disorders. Am J Speech Lang Pathol. 2010; 19(2):167–177

[25] van der Merwe A, Steyn M. Model-driven treatment of childhood apraxia of speech: positive effects of the speech motor learning approach. Am J Speech Lang Pathol. 2018; 27(1):37–51

[26] Storkel HL. Implementing evidence-based practice: selecting treatment words to boost phonological learning. Lang Speech Hear Serv Sch. 2018; 49(3):482–496

[27] McLeod S, Doorn JV, Reed VA. Normal acquisition of consonant clusters. Am J Speech Lang Pathol. 2001; 10(2):99–110

[28] Langer EJ. The Power of Mindful Learning. Boston, MA: The Perseus Book Group; 2016

[29] Samuelsson IP, Carlsson MA. The playing learning child: towards a pedagogy of early childhood. Scand J Educ Res. 2008; 52(6):623–641

[30] Hirsh-Pasek K, Golinkoff RM, Eyer DE. Einstein Never Used Flash Cards: How Our Children Really Learn—and Why They Need to Play More and Memorize Less. New York: MJF Books; 2008

[31] Sullivan KJ, Kantak SS, Burtner PA. Motor learning in children: feedback effects on skill acquisition. Phys Ther. 2008; 88(6):720–732

[32] Fullerton EK, Conroy MA, Correa VI. Early childhood teachers' use of specific praise statements with young children at risk for behavioral disorders. Behav Disord. 2009; 34(3):118–135

[33] Maas E, Robin DA, Austermann Hula SN, et al. Principles of motor learning in treatment of motor speech disorders. Am J Speech Lang Pathol. 2008; 17(3):277–298

[34] Taps J. An innovative educational approach for addressing articulation differences. Perspectives on School-Based Issues. 2006; 7(4):7–11

[35] Edeal DM, Gildersleeve-Neumann CE. The importance of production frequency in therapy for childhood apraxia of speech. Am J Speech Lang Pathol. 2011; 20(2):95–110

[36] Hansen CC, Zambo D. Loving and learning with Wemberly and David: fostering emotional development in early childhood education. Early Child Educ J. 2007; 34(4):273–278

[37] Bryck RL, Fisher PA. Training the brain: practical applications of neural plasticity from the intersection of cognitive neuroscience, developmental psychology, and prevention science. Am Psychol. 2012; 67(2):87–100

[38] Van Horne AJO, Fey M, Curran M. Do the hard things first: a randomized controlled trial testing the effects of exemplar selection on generalization following therapy for grammatical morphology. J Speech Lang Hear Res. 2017; 60(9):2569–2588

[39] Coon D. Introduction to Psychology: Exploration and Application. St. Paul, MN: West Publishing Company; 1989

[40] Peters A, Rosene DL. In aging, is it gray or white? J Comp Neurol. 2003; 462(2):139–143

[41] Peters A. The effects of normal aging on myelinated nerve fibers in monkey central nervous system. Front Neuroanat. 2009; 3:11

[42] Bureau of Labor Statistics. U.S. Department of Labor, The Economics Daily, Employment in families with children in 2016. On the Internet at https://www.bls.gov/opub/ted/2017/employment-in-families-with-children-in-2016.htm/. Accessed May 17, 2019

[43] Karsenti T, Collin S. The impact of online teaching videos on Canadian pre-service teachers. Campus-Wide Inf Syst. 2011; 28(3):195–204

[44] Roberts MY, Kaiser AP. The effectiveness of parent-implemented language interventions: a meta-analysis. Am J Speech Lang Pathol. 2011; 20(3):180–199

[45] Breitenstein SM, Gross D, Christophersen R. Digital delivery methods of parenting training interventions: a systematic review. Worldviews Evid Based Nurs. 2014; 11(3):168–176

[46] Greenberg JH, Ferguson CA, Moravcsik EA. Universals of Human Language. Stanford, CA: Stanford University Press; 1978

[47] Gierut JA, Champion AH. Syllable onsets II: three-element clusters in phonological treatment. J Speech Lang Hear Res. 2001; 44(4):886–904

[48] Zhang J, Meng Y, He J, et al. McGurk effect by individuals with autism spectrum disorder and typically developing controls: a systematic review and meta-analysis. J Autism Dev Disord. 2019; 49(1):34–43

[49] Derrick D, Bicevskis K, Gick B. Visual-tactile speech perception and the autism quotient. Front Commun. 2019; 3

[50] Peeva MG, Tourville JA, Agam Y, Holland B, Manoach DS, Guenther FH. White matter impairment in the speech network of individuals with autism spectrum disorder. Neuroimage Clin. 2013; 3:234–241

[51] Gopin CB, Berwid O, Marks DJ, Mlodnicka A, Halperin JM. ADHD preschoolers with and without ODD: do they act differently depending on degree of task engagement/reward? J Atten Disord. 2013; 17(7):608–619

8

9 Promoting Early Literacy Skills When Treating Speech Sound Disorders

A moving child is a learning child.
—Gill Connell and Cheryl McCarthy

Parents often ask if a preschooler with a speech sound disorder is at greater risk for future literacy difficulties. The answer is not simple. For instance, you cannot be sure of who among your preschool students will still present with speech impairment at elementary age, which indicates an increased risk of literacy difficulties.[1] There can also be intervening factors. It is possible the child has an undiagnosed history of dyslexia in the family, which would significantly elevate risk for literacy difficulties.[2]

Recent research indicates that preschoolers with a sole diagnosis of speech sound disorders are at only a *slightly* increased risk for poorer phonemic awareness and spelling at 5.5 years and poorer word reading at 8 years.[2] This does not mean that a speech-language pathologist should be complacent.

9.1 Red Flags: What Are Concurrent Risk Factors for Future Literacy Deficits?

Look for high-risk factors that include a family history of reading disorders,[2] a diagnosis of concurrent language impairment,[2,3] or a diagnosis of childhood apraxia of speech.[4] Additional indicators are poor performances in any of the following areas: receptive vocabulary,[5] phonological awareness skills,[6] print/alphabet knowledge,[7] phonological memory,[8] phonological processing,[9] and narrative skills.[10] Furthermore, the presence of multiple risk factors predicts increased risk for reading disorders, especially concomitant language impairment or a family history of dyslexia.[2]

9.2 Red Flags: Can Speech Errors Indicate Later Literacy Deficits?

Interestingly, in predicting the presence of later literacy difficulties, recent research indicates that the severity of the speech sound disorder has very little, if any, effect on development of literacy skills. Study also indicates that although atypical speech errors predict poorer word reading at age 5.5 years, these differences are remedied by 8 years.[2] Nevertheless, there is a body of evidence indicating that atypical errors may have some prognostic value in indicating literacy deficits.[5,11,12,13]

9.3 Atypical Errors

For speech-language pathologists, the ability to readily identify typical versus atypical error patterns is of crucial importance in both evaluating and treating speech sound disorders efficiently. Considering that there is evidence to suggest that atypical error patterns at preschool age may indicate increased risk for literacy deficits in elementary school, there is clinical value in being able to differentiate between typical and atypical error patterns.[5,11,12,13]

Please refer to Preston's extensive list of atypical error patterns in Chapter 7, in which research found that greater than 10% of errors being atypical at the preschool level indicated increased risk for literacy deficits at elementary age.[12] In the absence of risk factors aforementioned, a large number of atypical errors may indicate a need for further assessment of phonological awareness skills. A widely used, norm-referenced assessment in research and practice for children aged 4 to 24 years is the *Comprehensive Test of Phonological Processing—Second Edition*.[14]

9.4 Polysyllabic Words and Omissions

Recent research indicates that children who misproduce three to four syllable polysyllabic words are at increased risk for literacy deficits. Specifically, polysyllabic errors that indicated the greatest risk for literacy delays were omissions, alterations in phonotactics (syllables migrating to another place in a word), or alterations in timing (inappropriately placed pauses within words).[8]

Additionally, research indicates omitting sounds to be a red flag in that children with frequent sound omissions were more likely to present with concurrent language impairment.[15] This presence of language impairment, by default, indicates

Table 9.1 Putting research into practice: Identifying red flag speech errors that indicate further testing of phonological awareness (refer to Chapter 7)

Stimulus Item → Child's Production	Identify the type of Error: Distortion, Typical Phonological Process, Assimilation, Atypical Error, Polysyllabic Word Error, Omission	Error indicates risk for later literacy difficulties (Y/N)? Why or why not?
Mouse: /maʊs/ → /maʊt/		
Lemonade: /ˈlɛməˈneɪd/ → /ˈwɛməˈneɪd/		
Watermelon: /ˈwɔtərˌmɛlən/ → /ˈtərˌmɛwən/		
Door: /dɔr/ → /gɔr/		
Spoon: /spun/ → /sun/		
Gate: /geɪt/ → /geɪ/		
Lake: /leɪk/ → /leɪt/		
Bakery: /ˈbeɪkəri/ → /ˈkərbi/		
Van: /væn/ → /fæn/		
Swing: /swɪŋ/ → /fwɪŋ/		
Lemonade: /ˈlɛməˈneɪd/ → /ˈnɛməˈneɪd/		
Grapes: /greɪps/ → /gweɪps/		

Is It Important to Include Literacy Activities for Children with Distortion Errors?

Recent research indicates that if /s/ and /r/ sounds are mispronounced, they are likely to be misperceived.[16] These are highly frequent sounds that play a pivotal role in grammatical morpheme development. Despite indications that distortions at preschool age are less indicative of linguistic deficits than omissions,[13] distortions that persist into elementary age can negatively impact literacy skills.[1]

For these reasons, be safe and not sorry. Embed literacy rich activities and literacy intervention strategies across activities at preschool age. Research indicates that phonological awareness skills can be effectively targeted when treating speech sound disorders.[17,18] It is a wise investment as plasticity in the brain is greater at a younger age, resulting in increased neuronal change in preventing later deficits.[19,20]

increased risk for later reading difficulties. Taken together, these two studies support the assertion that omissions indicate a compromised linguistic system in which phonological representations are entirely absent. Whereas distortions indicate a stronger linguistic system due to phonological representations being at least partially present.[15]

Please see ▶ Table 9.1 for practice identifying atypical errors, omissions, and polysyllabic errors that indicate further testing of phonological awareness skills.

9.5 Early Literacy Intervention

In this chapter, you'll learn how to strengthen early literacy skills by incorporating speech perception using the child's treatment target. You'll also learn strategies to improve phonological awareness skills, phonemic awareness skills, print knowledge, and narrative skills through explicit instruction embedded within speech sound disorder therapy.[21]

Keep in mind that density of accurate production of speech targets must not be compromised when incorporating literacy strategies in therapy.[22] The child's limited time in therapy should be an active learning process in which preschoolers are both heard and seen through verbal and nonverbal participation.

If speech improvement occurred as a natural result of a child listening to a correct model, the child would not be in therapy. The child is exposed to numerous correct speech models throughout the day, across people, and across settings, with phonological processes and distortions further habituating with each incorrect production. For this, emphasize frequency of correct productions to develop new motor patterns.

When providing literacy intervention, refer to *Chapters 6: Dynamically Prompting and Errorlessly Fading Multimodal Cues* for methodology. The process for literacy intervention is very much the same as treating speech sound disorders. Our interest is not in what the child is able to do, but rather in what the child is able to do with a maximum level of support or the child's *zone of proximal development*.[23] Working at the child's highest level will result in optimal gains to occur at a time when brain plasticity is at a greater level. In therapy, we are not testing the child but rather teaching so scaffolds will gradually be removed while continually ensuring a minimal 80% accuracy rate in the practice of newly learned behavior.

Therefore, we will be applying principles of dynamic, tactile, temporal, visual, and verbal cueing. This will allow us to insert and remove scaffolds and to provide cues as necessary to ensure a minimal 80% success level. Importantly, these cues incorporate multiple modalities to make newly introduced abstract literacy concepts salient for preschoolers.

In the initial stages, use the *same* language repetitively so the child can focus on the literacy skill and not the semantics of learning a diverse vocabulary. Additionally, using academic literacy vocabulary repetitively allows the child to assume an internal locus of control in being able to independently state the concepts and self-teach.

Early childhood literacy expert Professor Anne van Kleeck defines academic talk as "the broad pattern of language use that is employed when engaged in teaching and learning, allowing teachers and other adults to transmit, and children to develop and display ideas and knowledge." Professor van Kleeck advocates for embedding academic talk into intervention at the preschool level, particularly in treating children with concurrent language impairment. She also recommends academic talk when working with children from culturally and linguistically diverse populations to prepare them for vocabulary commonly used within the elementary level curriculum.[24]

In Chapter 5, we discussed academic discourse and the use of simple definitions, or "callouts," with Tier 2 vocabulary. Tier 2 vocabulary is academic, inferential, critical thinking vocabulary that can be used across subject matters. In this chapter, we will go into even greater depth with increasing phonological awareness skills, narrative development, and story grammar knowledge using Tier 2 vocabulary.

Finally, in the last stages, the child assumes an internal locus of control in taking responsibility for correct production of literacy skills. With an array of multimodal cues provided in the initial stages of therapy, the child will be able to draw upon a greater diversity of cues when needed as independence is established.

9.6 Speech Perception

First, we will briefly look at assessing the child's *speech perception*, which can be defined simply as how sounds are heard, interpreted, and understood. Importantly, recent research indicates speech perception is less predictive of later literacy deficits than originally postulated. Phonemic awareness at preschool age has a much higher predictive value for school age reading performance than speech perception.[1]

ASHA currently recommends assessment of speech perception as a component of the speech evaluation.[25] See Video 9.1 and refer ▶ Table 9.2. In this digital clip, you'll see Ms. Becca reference ▶ Fig. 9.1, Sounds Right versus Sounds Wrong, as Santiago assesses a puppet's production of sounds. He will also self-assess his own productions in assuming the role of teacher.

Santiago gets to play the role of teacher and tell Ms. Becca if the target words are said "right" or "wrong" by pointing to a smiley face or a sad face. Approximately half of the time, we will say the child's treatment target word incorrectly and half the time correctly in a randomly mixed sequence format.

We prefer to present words in a randomly mixed sequence (right-wrong-right-right-wrong-wrong) from the initial stages to ensure flexibility in the child's response. For optimal learning to occur we also select an 80% minimal accuracy level, in which we may add vocal and facial cues or exaggerate the

9

Table 9.2 Evaluating literacy activities

Video Number:_____					
Please indicate your level of agreement to the following statements in reference to the literacy digital clip presented.	Strongly Disagree	Disagree	Neutral	Agree	Strongly Agree
1) Literacy activity was fun, engaging, and developmentally appropriate	1	2	3	4	5
2) Used same language repeatedly to teach new concepts (e.g., rhyming defined consistently as when the "end of the words sound the same").	1	2	3	4	5
3) Used same multi-modal prompting repeatedly to teach new concepts (e.g., putting fists together and pulling apart for elision of compound words).	1	2	3	4	5
4) Incorporated 3-dimensional materials (over 2-dimensional) whenever possible.	1	2	3	4	5
5) Materials were strategically placed so that the child could focus attention on newly presented concepts and producing treatment targets accurately.	1	2	3	4	5
6) The child requested using the treatment target numerous times.	1	2	3	4	5
7) Cueing was dynamically provided though fading and provision of prompts to promote independence, while ensuring a minimal 80% success rate.	1	2	3	4	5
8) Literacy cues were multi-modal, incorporating movement in space, verbal, visual and tactile feedback as necessary.	1	2	3	4	5
9) Child both nonverbally and verbally participated in learning the literacy concept while practicing treatment targets.	1	2	3	4	5
10) Incorporated Tier 2 literacy vocabulary meaningfully, as applicable, to encourage academic discourse development.	1	2	3	4	5
11) "Call outs" or simple definitions were provided to define Tier 2 academic vocabulary.	1	2	3	4	5
12) Explicit references were made to print to label, answer questions, solve problems, read, report results.	1	2	3	4	5
13) Pacing was appropriate to the individual child to maintain attention, while challenging the child to process and formulate ideas.	1	2	3	4	5
14) Therapist conveyed joy and enthusiasm, treating phonological awareness activities of playing with sounds/words like playing with toys.	1	2	3	4	5

9

Table 9.2 (*Continued*) Evaluating literacy activities

Video Number:_____					
Please indicate your level of agreement to the following statements in reference to the literacy digital clip presented.	Strongly Disagree	Disagree	Neutral	Agree	Strongly Agree
15) Therapist was able to break an activity into multiple steps to have the child narrate how to complete a procedure to request access to an activity in response to *how* questions, as applicable.	1	2	3	4	5

Strengths:

Weaknesses:

Suggestions for Improvement:

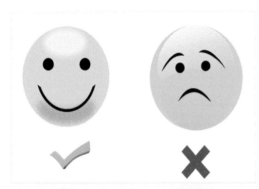

Fig. 9.1 "Sounds Right" versus "Sounds Wrong": Smiley and sad face for preschooler to indicate speech perception.

error as necessary based on the child's performance. Refer ▶ Table 9.2 when viewing literacy intervention therapy sessions presented throughout this chapter.

9.7 Improving Phonological Awareness and Phonemic Awareness Skills

Phonological awareness is a broad, umbrella term that involves identifying and manipulating sounds, syllables, and words in oral language. Phonemic awareness specifically refers to the ability to identify and manipulate individual sounds.

Pre-literacy skills that I have researched and effectively used with neurotypical preschoolers required verbal participation with concurrent use of gestures and movement. With each intervention,

preschoolers consistently demonstrated an approximate 25% group average improvement on the *Phonological Awareness Test-Second Edition*[26] after attending only six 40-minute group sessions in phonological awareness skills.[27]

Phonological skills that we taught multimodally using movement included print referencing (tapping words as spoken), counting syllables in words (with clapping syllables as spoken), and identifying phonemes in the beginning and end of words (using the ASL "I love you sign" with their hands pretending to be a swinging "monkey"). The head (thumb) represents the beginning sound and the tail (pinky) represents the ending sound. In all areas of phonological awareness intervention, the learner's nonverbal movements are as important as the verbal in ensuring that active learning is occurring and the learning could occur more memorably and efficiently.[28]

9.8 Identifying Phoneme across Positions in a Word

In the next digital clip (Video 9.2), you'll see another phonemic awareness activity in which Xavier identifies the /g/ sound as being in the beginning or end of the word. He is being introduced to the swinging monkey gesture prompt for the first time.

Alicia opted to not include "please" at the end of the phrase because Xavier glided the /l/ with a maximum level of prompting and she did not want to reinforce gliding. (In Video 9.2, we did not use real three-dimensional objects, which are generally preferred, because they would have been too heavy for the magnetic fishing pole.)

How to be Ineffective by Not Incorporating Movement in Literacy Instruction

In one study, our neurotypical preschoolers were asked to identify the first and last sounds when hearing the spoken word (e.g., "Pot: What is the beginning sound in the word? What is the ending sound in the word?"). Baseline data and postintervention data on the *Phonological Awareness Test-Second Edition* were compared.

When not using movement, the neurotypical preschoolers did *not* attain the expected approximate 25% group average improvement that I had grown accustomed to each year. In fact, they even performed 13% worse on identifying initial consonants and only 10% better in identifying final consonants.[29] The difference in this ineffectual intervention could have been that the preschoolers did not use body movement in learning the literacy skills as they had in the other studies. Instead of having the children use body movement to discover the beginning and end sounds, I had them sort objects in "beginning" or "ending" boxes based on the targeted sound's position in a word.

My hypothesis was that the exclusion of the child using movement contributed to the lackluster gains. The following year, I replicated the study *exactly* by using all of the same materials and activities. I also used an age matched and baseline performance matched neurotypical intervention comparison group. I controlled all intervention variables except the addition of movement. This was a physical hand cue in which children made the "I love you" sign to indicate their thumb ("the monkey's head") to be the beginning sound and their pinky ("the monkey's tail") to be the ending sound (see ▶ Fig. 9.2 and ▶ Fig. 9.3).

The hand cue was modelled for the preschoolers, giving them the option to spontaneously use the cue themselves. After six sessions, the neurotypical preschool age intervention group demonstrated a 20% average improvement in identifying beginning sounds and a 24% improvement in identifying ending sounds. This is only one small study, but it indicates movement to be an active ingredient in effective literacy intervention with preschoolers.[28]

Putting Research into Practice: Incorporating Movement into Phonemic Awareness Instruction

Develop a beginning and ending phoneme activity using three-dimensional materials. You are welcome to use ▶ Fig. 9.2. My original thought was to use a dog icon; however, I had the wonderful fortune to meet Professor Thora Másdóttir from the University of Iceland at the ASHA 2017 annual convention in Los Angeles. As I presented my highly *ineffective* nonmovement, sorting phoneme awareness intervention poster, Dr. Másdóttir recommended I use a monkey gesture for my next study. Unlike a dog, it swings and always has a long tail.

I share this story because we can always improve upon our intervention strategies and should continually approach intervention with a growth mindset.[30] I'm not a good therapist or clinical educator if I myself am not evolving each year in learning from others.

Adopt a growth mindset in looking to improve upon the evidence-based strategies presented throughout this book. You bring a lot to the table. I know that the generosity of parents and graduate students in altruistically sharing their children and talents were not done in vain. This book is a give and take. It is parents, graduate students, and myself putting it all on the table so you can tinker with rich material by applying your unique gifts to further evolve practice.

Beginning versus Ending Sound Motor Cue

What is a motor cue that you could use? You could use the thumb and pinky monkey gesture or develop your own. Think about how you can saliently and meaningfully teach abstract phonological awareness skills through movement. When movement cues are authentically meaningful to you, you will communicate them more strongly verbally and nonverbally. As a result, children will experience cues in a meaningful manner, thereby learning them more quickly and deeply.

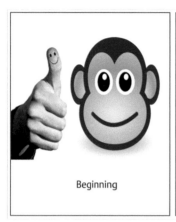
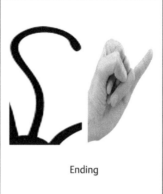

Fig. 9.2 Beginning sound (monkey's head) and ending sound (monkey's tail): Sorting icons based on position in words.

Beginning

Ending

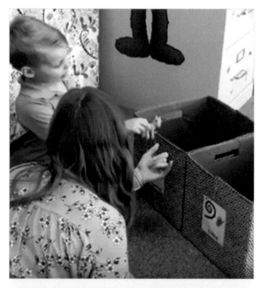

Fig. 9.3 The swinging monkey's head (thumb) versus the monkey's tail (pinky) as a motor cue for beginning versus ending sounds.

Also, see Video 9.3 in which Elowen uses the monkey gesture cue with Ms. Holly.

9.9 Rhyming

Rhyming at the preschool level is simply when two or more endings of words sound alike. Identifying rhyming words has been seen as a crucial underlying foundational skill predictive of other areas of phonological awareness development.[31]

In Video 9.4 you'll note that Becca uses a maximum level of support strategy in helping rhyme identification through exaggerating the voice, making exaggerated facial expressions, and providing phonemic support to help Santiago's ability to generate the rhyming number.

9.10 Blending

Blending is a phonemic awareness skill in which a child is presented with individual phonemic sound components that make up a word, with the child combining the sounds to form the word. It has been identified as both predictive of later literacy skills and as a challenging skill for preschoolers who have speech sound disorders.[5,8]

In Video 9.5 you'll note Becca dynamically cueing Santiago by shortening the duration between phonemes to prompt success with a maximum level of prompting. Later, she'll increase the amount of time between phonemes. You'll also see her use genie arms in unison with Santiago and echoed speech to ensure his active engagement in blending the phonemes together. Note how similar this process is to maximum prompting in treating speech sound disorders to ensure accuracy.

Also see Video 9.6 in which Emory uses the genie arm technique to blend sounds in words.

9.11 Elision

Elision is when children are presented a word and asked to delete parts (i.e., words, syllables, sounds) of words and identify the remaining part. It can occur when deleting a word within a compound word (e.g., cupcake – cup = cake), deleting a syllable from a word (e.g., baby – ba = by), or deleting a phoneme from a word (e.g., fish – f = ish). At the preschool level, difficulty with elision is highly predictive of literacy deficits at school age.[8]

9

In Video 9.7, Ms. Becca is implementing a most-to-least prompting hierarchy in which she provides multimodal cueing using her fists, while slowly fading the visual support, to errorlessly teach this very challenging skill at the preschool level for the very first time.

See also Video 9.8 in which Ms. Torey effectively teaches Cooper elision for the very first time using the fist multimodal cueing strategy.

9.12 Syllable Counting

Syllable Counting is a component of phonological awareness in which students are able to understand that words are divided into syllables. When counting syllables, preschoolers indicate that they understand that sounds can be combined into parts and that words can be broken up into parts.

In Video 9.9, notice how Ms. Mary Lyn, teaching this new skill to Anthony, provides a maximal level of prompting to ensure accuracy using multimodal clapping cues.

See also Video 9.10 in which Ms. Katelyn counts syllables in the literacy rich activity with Deenie. Regardless of limitations, it is important that all children engage in educationally rich, developmentally age-appropriate activities. Deenie experiences the syllables with each spin of the boat.

> ### Putting Research into Practice: Counting Syllables with Hand Claps
>
> Create an engaging activity that involves clapping hands to count syllables. Also, create a graphing component in which the preschooler can record the number of syllables in each word.

9.13 Alphabet Print Knowledge and Letter Sound Awareness

Print knowledge refers to labelling letters, identifying letter sounds, and indicating knowledge of print concepts, such as symbols, signs, numbers, letters, words, sentences, author, and title. Research indicates that pairing letter name with sound identification does not detract from phonological awareness instruction. Pairing, therefore, would be a recommended practice to increase meaningful exposure to print.[32]

Additionally, explicit print referencing is indicated as an evidence-based practice in impacting children's literacy development.[33] This explicit reference to print can be integrated into any activity. Common examples are "going for a word hunt" in searching for environmental print and "finding the title and author on the cover."

In Video 9.11 Becca is improving alphabet/print knowledge in the context of making alphabet soup.

See Video 9.12 for an example of print referencing tickets to locate country's flags from a challenging oculomotor skills. In video 9.13, you'll see Jillian not only have to have print knowledge but also apply that knowledge solving problems in stamping locations visited on her passport.

9.14 Narrative Development

In 2004, Law and colleagues' meta-analysis indicated a dismal lack of evidence for speech-language therapy significantly impacting comprehension for children with receptive language difficulties.[34] However, recent storytelling and retelling interventions are indicating promising gains in language comprehension for diverse populations of preschoolers.[35,36,37]

Storytelling and retelling are complex processes that challenge the child in terms of word retrieval, academic discourse, use of conjunctions, and organization of newly presented information. There is also a challenge for the child's working memory to use sentences of increased length and complexity. Research also suggests engaging in morphology and syntax at an optimal level will have cascading effects on earlier developing grammatical and syntactical structures.[38,39]

In Video 9.14 and Video 9.15, you'll see a most-to-least prompting hierarchy to increase expressive language for children with limited verbal output. Both Madison and Mikey, at age 4 years, began the five-session summer program largely speaking in two to three word utterances. We wanted both of them to develop complex sentences using a most-to-least prompting hierarchy similar to the hierarchy implemented in speech sound disorder therapy. For both children, the treatment target was "We have toys so we can play." With increased independence, each child is independently able to produce the complex sentences and responses become more generative and diverse. In the first clip, you'll see Madison receiving a moderate level of verbal and gestural cueing during her third day of therapy.

9

In the next clip, the therapist has faded verbal cueing, yet continues to provide gestural cueing for Mikey.

Apply the hierarchy presented in *Chapter 6* to language intervention in a most-to-least support methodology. The final step will be for both Madison and Mikey to produce complex sentences independently and spontaneously as they assume an internal locus of control in which they are their own teachers.

9.15 Increasing Language Length and Complexity

In Video 9.16, you'll see a child learn the structure of explaining *how* to complete a sequence using conjunctions *first, then,* and *lastly.* Building automaticity of this sequence will empower the child to convey simple narratives in an organized manner more easily, thereby freeing up capacity for the child to focus on retrieval and execution of ideas.

The prompting strategy is consistent with the prompting strategy used in speech sound disorder therapy. A most-to-least prompting hierarchy dynamically fades support as the child demonstrates increased independence and dynamically provides support when assistance is needed. This empowers the child to produce language at the most complex level possible, resulting in greater change due to impact on earlier structures through a cascading effect.

With this errorless learning approach, prompt as needed, generally within 3 to 5 seconds. However, there will be much variation in wait time prior to prompting. In some children with attentional deficits, prompts will have to be provided almost instantly to maintain attention. In other children, who have maintained attention, allow them to struggle independently with word retrieval and increasing utterance length and complexity.

You'll sense neurological connections being made during these effortful pauses. The child's visible demonstration of pride is immeasurable when the child steps out of the comfort zone in independently producing a higher level complex utterance. This growth of achieving what was previously incapable develops self-confidence, self-efficacy, and grit. Always respond with objective feedback in nurturing the child's *growth mindset* that highlights effort instead of a *fixed mindset* that praises ability.[30]

Putting Research into Practice: Having Children Mand by Describing a Process with Complex Sentences

In reading, there are often causal relations that are expressed through conjunctions in complex sentences. Develop an engaging multistep activity that will have the child say a complex cluster treatment target in a complex linguistic context of responding to a *how* question.

Adult: How do we paint?

Child: First we *spr*ead the brush into the paint. *Then,* we *spr*ead the paint around. *Lastly,* we *spr*ead the paint on the paper *because* that's how we paint.

9.16 Learning Elements of the Story

Narrative development is not only a crucial method to dramatically increase utterance length and complexity and knowledge of story grammar, but also perhaps more importantly an emotional protective factor. For preschoolers, the ability to narrate their concerns regarding social and academic challenges can contribute to the child's overall well-being at present and later on into school age.[40]

In improving narrative skills, I was inspired by the commercially available narrative intervention program *Story Champs: A Multi-Tiered Language Intervention Program.*[41] This intervention is empirically supported, demonstrating significant gains in language skills, narrative skills, and knowledge of story grammar in diverse groups of preschoolers.[36,37,42,43] Having effectively used all of the *Story Champ* stories with my caseload, I found myself running out of stories to tell and retell.

I therefore created my own stories using basic elements of the story with engaging gestures and visual icons. Elisa DeLuca, a Wayne State University speech-language pathology graduate student, assisted me. Elisa was also working as a ballet instructor and choreographer and I teach yoga. Hence, we thoroughly enjoyed the process of creating engaging and meaningful gestures that most clearly spoke to us and our preschoolers. Whether

9

Putting Research into Practice: Creating Stories Using Elements of the Story

Create a story with each story card representing an element of a story, using the sequential format of the elements of the story: character→ setting→ problem→ emotion→ action→ consequence.

Write an engaging story for preschoolers with the following elements:

Character: Who the story is about. It can be a person, an animal, or an object personified.

Setting: Location and/or time (past, future, present) of an event

Problem: Conflict or big event (could be positive or negative)

Emotion: How the character(s) feel as a result

Action: What the character(s) does in response to the problem or event

Consequence: The resolution of how an event unfolds

Make sure to use "labeled for reuse" pictures from image searches on the internet (or simply hand draw your own) with accompanying text. You are welcome to use the gestures and icons presented in the video or create your own.

Elisa and I developed approximately 50 stories for preschoolers together. In making stories, use events that matter to preschoolers, such as going on big, scary water slides, getting lost at a zoo, or being too short for rides at an amusement park. My library continues to expand yearly with new short stories and they are quite easy to write when using the elements of the story as a guide.

---

providing speech, literacy, or language intervention, create gestural prompts that are meaningful to you. If you don't authentically buy into your gestural prompts, children won't either.

The next clip will once again demonstrate the importance of the child learning through active participation both nonverbally, through movement, and verbally, through echoed speech. The child is learning the *schema*, or organizational outline, for six elements of the story. When this schema becomes automatic, the child will be empowered to comprehend and express stories more easily. In Video 9.17, Alicia is teaching Xavier the gestures and elements of the story for the very first time with a maximum level of support.

For another example of learning the elements of the story for the first time, see Ms. Becca with Harris in Video 9.18. In Kelly's Corner Video 9.19 the value of learning the elements of of the stories in improving literacy skills from preschool through adulthood is discussed.

9.17 Chapter Summary

In this chapter we covered literacy activities to improve phonological awareness skills, print knowledge, and narrative development. Our approach to literacy intervention is much like our approach to speech sound disorder treatment in terms of selecting the most complex treatment targets and exposing the child to academic talk to ignite maximum neurological change. We

highlighted the need, on a moment to moment basis, to dynamically provide temporal, tactile, visual, and verbal cueing based on the child's need to support a minimal 80% accuracy level. Doing so avoids negative practice, while reinforcing new learning.

An ongoing emphasis is that the child is participating actively using both words and movement to learn abstract phonological awareness concepts and develop narrative skills more efficiently and deeply. Always challenge the child to perform at the child's highest level of capability with support, or at his or her *zone of proximal development*, while fading support to create an internal locus of control.[23]

Lastly, it is crucially important that emphasis remains on the child *producing* targets accurately at a high level of density for optimal improvements in speech to occur when integrating literacy intervention into speech therapy. Learning should be both seen and heard as the child actively participates both verbally and nonverbally.[44,45]

References

[1] Nathan L, Stackhouse J, Goulandris N, Snowling MJ. The development of early literacy skills among children with speech difficulties: a test of the "critical age hypothesis.". J Speech Lang Hear Res. 2004; 47(2):377–391

[2] Hayiou-Thomas ME, Carroll JM, Leavett R, Hulme C, Snowling MJ. When does speech sound disorder matter for literacy? The role of disordered speech errors, co-occurring language impairment and family risk of dyslexia. J Child Psychol Psychiatry. 2017; 58(2):197–205

9

[3] Raitano NA, Pennington BF, Tunick RA, Boada R, Shriberg LD. Pre-literacy skills of subgroups of children with speech sound disorders. J Child Psychol Psychiatry. 2004; 45(4):821–835

[4] McNeill BC, Gillon GT, Dodd B. Phonological awareness and early reading development in childhood apraxia of speech (CAS). Int J Lang Commun Disord. 2009; 44(2):175–192

[5] Preston J, Edwards ML. Phonological awareness and types of sound errors in preschoolers with speech sound disorders. J Speech Lang Hear Res. 2010; 53(1):44–60

[6] Anthony JL, Aghara RG, Dunkelberger MJ, Anthony TI, Williams JM, Zhang Z. What factors place children with speech sound disorders at risk for reading problems? Am J Speech Lang Pathol. 2011; 20(2):146–160

[7] Murphy KA, Justice LM, O'Connell AA, Pentimonti JM, Kaderavek JN. Understanding risk for reading difficulties in children with language impairment. J Speech Lang Hear Res. 2016; 59(6):1436–1447

[8] Masso S, Baker E, McLeod S, Wang C. Polysyllable speech accuracy and predictors of later literacy development in preschool children with speech sound disorders. J Speech Lang Hear Res. 2017; 60(7):1877–1890

[9] Hakvoort B, de Bree E, van der Leij A, et al. The role of categorical speech perception and phonological processing in familial risk children with and without dyslexia. J Speech Lang Hear Res. 2016; 59(6):1448–1460

[10] Wellman RL, Lewis BA, Freebairn LA, Avrich AA, Hansen AJ, Stein CM. Narrative ability of children with speech sound disorders and the prediction of later literacy skills. Lang Speech Hear Serv Sch. 2011; 42(4):561–579

[11] Holm A, Farrier F, Dodd B. Phonological awareness, reading accuracy and spelling ability of children with inconsistent phonological disorder. Int J Lang Commun Disord. 2008; 43(3):300–322

[12] Preston JL, Hull M, Edwards ML. Preschool speech error patterns predict articulation and phonological awareness outcomes in children with histories of speech sound disorders. Am J Speech Lang Pathol. 2013; 22(2):173–184

[13] Brosseau-Lapré F, Roepke E. Speech errors and phonological awareness in children ages 4 and 5 years with and without speech sound disorder. J Speech Lang Hear Res. 2019; 62(9):3276–3289

[14] Wagner RK, Torgesen JK, Rashotte CA, Pearson NA. Comprehensive Test of Phonological Processing. 2nd ed. Austin, TX: Pearson; 2013

[15] Macrae T, Tyler AA. Speech abilities in preschool children with speech sound disorder with and without co-occurring language impairment. Lang Speech Hear Serv Sch. 2014; 45(4):302–313

[16] Hearnshaw S, Baker E, Munro N. The speech perception skills of children with and without speech sound disorder. J Commun Disord. 2018; 71:61–71

[17] Denne M, Langdown N, Pring T, Roy P. Treating children with expressive phonological disorders: does phonological awareness therapy work in the clinic? Int J Lang Commun Disord. 2005; 40(4):493–504

[18] Moriarty BC, Gillon GT. Phonological awareness intervention for children with childhood apraxia of speech. Int J Lang Commun Disord. 2006; 41(6):713–734

[19] Gierut JA. Phonological complexity and language learnability. Am J Speech Lang Pathol. 2007; 16(1):6–17

[20] Storkel HL. Implementing evidence-based practice: selecting treatment words to boost phonological learning. Lang Speech Hear Serv Sch. 2018; 49(3):482–496

[21] Kaderavek JN, Justice LM. Embedded-explicit emergent literacy intervention II: goal selection and implementation in the early childhood classroom. Lang Speech Hear Serv Sch. 2004; 35(3):212–228

[22] Edeal DM, Gildersleeve-Neumann CE. The importance of production frequency in therapy for childhood apraxia of speech. Am J Speech Lang Pathol. 2011; 20(2):95–110

[23] Vygotsky LS, Cole M. Mind in Society: The Development of Higher Psychological Processes. Cambridge, MA: Harvard University Press; 1978

[24] van Kleeck A. Distinguishing between casual talk and academic talk beginning in the preschool years: an important consideration for speech-language pathologists. Am J Speech Lang Pathol. 2014; 23(4):724–741

[25] ASHA. Speech sound disorders-articulation and phonology: comprehensive assessment. https://www.asha.org/PRP SpecificTopic.aspx?folderid=8589935321&section= Assessment/. Accessed April 4, 2019

[26] Robertson CR, Salter W. Phonological Awareness Test-Second Edition. East Moline, IL: Linguisystems; 2007

[27] Vess K, Hunter S. Integrated ASD literacy peer groups: the impact on literacy skills of typically developing preschoolers. Poster presented at: Annual American Speech, Language and Hearing Association Convention; November, 2014; Orlando, FL

[28] Vess K, Abou-Arabi M, De Luca E. Accelerating preschoolers' phonemic awareness skills through kinesthetic hand prompting. Poster presented at: Annual American Speech, Language and Hearing Association Convention; November, 2018; Boston, MA

[29] Vess K, Bradley L. Accelerating early literacy development through use of phonological awareness and print referencing strategies. Poster presented at: Annual American Speech, Language and Hearing Association Convention; November, 2017; Los Angeles, CA

[30] Dweck CS. Mindset: The New Psychology of Success. New York: Ballantine; 2016

[31] Anthony JL, Lonigan CJ. The nature of phonological awareness: converging evidence from four studies of preschool and early grade school children. J Educ Psychol. 2004; 96(1):43–55

[32] Olszewski A, Soto X, Goldstein H. Modeling alphabet skills as instructive feedback within a phonological awareness intervention. Am J Speech Lang Pathol. 2017; 26(3):769–790

[33] Justice LM, Kaderavek JN, Fan X, Sofka A, Hunt A. Accelerating preschoolers' early literacy development through classroom-based teacher-child storybook reading and explicit print referencing. Lang Speech Hear Serv Sch. 2009; 40(1):67–85

[34] Law J, Garrett Z, Nye C. The efficacy of treatment for children with developmental speech and language delay/disorder: a meta-analysis. J Speech Lang Hear Res. 2004; 47(4):924–943

[35] Isbell R, Sobol J, Lindauer L, Lowrance A. The effects of storytelling and story reading on the oral language complexity and story comprehension of young children. Early Child Educ J. 2004; 32(3):157–163

[36] Spencer TD, Kajian M, Petersen DB, Bilyk N. Effects of an individualized narrative intervention on children's storytelling and comprehension skills. J Early Interv. 2014; 35(3):243–269

[37] Petersen DB, Spencer TD. Using narrative intervention to accelerate canonical story grammar and complex language growth in culturally diverse preschoolers. Top Lang Disord. 2016; 36(1):6–19

[38] Van Horne AJO, Fey M, Curran M. Do the hard things first: a randomized controlled trial testing the effects of exemplar selection on generalization following therapy for grammatical morphology. J Speech Lang Hear Res. 2017; 60(9):2569–2588

9

[39] Thompson CK. Complexity in language learning and treatment. Am J Speech Lang Pathol. 2007; 16(1):3–5

[40] Lyons R, Roulstone S. Well-being and resilience in children with speech and language disorders. J Speech Lang Hear Res. 2018; 61(2):324–344

[41] Spencer TD, Petersen DB. Story Champs: A Multi-tiered Language Intervention Program. Laramie, WY: Language Dynamics Group; 2012

[42] Spencer TD, Petersen DB, Adams JL. Tier 2 language intervention for diverse preschoolers: an early-stage randomized control group study following an analysis of response to intervention. Am J Speech Lang Pathol. 2015; 24(4):619–636

[43] Spencer TD, Petersen DB, Restrepo MA, Thompson M, Arvizu MNG. The effect of Spanish and English narrative intervention on the language skills of young dual language learners. Top Early Child Spec Educ. 2018; 38(4):204–219

[44] Callcott D, Hammond L, Hill S. The synergistic effect of teaching a combined explicit movement and phonological awareness program to preschool aged students. Early Child Educ J. 2015; 43(3):201–211

[45] Pieretti RA, Kaul SD, Zarchy RM, O'Hanlon LM. Using a multi-modal approach to facilitate articulation, phonemic awareness, and literacy in young children. Comm Disord Q. 2015; 36(3):131–141

9

10 Researching Your Practice to Hone Your Craft

Constantly think about how you could be doing
things better and question yourself.

—Elon Musk

What doesn't kill you makes you stronger. As a speech-language pathologist, you are in an amazing position. Odds are, you have a large caseload. Although a large caseload can be daunting, it provides you with the potential participants to research which evidence-based best practices are merely good and which are excellent. You should only proceed, however, with the best interests of the child foremost and with parents' informed consent and permission to release and present findings. My administration is highly supportive of research and even provides free legal counsel to approve my permission slips. Work closely with your employer to develop informed consent and permission to release data forms.

Research, in addition to improving your practice, can be exciting. I'm not embarrassed to admit that while awaiting results of comparing treatment variables, I'm like a child on Christmas Eve waiting to open presents under the tree. I'm always eager to discover if a variable is effective or ineffective and what impact it can have on outcomes. Implementation of a discovery will lead to more discoveries and excite further research. I believe you will find that avoiding complacency by researching your practice will make your work much more exciting and rewarding.

In accepting a dual role of both a clinician and researcher, you must acknowledge the presence of *researcher bias*. *Researcher bias* is the impact on the results by what we believe to be true, whether or not it is actually true.[1] During intervention and testing, if you believe one strategy to be more effective over another, you may unintentionally send expectations of success or failure to the child. The child may therefore perform better or worse based on your bias.

10.1 Controlling Variables in Researching Your Practice

What can speech-language pathologists learn from successful corporations like Google, Yahoo, Amazon, Netflix, Facebook, Twitter, Expedia, and Airbnb? These corporations, despite their differences, routinely do *A/B Testing* on their websites. In *A/B Testing*, also referred to *as split testing*, all variables are controlled for except for two (Variable A and Variable B) to determine which version is more effective in increasing the viewer's level of interaction and duration on a website.

Why is the use of A/B Testing by corporations on their websites of interest to us? Our work, like that of these major corporations, matters. We may not be dealing with a billion dollar enterprise but we are dealing with someone's life. The stakes are high. The intervention we do today may help determine if a child grows up to have friends, attends college, or works and lives independently.[2]

Recent research indicates that therapy enables us to create neurological connections, rewiring and reorganizing the brain when plasticity is at its greatest level.[3] We can accomplish this important task by deliberately applying only the most effective evidence-based practices. How do we ensure that our therapy will have an optimal impact? We can judiciously research our practice by using A/B Testing in our work.

How does A/B Testing typically work? On a simplistic level, a viewer is randomly assigned to one of two websites. For instance, one website has a blue search engine button (A), and the other has a green search engine button (B). Over time, corporations hone their craft by gradually and consistently implementing small changes based on statistically significant viewer responses, such as a search engine button color.

Even though A/B Testing is simple, it can help us make important, impactful decisions in therapy. In comparing evidence-based strategies against each other by examining only one variable, the risk for ineffective practice is minimalized and we can more clearly attribute change to a single variable.

Applying research terminology, A/B Testing compares two *independent variables*: Variable A and Variable B. For our intervention research purposes, both variables compared should be empirically and theoretically supported. These *independent variables* are factors that can be manipulated to impact *the main effect*. The *main effect*, also known as the *dependent variable*, is the measurable outcome of the independent variables. In designing research experiments, my best advice is to try to keep everything the same except for the independent variables.

10.2 How to Conduct A/B Testing in Experimental Research

Experimental Research is the most scientifically sophisticated research method in that participants are *randomly* assigned to groups. In A/B Testing we can only examine the relative impact that manipulated independent variables have in comparison to one another on a dependent variable or dependent variables.

We can only determine a relative impact, not an absolute impact, as denying therapy to preschool age clients by having them serve as a control group or providing a placebo intervention would obviously be unethical. In particular, we would not want to deny intervention for preschoolers, considering the optimal level of plasticity in the brain at younger ages.

An advantage of alternate intervention research over the traditional control versus treatment group methodology is that alternate intervention research controls for *attention effects. Attention effects* is a phenomenon in which children in the treatment group make gains simply as a result of added attention, which children in the control group do not receive.

For these reasons, an A/B Testing intervention approach is recommended by which children are randomly assigned to one of two evidence-based intervention strategies or conditions. As far as duration of the intervention is concerned, meta-analytic research indicates that speech and expressive language intervention gains become evident following an 8-week time span.[4] In terms of treatment intensity, be certain that the *dosage* in frequency and duration of intervention intensity remains constant across A/B conditions and interventions.[5,6]

Details matter. I feel that I can conclusively state that they will make you an effective interventionist. Strive to be able to explain *every* detail of your therapy in terms of its evidence base and theory. Blindly adopting a comprehensive approach is operating on autopilot and you will unknowingly engage in ineffectual practices. Our current time constraints and growing caseloads necessitate that these ineffective practices be readily identified and cut.

As a therapist, your goal is to deliver a comprehensive approach that includes *only* the most effective practices. When explaining to graduate students how to create comprehensive approaches that include only the very best evidence-based practices, I often use the analogy of creating "best practice stew." Through diligently researching our practice, we are continually developing special "best practice stew" recipes for speech sound disorders, language delays, literacy interventions, and treating minimally verbal children that only include the most effective evidence-based strategies as our active ingredients.

Your responsibility to your client is to provide best practice therapy based on the best research currently available. You also need to continually hone in on the details of your practice in order to tease out effective intervention strategies from ineffective ones. Continue to search for effective strategies that have the biggest impact. See examples of intervention research questions that I've studied with graduate students using the A/B Test Design in ▸ Table 10.1 to further develop your practice.

10.3 Grouping Participants for Research

In completing AB test research, the following are common examples in grouping of participants.

10.3.1 Pre-test, Post-test Random Assignment Design

A pre-test, post-test random intervention assignment design of two groups of children assigned to evidence-based strategies or conditions is the most scientifically rigorous intervention design. In this scenario, randomly assign children to Intervention A or Intervention B to compare gains, with groups being comparable due to random assignment.

Children could also be randomly assigned to a condition. For instance, children could be assigned to conditions of differing physical distance from a communicative partner. A preverbal child could remain proximally seated next to a communicative partner to exchange a sentence strip (Condition A) or be required to travel 5 feet to exchange a sentence strip (Condition B) in the context of requesting desired objects and actions within a naturally rewarding activity. The dependent variable of verbal output in terms of consonantal vocalizations, word approximations, and words spoken could be compared across conditions.

10

Table 10.1 Putting research into practice: Answering research questions using the A/B Test Design

Below are questions that we've researched, using an A/B Test Design approach. This research has improved our practice in treating speech sound disorders, increasing verbal output, increasing language length and complexity, and improving literacy skills:

1-Do preschoolers make greater standardized testing speech articulation gains (dependent variable) by requesting with treatment targets at the single word level (A) or treatment targets embedded into carrier sentences (B) in therapy?

2-Do preschoolers make greater standardized testing speech articulation gains (dependent variable) with 2-element blend (A) or 3-element blend (B) therapy treatment targets?

3-Do preschoolers make greater improvement in Percent Consonant Correct (dependent variable) using a variety of complex consonant cluster exemplar targets (A) or one complex consonant cluster treatment target (B) in therapy?

4-Does a child's number of words spoken increase (dependent variable) when using Picture Exchange Communication Systems (A) or Common Core Vocabulary Boards (B) to mand?

5-Do preschoolers with ASD perform better on single word standardized tests (dependent variable) when spontaneously labeling (A) or imitatively labeling (B)?

6-Do minimally verbal preschoolers with ASD produce more words and pleasurable vocalizations (dependent variables) within seated activities (A) or movement activities (B)?

7-Do minimally verbal preschoolers with ASD produce more words and vocalizations (dependent variable) with immediate natural reward delivery (A) or 3–5 second delay prior to reward provision (B)?

8-Do preschoolers make greater improvement in phonological awareness skill test performance (dependent variable) without performing accompanying motor gestures (A) or with performing accompanying motor gestures (B) in therapy?

9-During movement songs, do preschoolers with ASD demonstrate an increase in number of motor imitation acts (dependent variable) in response to live, human, modeling of actions with music (A) or in response to live, human, modeling actions with music and addition of a visual SmartBoard presentation demonstrating actions (B)?

10.3.2 Randomized Block Design

A randomized block design involves creating subgroups so that participants can be compared to similar participants. *A randomized block design* may be indicated with a high level of variability within a group, such as disorder, age, and severity level. For instance, we were studying the impact of our integrated literacy peer groups on phonological awareness skills. The group was of mixed etiology, including both preschoolers with autism spectrum disorder (ASD) and their neurotypical peers.

An example of applying a *randomized block design* is as follows. Children can be first divided into two subgroups, based on etiology, a Preschoolers with ASD Group and a Neurotypical Group. Each child can next be randomly assigned to either literacy intervention strategy group A or B. Children with ASD can be randomly assigned to *Intervention Strategy A-Children with ASD* or assigned to *Intervention Strategy B-Children with ASD*. Children who are neurotypical can also be randomly assigned to *Intervention Strategy A-Children who are Neurotypical* or to *Intervention Strategy B-Children who are Neurotypical*.

While using *randomized block design* in this scenario, children are compared to children with the same etiology. Thus, the influence of the presence or absence of a disorder is removed, thereby limiting *confounding variables*. *Confounding variables* are extra variables that could impact the dependent variable. Randomized block design enables us to study the impact of the independent variables, not the confounding variables related to the disorder, on the dependent variable more clearly.

10.3.3 Quasi-Experimental Study

A *quasi-experimental study* is similar to a true experimental study. Its subjects, however, are not distributed based on random assignment, making it *quasi-experimental*, which is literally, "*resembling experimental*." I collaborated with graduate students in a quasi-experimental study in which preschoolers were *not* randomly assigned to each treatment variable. Instead, assignments were based on individual testing performances and whether a 2-element or 3-element treatment target would be a more appropriate treatment target for each individual child.

In this study, if a child presented with two phonological processes of stopping fricatives and gliding liquids, the graduate students would likely select a 2-element /sl/ blend as a treatment target to increase the saliency of focusing on just those two phonological processes. If the child presented with three phonological processes (such as stopping fricatives, fronting velars, and gliding liquids), the graduate student would select a target of /skɹ/ to address all three phonological processes concurrently.

Quasi-experimental studies can give us insight into trends for further, more stringent randomly designed, larger scale research studies. In analyzing data from quasi-experimental studies, treatment groups must be analyzed to ensure that differences between groups are attributed to the independent variable and are not due to group differences.

In quasi-experimental studies of speech sound disorders at the preschool level, it is pertinent to check that treatment groups are equivalently matched in terms of baseline performance, age, severity of impairment, etiology, and presence of concurrent social, language, cognitive, or motor delays.

10.3.4 Crossover Design

A *crossover* or *repeated measures design* is indicated when random assignment is not possible due to a small number of participants. In a *crossover* or *repeated measures design*, the children in the group are compared against themselves across conditions or interventions. A crossover design is not considered an experimental design but rather a *pre-experimental design* in that it does not have a comparison group.

A weakness of a *crossover design*, also referred to as an *alternating treatment design*, is that a history of exposure to one independent variable would likely impact a child's response to the second independent variable, resulting in an *interaction effect*. An *interaction effect* is the cumulative impact of exposure to two independent variables in which the relative impact of each independent variable on the dependent variable is not clear. Also, perhaps, only one independent variable is responsible for the cumulative impact, leaving the researcher unable to identify which one.

The *order effect* is the difference in participants' responses as a result of the order in which independent variables are presented to them. In a crossover design, the order effect can impact the results. Because of this, it is important to alternate the sequence in which independent variables are presented.

Lastly, unlike comparison group experimental research, in which intervention variables are introduced at the same time, crossover design requires intervention to be delivered at separate times, resulting in greater risk for *maturational effects*. *Maturational effects* are developmental changes that occur over time, regardless of the intervention. The longer a study, the greater the maturational effect can be indicated in changes. Here, normative linguistic data over time, such a Mean Length of Utterance,[7] could be referenced to better understand the role that maturation contributed to dependent variable change.

10.4 Forming a Research Question

Turn your passions, insights, and knowledge of your clients into important questions that drive your research. The worst advice is to review all published research currently available to formulate a hypothesis based on a question that is currently unanswered. The premise that there are only a few questions unanswered is absurd and perhaps some questions are not researched due to a lack of relevance.

Truth is our research base is limited. Recent meta-analyses indicate that a majority of speech sound disorders intervention research currently published are case studies.[8,9] Case studies can provide direction for further research but simply lack the scientific rigor in generalization and transference to inform clinical practice.

For direction in forming a research question, ask, "What single thing could we do differently today to produce better outcomes for our clients?" This question will put you on the right track in asking questions that truly matter. After having your question, reference research available to further refine it. Important questions create meaningful research.

Look in all directions in gathering research on your topic. You will know your discipline more deeply and holistically from referencing neurological, medical, kinesiological, occupational therapy, physical therapy, psychological, linguistic, pedagogical, and applied behavioral fields, to name a few. You may have noticed in this chapter that we are applying artificial intelligence web marketing A/B research methodology to improve our practice.

In identifying variables that specifically matter in efficacy research, I encourage you to reference a well-organized and detailed chart by Baker and colleagues titled *Phonological Intervention Taxonomy*, presented in the *American Journal of Speech-Language Pathology*.[10] Some influential variables presented to research include the following: treatment targets, linguistic context, cueing methodology, level of prompting, provision of feedback, intervention context, materials, activity type,

10

Table 10.2 Putting research into practice: Asking good questions in A/B Testing intervention research across linguistic domains

Domain: Define Dependent Variable as a Measurable Outcome	Define Treatment or Condition (Independent Variable A)	Define Treatment or Condition (Independent Variable B)	How will you assign participants?	What other variables must be kept the same that could present as confounding variables?
Augmentative and Alternative Communication:				
Literacy:				
Morphology:				
Phonology:				
Pragmatic:				
Semantics:				
Syntax:				

intensity, frequency, density of productions, personnel training, parent involvement, and type of evaluation.

For practice in designing experiments, refer ▶ Table 10.2. Clearly define your measurable outcome (dependent variable) and the conditions or strategies that will serve as your independent variables to compare (A and B). Lastly, how will you keep all other variables the same and assign your participants?

10.5 Obtaining Informed Consent

In university settings, you have access to an Internal Review Board to approve your informed consent form, which indicates that patients are knowledgeable and their rights are protected in the research. However, in schools, private practice, and nonacademic clinical settings, you most likely won't have access to an Internal Review Board. In these noncollegiate settings, you will need to work very closely with your administration and its legal team to ensure that your process of informed consent is valid and ethical.

In drafting a participant informed consent form for administrative and legal review, be sure to reference the following general aspects of informed consent[1]:

Regarding voluntary participation, patients must be informed that:
1. They are participating in research.

2. There is absolutely no adverse consequence for not participating in research.
3. They can discontinue participating at any time.

Regarding the intervention itself, explanation should be provided as to the following:
1. The purpose, procedures, and duration of the intervention
2. The benefits and risks that can be reasonably anticipated

10.6 Pilot Your Instruments

Select appropriate assessments based on the test's quality in terms of *validity*, which is the accuracy in assessing your dependent variable. Also, look at *reliability*, which is the test's consistency of results. The test selected must also be appropriate to your participants' current performance level. This can be quite challenging in assessing diverse populations of preschoolers with communicative disorders, such as preschoolers with ASD.

An example illustrating a mismatch between a quality instrument selected and populations assessed was our research on accelerating the phonological awareness skills of preschoolers. Our goal was to use one well-normed standardized assessment to assess diverse treatment groups in order to draw comparisons later.

My graduate intern and I had one (very much treasured) day off of work in which we could obtain baseline data for neurotypical peers that would attend our integrated literacy peer groups for preschoolers with ASD. We had a well-normed popular phonological awareness test at our disposal and were ready for a full day of baseline testing. The problem was that a majority of the neurotypical children were achieving 100% accuracy on the subtests of interest. Conversely, our students with ASD were uniformly scoring 0% on those same subtests.

Our testing with the neurotypical preschoolers indicated a *ceiling effect*. With a *ceiling effect*, test items are too easy to truly assess the child's current level of performance. Conversely, using the very same standardized measurement with preschoolers with ASD indicated a *floor effect*. With a *floor effect*, test items are too difficult to assess the child's current performance levels. In both cases, we ended with limited information regarding the children's actual literacy skills at baseline.

Hindsight is 20/20 but *piloting* of this assessment by administering it to a few randomly selected children prior to committing to a full day of testing would have resulted in more appropriate instrument selection and more constructive use of our very limited resource of time.

In any case, with extreme scores in baseline testing, *regression toward the mean*, also referred to as *statistical regression*, is also a threat. *Regression toward the mean* occurs when outlier performances, at the highest and lowest ends of the spectrum, move toward average over time regardless of the independent variable. Having an exceptionally superior or horrible performance during baseline testing, odds are a closer to average performance will surface during post-testing.

10.7 Putting Research into Practice: Examining Alternate Interventions for Fidelity and Control of Extraneous Variables

Video 10.1, Video 10.2, Video 10.3, and Video 10.4 demonstrate our current study researching an intervention strategy in which preschoolers with speech sound disorders were randomly assigned to Variable A Linguistic Context Complex Sentence or Variable B Linguistic Context Paragraph. Our dependent variables in this research are number of errors on standardized speech testing, Percent Consonants Correct, and Mean Length of Utterance change from baseline to post-intervention.

Review Video 10.1, Video 10.2, Video 10.3, and Video 10.4. Are there any aspects of the intervention that lacked *fidelity*, which is adherence to administration of the independent variables? The preschoolers received the same activities, the same interventions, in that each intern had a balance of children requesting with a complex sentence or a paragraph as a linguistic context. Interns rotated across activities with their students, resulting in every child engaging in the very same activities. Can you find *confounding variables* among the four videos that could impact the dependent variables?

In Video 10.1, see Ms. Holly with Tierce, requesting using a complex sentence linguistic context.

In Video 10.2, see Ms. Katelyn with Marabeth, requesting using a paragraph linguistic context.

In Video 10.3, see Ms. Torey with Jillian, requesting using a complex sentence linguistic context.

In Video 10.4, see Ms. Torey with Conrad, requesting using a paragraph linguistic context. See video 10.5 in which I summarize the simple design and A/B variables compared in this study.

10.8 Analyzing Your Data

The beauty in the simplicity of A/B Testing with random distribution research design is that all variables are controlled except for the independent variables. For this you can assess your data rather simply and therefore advance your practice more efficiently. This means that generally you will not have to do complex regression analysis by controlling for the contributing impact of multiple variables. This eliminates the need for expensive statistical software and advanced training.

First, make sure your organization has an increased privacy level with Google as mine does to use Google Sheets. In inputting the data into Google Sheets, each child can be assigned a number with intervention variable A or B (e.g., "Child 1A, Child 2A, Child 1B, Child2B, etc...") in place of a name to protect confidentiality. To protect data, the name to number correspondence should be known only to you, the principal investigator of your research. Please see ▸ Table 10.3 along with ▸ Table 10.4 which illustrate how to complete simple t-test data analysis using Google Sheets and the internet free of cost.

10

Table 10.3 Fictional data sample for illustrative purposes of how to use Google Sheets for simple statistical analysis

	A	B	C	D
	Variable A Group: Trisyllabic Word Target	Decrease in Number of Speech Test Errors	Variable B Group: 3-Element Consonant Cluster	Decrease in Number of Speech Test Errors
1				
2	Child 1A	5	Child 1B	9
3	Child 2A	5	Child 2B	8
4	Child 3A	7	Child 3B	5
5	Child 4A	8	Child 4B	10
6	Child 5A	4	Child 5B	8
7	Child 6A	6	Child 6B	6
8	Child 7A	3	Child 7B	8
9	Child 8A	5	Child 8B	9
10	Child 9A	6	Child 9B	10
11	Child 10A	4	Child 10B	10
12		=AVERAGE (B2:B11)		=AVERAGE (D2:D11)
13	=TTEST (B2:B11; D2:D11, 2, 3)	=STDEV (B2:B11)		=STDEV(D2:D11)
14				

Table 10.4 How to complete simple t-test data analysis using Google Sheets (refer ▶ Table 10.3)

Below is a simple data analysis comparing A/B variable treatment groups using *Google Sheets*. Reference ▶ Table 10.1. This method assumes that both groups are equivalently matched in number of participants and averages.
Step 1: Input data child's data next to the child's code name (e.g., Child 1A, Child 1B) for both the Variable A Group in one column and Variable B Group in another column.
Step 2: Obtain means for both groups. In the formula bar type **=AVERAGE (B2:B11) =AVERAGE (D2:D11)**
Step 3: Assess for statistical probability. Compare both group averages using a two-tailed probability test for each group by typing **=TTEST (B2:B11; D2:D11, 2, 3)** in the formula bar. A probability of .05 ($p=.05$) or below typically indicates meaningful difference, not by chance.
Step 4: Assess standard deviation. Standard deviation measures how spread out data is from the mean.[a] Find the standard deviation in each group by typing **=STDEV(B2:B11)** for the Variable A group and **=STDEV(D2:D11)** for Variable B Group in the formula bar.
Step 5: Assess effect size. Use "Cohen's d" if groups are the same size and "Hedge's g" if comparison groups are different in number. A reputable calculator on the web is https://www.socscistatistics.com/effectsize/
Step 6: Assess group equivalence. Obtain and report group averages (see Step 2) regarding variables that would impact response to intervention at preschool age such as child's age, baseline testing performance, etiology, and concurrent impairments. Great variation between groups would indicate need for additional statistical testing.[b]
Step 7: Minimally complete steps 2–6 for basic interpretation of your findings. Consult a statistician to review your data analysis prior to publishing your work.

a. A higher standard deviation indicates that data points are more dispersed from the mean. Data with a higher standard deviation are less reliable than data with a lower standard deviation.
b. When significant variation between Variable A and Variable B intervention groups is present, more advanced statistical testing is indicated to control for between group differences, such as a Welch's t-test. A Welch's t-test Calculator is available at http://www.statskingdom.com/150MeanT2uneq.html

10.9 Consider Both Successes and Failures to Understand Why

In research, failures are as important as successes. Numbers speak the truth while perceptions and ego often lie. My research these past 18 years, successful and otherwise, has enabled me to eliminate many wasteful and ineffective practices and strategies.

Failures inform as to *why* intervention variables are successful or unsuccessful. In controlling for all variables except for one, we find what successful variables have in common that ineffectual variables uniformly lacked. From there, we can then take that hypothesis and directly test it with A/B Testing to scientifically answer why an intervention was successful or why it failed.

For instance, in our work on improving phonological awareness skills with preschoolers, we have consistently found that the integration of movement has impacted results in improving a number of phonological awareness skills that we've studied over the years. To experimentally study the impact of movement with an A/B test, we compared teaching performance of a phonemic awareness skill of identifying initial and final phonemes in a word (dependent variable) with movement (Variable A) and without movement (Variable B). Variable A indicated positive gains, whereas Variable B indicated lackluster results with negative to minimal change. All variables were controlled for with equivalently matched groups based on baseline test performance, age, etiology and random assignment.

While integrating research into therapy, assume the role of a chef. Each effective intervention strategy or condition is shelved in your pantry as a "go-to" ingredient. Conversely, ineffective strategies should be trashed. When providing therapy, create your own best practice stews, which combine the most efficacious strategies to treat speech sound disorders, language impairments, behavioral difficulties, and literacy deficits.

10.10 Evaluating Others' Research

Statistically significant can be quite insignificant. When referencing *experimental research*, always evaluate both *effect size* and *statistical significance*. The *effect size* is simply the difference in group means (averages) between two groups or two conditions. *Effect size* is easily understood as a percentage of a standard deviation on a bell curve.

Consider both statistical significance and effect size when evaluating intervention research. A treatment group study could report a statistical difference due to a large number of participants with the effect size, actually indicating the difference to be trivial.

An example of this problem is the study of more than 22,000 people on a daily aspirin regiment to prevent heart attacks. The study was terminated early due to highly statistically significant findings ($p = 0.00001$) that indicated daily aspirin intake was associated with a reduction in heart attacks.[11]

Closer examination of the study however indicated the effect size to be trivial: a difference of less than 1% (0.77%) for those taking aspirin daily with a squared r ($r^2 = 0.001$) reported. (r^2 is Pearson's correlation coefficient r squared, which indicates percentage of variance that can be attributed to that variable.) Therefore, this research suggests that 0.1% of the variability in myocardial infarctions between treatment and nontreatment groups can be attributed to daily aspirin consumption.[12]

Yet, as a result of this "statistically significant" study, many patients were advised by their doctors to take aspirin daily. Adverse side effects of aspirin consumption such as gastrointestinal issues, heartburn, nausea, rashes, and bleeding likely outweigh the reward of an extremely minimal decrease in heart attack rate.

10.11 Nonstatistically Significant Does Not Necessarily Indicate Insignificance

Conversely, there can be a large effect size, such as $d = 0.8$, with a lack of statistical probability, such as $p = 0.10$, due to a limited number of participants that could logically impact clinical practice. For instance, suppose there is an A/B Testing intervention design for 10 preschoolers ($N = 10$) with childhood apraxia of speech (CAS). They are randomly assigned to Treatment Target Group A ($n = 5$) or Treatment Target Group B ($n = 5$).

In this fictional, well-designed study, the only difference between the two groups is the treatment target. Therapy approach, activities, dosage, location, time, density in production, personnel training, parent involvement, and interventionists remain the same. Only the treatment target verb differs. Group A is assigned a 3-element verb treatment target in the request phrase, "Can you *scrape* (/skɹeɪp/) it to me please?" Group B is assigned a trisyllabic verb treatment target in the same request phrase, "Can you *recycle* (/ɹiˈsaɪkəl/) it to me please?" to request natural rewards and actions over an 8-week period. Both verbs contain the later developing phonemes /s/, /k/, and /r/. Group A presents these sounds in a 3-element consonant cluster, monosyllabic verb, whereas group B presents the same sounds as singletons in a trisyllabic verb.

Baseline and post-treatment Percent Consonants Correct are collected for both Group A and Group B. Suppose that Group A (3-element cluster) demonstrated a large effect size of $d = 0.8$ in improvement in Percent Consonants Correct in connected speech over Group B (a trisyllabic word). However, results are at a statistical probability level of $p = 0.10$, thereby not making it statistically significant at a widely accepted minimal $p = 0.05$ level. In this case a *null hypothesis (H0)* would be accepted, which means that any difference is due to chance, not an identifiable cause.

Considering the large effect size, however, and small number of participants, this study could be referred to as an *underpowered* study. *Underpowered* studies lack statistical probability due to an insufficient sample size ($N = 10$) in which the *null hypothesis* that indicates there is no significant difference between the two groups, is accepted due to a lack of statistical probability ($p = 0.10$) despite evidence of a large effect size ($d = 0.8$).

Considering the large effect size of this fictionally underpowered study, due to the rarity of the disorder, results should *not* be interpreted as an absence of evidence. It could still be beneficial to thoroughly review this nonstatistically relevant research as it could logically inform further investigation, research, and even provide some direction in guiding your own clinical practice with closer examination of the target's impact on outcomes.

Why is a statistically significant level of *probability* ($p = 0.05$) so important? This statistical level of significance suggests to accept the *alternate hypothesis (H1)*. The *alternate hypothesis (H1)* indicates that changes in the dependent variable are due to the impact of independent variable and not due to chance.

This level of probability ($p = 0.05$) is widely used to indicate the difference between two groups is not due to *sampling variability. Sampling variability* is the difference between your sample and the actual, real population it purports to represent.

Generally, a larger sample would indicate less sampling variability as a larger sample would more likely represent the real population. As a general rule, as sample size increases, effect sizes decreases.[13] Also, too large sample size would be a wasteful use of resources. These resources should instead be economically applied to other research projects for furthering our knowledge base.

10.12 Evaluating Descriptive Research

Correlational research studies relationships among two or more variables by examining how a *predictor* variable impacts the *predicted* variable. It can help us understand aspects of human behavior within subgroups. This type of research is often referred to as *cohort* studies. In these we learn characteristics or risk factors inherent to a specific population.

For example, 65 children and adolescents with ASD who were minimally verbal were recently studied. Findings indicated that minimally verbal children with ASD were statistically likely to present with comorbid psychopathology and maladaptive behavior.[14] Correlation never implies causation.[15]

We do not know *why* these children present with increased risk for psychopathology and maladaptive behaviors. Recent research indicates that multiple variables are interacting and there could be neurological variables, of which we are currently unaware, causing this psychopathology.[16] Nonetheless, this information is useful in proactively treating the minimally verbal child with ASD, by understanding the high risk for clinical behavioral challenges.

In evaluating strength of *relationships*, a *Pearson Correlation Coefficient* is often referenced, which is denoted as r. It can occur on a continuum from -1 (a perfectly negative correlation) to $+1$ (a perfectly positive correlation). A *negative correlation* is a relationship in which when one variable increases, the other variable decreases. A *positive correlation* is a relationship in which when one variable increases, the other variable increases as well. A correlation coefficient of 0 indicates absolutely no relationship between the two variables.

In correlational research, Cohen recommends interpreting r with the following guidelines: a small/weak association ($r = 0.10$), moderate correlation ($r = 0.30$), or a large correlation ($r = 0.50$).[17] An r-squared measurement (denoted as r^2) is used to determine percentage of variance between groups that can be accounted for by a specified variable.

To gauge variance accounted by a specific variable, simply square r by multiplying r by itself. For instance, if a report indicates an $r = 0.50$, which is a large correlation between variables, we could square r and report percentage of variance between groups that can be attributed to that variable to be 25% ($r^2 = 0.25$).

10.13 Publication Bias

Finally, it is important as a reader and researcher to realize that publication bias exists. In the field of social sciences statistically significant findings are much more likely to be both submitted and published than nonstatistically significant findings. Current research estimates that statistically significant results are 60% more likely to be submitted for publication and 40% more likely to be published than nonstatistically significant results.[18]

As a consumer of research, being aware of the fact that publications are largely dependent on statistical significance and that tenure and advancement in academia are largely contingent on getting published, it would be logical to question the objectivity of a researcher.

Furthermore, research indicates that there is more scientific bias in academic environments where competition and pressure to publish is high. This contributes to a higher frequency of statistically significant results occurring in states that had higher publications per capita.[19] This link between more productive locations and the production of greater numbers of highly statistical results should caution readers to approach published research with some level of skepticism. Consider the ominous environmental influence of "publish or perish."

10.14 Role of Neuroscience in Future Intervention

Neurological data presented in the future will give young children an unfiltered voice that will drastically improve practice. It is expected that neurological measures, such as electroencephalograms (EEGs), electromyography (EMG), event related potentials (ERPs), positron emission tomography (PET) scan, and functional magnetic resonance imaging (fMRI), will improve in accuracy and reliability in analyzing brain activity. It is naturally also expected that over time scans will be more comfortably and safely applied to children with minimal risk. With these technological advances, we will be able to understand disorders more accurately and effectively treat individual neurological differences with a clear vision of specific therapeutic behavior's impact on the brain.

Neurological data will help us to better understand not only where and why breakdowns are occurring but also, most importantly, what we can do about it. This can be accomplished by measuring both the brain's immediate and longer term neurological response to specific therapeutic methods. This has the potential to direct efforts that effectively rewire and reorganize the brain when neuroplasticity is at its highest level, which can dramatically impact lifelong outcomes.

Currently, work with adult populations is suggesting increased linguistic complexity results in increased widespread neuronal activity.[3] With medical advances, we will soon have more objective neurological studies of children to clearly evaluate the role of linguistic complexity in accelerating neurological development to ignite maximal change.

10.15 Chapter Summary

The concept that the *world is flat* applies to today's speech-language pathologist more than ever. Previously, one would need to be an active member of an academic institution to avoid spending a small fortune to access research. This is no longer the case.

Access to some of the most scientifically rigorous journals is freely available across disciplines. Also, reliable information is widely available with internet connection through reputable search engines such as Google Scholar.

Communication impairments have a multi-faced impact. Thus, they require a multi-faceted approach for evaluation and treatment. Working harder will not result in more effectively treating the high caseloads which pervade today. Working, however, smarter will.

Reading across disciplines empowers SLP's to more efficiently serve children by creating educationally-rich activities and using evidence-based strategies that simultaneously target multiple developmental domains.

Look beyond your practice and look within. The children you serve likely come from a very different back porch than children referenced in published research. As discussed in Kelly's Corner Video 10.5, clinical research matters. Regularly, ask "Variable A" versus "Variable B" clinical questions. Your findings will refine the details of your practice, resulting in lifelong change.

10

References

[1] Dollaghan CA. The Handbook for Evidence-Based Practice in Communication Disorders. Baltimore, MD: Paul H. Brookes Publishing; 2012

[2] Law J, Rush R, Schoon I, Parsons S. Modeling developmental language difficulties from school entry into adulthood: literacy, mental health, and employment outcomes. J Speech Lang Hear Res. 2009; 52(6):1401–1416

[3] Kiran S, Thompson CK. Neuroplasticity of language networks in aphasia: advances, updates, and future challenges. Front Neurol. 2019; 10:295

[4] Law J, Garrett Z, Nye C. The efficacy of treatment for children with developmental speech and language delay/disorder: a meta-analysis. J Speech Lang Hear Res. 2004; 47(4):924–943

[5] Allen MM. Intervention efficacy and intensity for children with speech sound disorder. J Speech Lang Hear Res. 2013; 56(3):865–877

[6] Kaipa R, Peterson AM. A systematic review of treatment intensity in speech disorders. Int J Speech Lang Pathol. 2016; 18(6):507–520

[7] Rice ML, Smolik F, Perpich D, Thompson T, Rytting N, Blossom M. Mean length of utterance levels in 6-month intervals for children 3 to 9 years with and without language impairments. J Speech Lang Hear Res. 2010; 53(2):333–349

[8] Baker E, McLeod S. Evidence-based practice for children with speech sound disorders: part 1 narrative review. Lang Speech Hear Serv Sch. 2011; 42(2):102–139

[9] Baker E, McLeod S. Evidence-based practice for children with speech sound disorders: part 2 application to clinical practice. Lang Speech Hear Serv Sch. 2011; 42(2):140–151

[10] Baker E, Williams AL, McLeod S, McCauley R. Elements of phonological interventions for children with speech sound disorders: the development of a taxonomy. Am J Speech Lang Pathol. 2018; 27(3):906–935

[11] Bartolucci AA, Tendera M, Howard G. Meta-analysis of multiple primary prevention trials of cardiovascular events using aspirin. Am J Cardiol. 2011; 107(12):1796–1801

[12] Sullivan GM, Feinn R. Using effect size—or why the p value is not enough. J Grad Med Educ. 2012; 4(3):279–282

[13] Slavin R, Smith D. The relationship between sample sizes and effect sizes in systematic reviews in education. Educ Eval Policy Anal. 2009; 31(4):500–506

[14] Plesa Skwerer D, Joseph RM, Eggleston B, Meyer SR, Tager-Flusberg H. Prevalence and correlates of psychiatric symptoms in minimally verbal children and adolescents with ASD. Front Psychiatry. 2019; 10:43

[15] Justice L. Causal claims. Am J Speech Lang Pathol. 2009; 18 (1):2–3

[16] Ibrahim K, Eilbott JA, Ventola P, et al. Reduced amygdala–prefrontal functional connectivity in children with autism spectrum disorder and co-occurring disruptive behavior. Biol Psychiatry Cogn Neurosci Neuroimaging. 2019; 4(12):1031–1041

[17] Cohen J. Statistical Power Analysis for the Behavioral Sciences. London: Lawrence Erlbaum; 1988

[18] Franco A, Malhotra N, Simonovits G. Social science. Publication bias in the social sciences: unlocking the file drawer. Science. 2014; 345(6203):1502–1505

[19] Fanelli D. Do pressures to publish increase scientists' bias? An empirical support from US States Data. PLoS One. 2010; 5(4): e10271

Appendix A

Speech and Language Evaluation: Parent Report	
Child's Name:	Child's Date of Birth:
Person Completing the Form:	Relationship to the child:
Mother's Name: Complete Address:	Mother's Name: Complete Address (if different):
Name and Ages of Brothers:	Name and Ages of Sisters:
Contact Phone (mother): Contact Email:	Contact Phone (father): Contact Email:
Child's Pediatrician: Practice/Hospital::	Emergency Contact: Phone:

MEDICAL HISTORY	Circle	Yes: Please explain
Were there problems during pregnancy or birth?	Yes No	
Was your child born before the due date or at a low birth weight?	Yes No	
Has your child ever undergone general anesthesia?	Yes No	
Has your child been hospitalized for an extended time?	Yes No	
Is your child currently diagnosed with a syndrome or a developmental delay?	Yes No	
Is there presently or a history of ear, nose, oral, dental, or throat problems? PE Tube Placement?	Yes No	
Has your child had a hearing test or screening? When?	Yes No	
Is there a family history of speech, language, literacy, learning, or attention impairments?	Yes No	

DEVELOPMENTAL HISTORY	Circle	Yes: Please explain
Was your child's crawling or walking skills delayed? Are you currently concerned about gross motor development?	Yes No	
Are you currently concerned about your child's fine motor development (e.g., using utensils, drawing)?	Yes No	
Does your child have difficulty with toileting?	Yes No	
Is your child experiencing difficulties with sleeping?	Yes No	
Is your child experiencing difficulties with eating (e.g., swallowing or picky eating)?	Yes No	
Does your child experience difficulties in group or classroom settings?	Yes No	
Does your child attend preschool, child care, or school?	Yes No	When?
Does Your child currently/previously receive private therapy (speech, occupational, physical)?	Yes No	

COMMUNICATION SKILLS	
Language: How your child uses words and sentences to communicate	Speech: How clearly your child communicates
What concerns you about your child's language?	What concerns you about your child's speech?
When is your child most...	When is your child's speech...
talkative?	most clear?
quiet?	least clear?
Who suggested that language be evaluated?	Who suggested that speech clarity be evaluated?
Did your child babble frequently prior to speaking first words?	What percentage of your child's speech do you understand? About___%

If no, please explain: When did your child first use… Single words___months 2-3 word utterances___months Sentences___years How many words are in your child's longest sentence? About___words. Write an example of a long sentence below: Does your child initiate communication with others? If no, please explain: Does your child respond appropriately to others' directions? If no, please explain: Does your child respond appropriately to others' questions? If no, please explain:	How much of your child's speech do you think those familiar with your child understand (e.g., teachers, relatives)? About__% How much of your child's speech do you think unfamiliar adults understand? About__% How much of your child's speech do you think other children understand? About__% How does your child respond when others don't understand? Do others (e.g., siblings) speak for your child?

TEMPERAMENT	Please circle the best or closest response.		
How sensitive is your child to distractions or small changes (e.g., food, clothes, lighting, sounds)?	Not at all sensitive	Medium Sensitivity	Highly Sensitive
How much movement does your child show during the day?	Low levels	Medium levels	High levels
How intense are your child's reactions to events (positive and negative)?	Low	Medium	High
How does your child adapt to intrusions, transitions, or changes?	Easily	Variable	With Difficulty
Does your child become frustrated with obstacles or limitations placed on his or her activities?	Not easily frustrated	Variable	Easily frustrated

How consistent are your child's patterns of hunger, eating, and elimination?	Regular	Variable	Irregular
When upset, how easily can your child be distracted, diverted, and calmed?	Easily soothed	Variable	Hard to soothe
Does your child initially approach or back away from new situations, people, pets, or objects?	Approach	Variable	Withdraw
In child group settings, does your child primarily play alone or play with others?	Plays with others	Variable	Primarily plays alone
Does your child often use natural gestures when talking for clarification?	Frequently	Variable	Rarely

CHILD'S LIFE: Please complete the following statements.

My child is motivated by:

My child's strength are:

My child needs to work on:

Is there anything your child's teacher or therapist should know about your family's background, religion, faith, or dietary restrictions? If so, please explain:

My child's favorite...

Activities:

Books:

Movies/TV Shows:

Songs:

Toys:

Child's name:_____ Date: _____ DOB:_____ Age in months:_____

Examiner:_____

CONSONANT CLUSTER SCREENER Say, *"We're going to play a game. You say what I say. Ready? Say, wagon."* Write exactly what the child said using IPA phonetic spelling. Score 1 point for accurate production and 0 for inaccurate production of the initial consonant blend only. After the child imitates all words, close the book. Say, *"Now we're going to say words super clearly like a teacher. You get to say these words with me."* Provide maximum cueing one to two times for each word incorrectly imitated, speaking in unison with the child. Score 1 point for accurate productions and 0 for inaccurate productions of the *initial consonant blend* only. If the sound is mildly distorted with maximum cueing, give it a 0.5. (It may be an appropriate cluster to target.) Automatically assign a 1 score to accurate productions when verbally imitated, which indicates stimulability.

Item	Child's Response	Accurate? Y=1/N=0	Stimulable? Y=1/N=0
Example: "Say, Wagon"	Wagon"	1--Do not score	1--Do not score
1. fries			
2. scribble			
3. drum			
4. queen			
5. three			
6. plane			
7. slide			
8. tree			
9. spray			
10. tweet			
11. star			
12. flashlight			
13. snake			
14. block			
15. grapes			
16. cloud			
17. straw			
18. spoon			

Item	Child's Response	Accurate? Y=1/N=0	Stimulable? Y=1/N=0
19. swing			
20. square			
21. pretzel			
22. shrimp			
23. skate			
24. crown			
25. smoke			
26. glue			
27. splash			
28. broom			
29. puke			
30. beautiful			
31. tiara			
32. cute			
33. meow			
34. hyena			
35. skewer			
36. juice			
% Correct: Total imitated correctly divided by 36 =			
% Stimulable: Total number stimulable correct divide by 36 =			

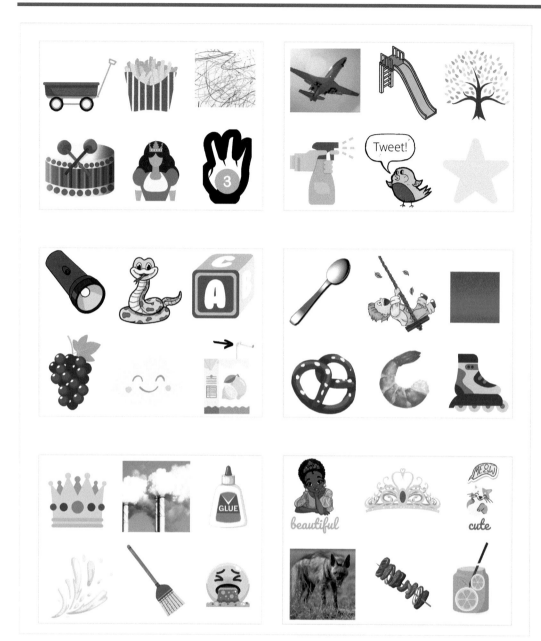

Child's Name:_____Date:_____DOB:_____

Directions: Score this form from the CONSONANT BLEND SCREENER. Score 1 for accurate 0 for inaccurate productions. Assign .5 for mild distortions. Calculate % Imitated and Stimulable.

3-Element Consonant Clusters and Affricate Blends: Score 0 or 1								Total # Correct/8 = %Correct
Cluster	skr(2)	dr(3) /dʒr/	tr(8) /tʃr/	spr(9)	str(17)	skw(20)	spl(27)	ski(35)	
Imitated									% Imitated
Max Pt									%Stimulable

Two Element S-Blends: Score 0 or 1							Total # Correct/7 = %Correct
Cluster	Sl(7)	St(11)	sn(13)	sp(18)	Sw(19)	sk(23)	sm(25)	
Imitated								% Imitated
Max Pt Stimulable								%Stimulable

Fricative Blends & Affricate /dʒ/						Total # Correct/5 = %Correct
Cluster	fr(1)	thr(5) /θr/	fl(12)	shr(22) /ʃr/	Ju(36)* /dʒ/	
Imitated						% Imitated
Max Pt Stimulable						%Stimulable

Two Element Voiced Stop Blends: Score 0 or 1							Total # Correct/6 = %Correct
Cluster	bl(14)	gr(15)	gl(26)	br(28)	bj(30)	mj(33)	
Imitated							% Imitated
Max Pt Stimulable							%Stimulable

Two Element Voiceless Stop Blends: Score 0 or 1											Total # Correct/10 = %Correct
Cluster	kw (4)	pl (6)	tw (10)	kl (16)	pr (21)	kr (24)	pj (29)	tj (31)	kj (32)	hj (34)	
Imitated											% Imitated
Max Pt Stimulable											%Stimulable

*The voiced affricate /dz/ is included for its complexity in targeting underlying /ʃ, ʒ, tʃ/.

Appendix B

Video 1.2. Answer Key for Jenna Completing *Consonant Cluster Screener* with Taylor

CONSONANT CLUSTER SCREENER Say, "*We're going to play a game. You say what I say. Ready? Say, wagon.*" Write exactly what the child said using IPA phonetic spelling. Score 1 point for accurate production and 0 for inaccurate production of the **initial consonant blend only.** After the child imitates all words, **close the book.** Say, "Now we're going to say words super clearly like a teacher. You get to say these words with me." Provide maximum cueing one to two times for each word incorrectly imitated, speaking in unison with the child. Score 1 point for accurate productions and 0 for inaccurate productions of the *initial consonant blend* only. If the sound is mildly distorted with maximum cueing, give it a 0.5. (It may be an appropriate cluster to target.) Automatically assign a 1 score to accurate productions when verbally imitated, which indicates stimulability.

Item	Child's Response	Accurate? Y=1/N=0	Stimulable? Y=1/N=0
Example: "Say, Wagon"	ˈwægən"	1--Do not score	1--Do not score
1. fries	fɹaɪd	1	1
2. scribble	ˈstɪɹbel	0	1
3. drum	drʌm	1	1
4. queen	Twin	0	1
5. three	Fwi	0	1
6. plane	pleɪn	1	1
7. slide	slaɪd	1	1
8. tree	tʃɹi	1	1
9. spray	spweɪ	0	1
10. tweet	Twik	1	1
11. star	stɑr	1	1
12. flashlight	ˈfwæ ʃlaɪt	0	1
13. snake	sneɪk	1	1
14. block	blɑk	1	1
15. grapes	dʒɹeɪps	0	1
16. cloud	klaʊd	1	1
17. straw	stʃɹɔ	0	1
18. spoon	Spun	1	1

Item	Child's Response	Accurate? Y=1/N=0	Stimulable? Y=1/N=0
19. swing	swɪŋ	0	1
20. square	tʃwɛr	0	1
21. pretzel	ˈpwɛtzəl	0	1
22. shrimp	ʃwɪmp	0	1
23. skate	steɪt	0	1
24. crown	tʃwaʊn	0	1
25. smoke	smoʊk	1	1
26. glue	glu	1	1
27. splash	plætʃ	0	1
28. broom	bwum	0	1
29. puke	pjuk	1	1
30. beautiful	ˈbutəfəl	0	1
31. tiara	tiˈjɑrə	1	1
32. cute	twut	0	1
33. meow	miˈiaʊ	1	1
34. hyena	haˈinə	1	1
35. skewer	ˈsuər	0	1
36. juice	dus	0	1
% Correct: Total imitated correct divided by (#1-36) by 36 =			
% Stimulable: Total number stimulable correct divide by 36 =			100%

Child's name: Jenna K.   Date: 7/16/2018 DOB: 5/9/2015   Examiner: Taylor McGraw

Directions: Score this form from the CONSONANT BLEND SCREENER. Score 1 for accurate 0 for inaccurate productions. Assign .5 for mild distortions. Calculate % Imitated and Stimulable.

3-Element Consonant Clusters and Affricate Blends: Score 0 or 1									Total #
Cluster	skr(2)	dr(3) /ʤr	tr(8) /tʃr/	spr(9)	str(17)	skw(20)	spl(27)	ski(35)	Correct/8 = %Correct
Imitated	0	1	1	0	0	0	0	0	25% Imitated
Max Pt	1	1	1	1	1	1	1	1	100% Stijulable

Two Element S-Blends: Score 0 or 1								Total #
Cluster	Sl(7)	st(11)	sn(13)	sp(18)	sw(19)	sk(23)	sm(25)	Correct/7 = %Correct
Imitated	1	0	1	0	0	0	1	25% Imitated
Max Pt Stimulable	1	1	1	1	1	1	1	100% Stijulable

Fricative Blends & Affricate /ʤ/						Total #
Cluster	fr(1)	thr(5) /θr/	fl(12)	shr(22) /ʃr/	ju(36)* /ʤ/	Correct/5 = %Correct
Imitated	1	0	0	0	0	20% Imitated
Max Pt Stimulable	1	1	1	1	1	100% Stijulable

Two Element Voiced Stop Blends: Score 0 or 1							Total #
Cluster	bl(14)	gr(15)	gl(26)	br(28)	bj(30)	mj(33)	Correct/6 = %Correct
Imitated	1	0	1	0	1	1	67% Imitated
Max Pt Stimulable	1	1	1	1	1	1	100% Stijulable

Two-Element Voiceless Stop Blends: Score 0 or 1										Total #
Cluster	kw (4)	pl (6)	tw (10)	kl (16)	pr (21)	kr (24)	pj (29)	tj (31)	kj (32)	hj (34)	Correct/10 = %Correct
Imitated	0	1	1	1	0	0	1	1	0	1	60% Imitated
Max Pt Stimulable	1	1	1	1	1	1	1	1	1	1	100% Stijulable

*The voiced affricate /ʤ/ is included for its complexity in targeting underlying /ʃ, ʒ, tʃ/.

Video 1.3. Errors in Landley's Connected Speech Sample

[du ju θɪŋk 'pɪgiz doʊ 'aʊt'saɪd? hɪr- wʌn. ænd aɪ 'wʌndər wɛr ðiz doʊ. aɪ θɪŋk ðɛr 'farmər wazd ðɛm ɔf bʌt nat ðɪs 'lɪtəl'pɪdi. aɪ θɪŋk nidz tu pʊt ðɛm ɪn hir. aɪ θɪn- ðɛr 'ganə goʊ ɪn hir. aɪ θɪŋk ðə 'lædʌ ju noʊ. ðeɪ tɪn doʊ ɪn hir. 'meɪbi ðɪs ʃʊd doʊ ɪn hir. ʌm səm'taɪmz. ʌm səm'taɪmz ðə 'farmər fidz ðɪs ɪn ə 'mɪnət. aɪ θɪŋk taʊ tʊd doʊ ʌp hir. ænd ðɪs taʊ ʃʊd doʊ ɪn hir. aɪ doʊnt noʊ wɛr hi ʃʊd doʊ. jæ. bʌt hi nidz tu bi ɪn ðə farm. ænd wɛr ʃʊd ðə maʊs goʊ? hiz 'gatə faɪnd ə weɪz tu slip.]

Note: The 3rd production of a word and subsequent productions as well as rhotic /ɛr/ and /ər/ are omitted (crossed out) from the count. Blue consonants are counted as accurate. Red are counted as errored.

$$\frac{\text{Total \# of Consonants (150)} - \text{Total \# of Inaccurate Consonants (10)} = 140/150 = 93\% \text{ PCC}}{\text{Total \# of Consonant (150)}}$$

Video 1.4. Sampson's Connected Speech Sample: Utterances Analyzed and Morphemes Spaced for MLU Count

First, to analyze MLU:

1. Place a space within words to indicate a bound morpheme. Also, take out spaces between words that count as one morpheme, such as proper nouns and reduplications (e.g., Mickey Mouse, night night).
2. Make sure to remove utterance numbers (or they will count toward total word count).
3. On either Microsoft Word and Google Docs, go to "Tools"→"Word Count."
4. Divide "Word Count" by number of utterances.
5. This sample has 199 words and morphemes, which is divided by 50 utterances:

$$\frac{199 \text{ (Number of Total Words and Morphemes)}}{50 \text{ (Number of Utterances)}} = 3.98 \text{ MLU}$$

6. Refer ▶ Table 1.4 for average recent MLU based on chronological age.

Why	Snake
Yeah	Maybe they' re so scary
I want to do this one	I don't know maybe in the bathtub
I don't know	What' s this
Oopsies!	I don't know maybe a sink
From the house maybe	Yeah maybe
What are these	One sink that goes down here
Look what is this	And where' s the bathroom
What is this piece	This is the bathroom
To wash your hand s	Somebody' s on it
This is a bathroom	I' m just pretend ing
I need to go poop	I' m just pretend ing somebody' s under it
Maybe he' s too big	Why not
Nope maybe not	No
Maybe this person	How do you do this
Awe no	I' m doing this
What is this	Here' s some melon
Maybe it' s in the house with the big bad wolf	Want this numnumnum
I don't know maybe to the bathroom	Watch me spin this
I need to go potty	Lamp look
Oopsies	Maybe it goe s on here
There she goes	Maybe it wiggle s
Maybe this one	And then this
I never saw big toy s before	Maybe I can play with this next time
No	MLU = 3.98
Nope	

Video 1.8. Sampson's Diadochokinetic Performance

$$\frac{\text{Total number correct (20)}}{20} = 100\% \text{ Accuracy}$$

Number of seconds to produce "pattycake" 20 times = 31 (30 seconds is considered average)[a]
To determine rate per second, divide total number of seconds (31) by 20 = 1.55 rate per second

$$\frac{\text{Total seconds (31)}}{20} = 1.55 \text{ DDK rate/sec (1.4–1.8 is considered within normal range, 3–5 years)}^{[a]}$$

$$\frac{\text{Number of Different Errored Productions of Pattycake (0)}}{20} = 0\% \text{ Variability}$$

Then, subtract % Variability from 100% to establish %Consistency:
100% minus 100%Variability = 100% Consistency
Observations regarding tongue, lip, cheek, and jaw movement: Efficient movement of articulators
Video 1.9. Kamdyn's Diadochokinetic Performance
To determine accuracy, divide total number correct by 20 = 0% Accuracy

$$\frac{\text{Total number correct (0)}}{20} = 0\% \text{ Accuracy}$$

Number of seconds to produce "pattycake" 20 times = 23 seconds (30 seconds is considered average)[a]
To determine rate per second, divide total number of seconds (23) by 20 = 1.15 rate per second:

$$\frac{\text{Total seconds (23)}}{20} = 1.15 \text{ DDK rate per sec (1.4–1.8 is considered within normal range, 3–5 years)}^{[a]}$$

$$\frac{\text{Number of Different Errored Productions of Pattycake (4)}}{20} = 20\% \text{ Variability}$$

100% minus %Variability = 80% Consistency

Observations regarding tongue, lip, cheek, and jaw movement: Inefficient movement of articulators with excess jaw movement to compensate for minimal labial and lingual movement. Pause between syllables indicating poor coordination of sequencing sounds. Deletion of middle syllable in all productions resulted in faster DDK rate.

Appendix C

Phonological Processes Based on Sampson's Standardized Speech Test Errors:

Stimulus Item *Orthographically* IPA	Sampson's Production *Orthographically* IPA	Phonological Process
teeth /tiθ/	teas /tis/	Consonant assimilation[a] (progressive)
rake /ɹeɪk/	wake /weɪk/	Gliding
fish /fɪʃ/	fiss /fɪs/	Depalatization
seal /sil/	see-awe /siɑ/	Gliding
zoo /zu/	sue /su/	Devoicing
cheese /ʧiz/	tease /tis/	Stopping, post-vocalic devoicing
leaf /lif/	yeaf /jif/	Gliding
thumb /θʌm/	fumb /fʌm/	Consonant assimilation[a] (regressive)
bathe /beɪð/	bave /beɪv/	Consonant assimilation[a] (progressive)
clown /klaʊn/	cown /kaʊn/	Cluster reduction
snake /sneɪk/	nake /neɪk/	Cluster reduction
thermometer /θərˈmɑmətə˞/	mometer /mɑmətə˞/	Weak syllable deletion

[a]Note that /θ, ð/ production varies based on influence of phonetic context.

Phonological Processes Based on Landley's Standardized Speech Test Errors:

Stimulus Item Orthographically IPA	Stimulus Item Orthographically IPA	Phonological Process(es)
gate /geɪt/	date /deɪt/	Fronting
king /kɪŋ/	teen /tin/	Fronting
ring /ɹɪŋ/	ween /win/	Gliding, Fronting
van /væn/	ban /bæn/	Stopping
jar /dʒɑr/	daw /dɔ/	Stopping, Gliding
watch /wɑtʃ/	watt /wɑt/	Stopping
them /ðɛm/	dem dɛm	Stopping
bridge /bɹɪdʒ/	bwidge /bwɪdʒ/	Gliding
grasshopper /'gɹæsˌhɑpɚ/	dwasshooper /'dwæsˌhɑpɚ/	Fronting, Gliding
fish /fɪʃ/	fis /fɪs/	Depalatization
jar /dʒɑr/	daw /dɔ/	Stopping, Gliding
rake /ɹeɪk/	wate /weɪt/	Gliding, Fronting

Phonological Processes Based on Kamdyn's Standardized Speech Test Errors:

Stimulus Item *Orthographically* IPA	Stimulus Item *Orthographically* IPA	Phonological Process(es)
pig /pɪg/	pid /pɪd/	Fronting
swing /swɪŋ/	fwin /fwin/	Coalescence, Fronting
knife /naɪf/	nice /naɪs/	Alveolarization
fish /fɪʃ/	fis /fɪs/	Alveolarization
seal /sil/	seaw /siɑw/	Gliding
sheep /ʃip/	seep /sip/	Depalatization
cheese /tʃiz/	sheeze /ʃiz/	Deaffrication
weaf /wif/	leaf /lif/	Gliding
lemonade /ˈlɛməˈneɪd/	nemonade /ˈnɛməˈneɪd/	Consonant assimilation (regressive)
computer /kəmˈpjutɚ/	puter /ˈpjutɚ/	Weak syllable deletion
snake /sneɪk/	sate /seɪt/	Cluster reduction, Fronting
them /ðɛm/	vem /vɛm/	Consonant assimilation[a] (regressive)
thermometer /θərˈmɑmətɚ/	mometer /ˈmɑmətɚ/	Weak syllable deletion

[a]Note that /θ, ð/ production varies based on influence of phonetic context.

Appendix D

Diploma Illustrating Five Prosocial Communication Rules

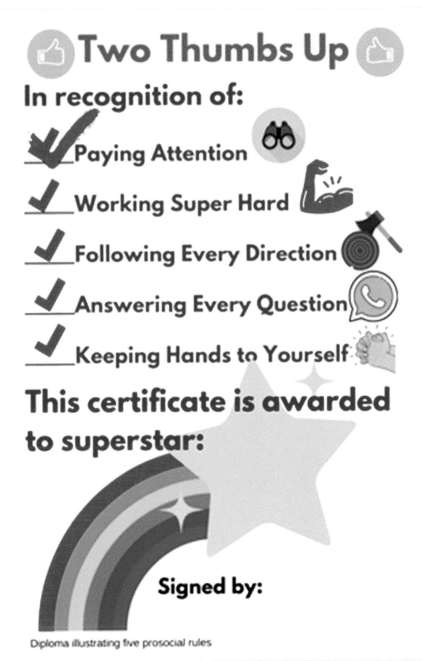

Diploma illustrating five prosocial rules

Appendix E

Request Treatment Target Cards: Simple → Complex → Generalization Stage

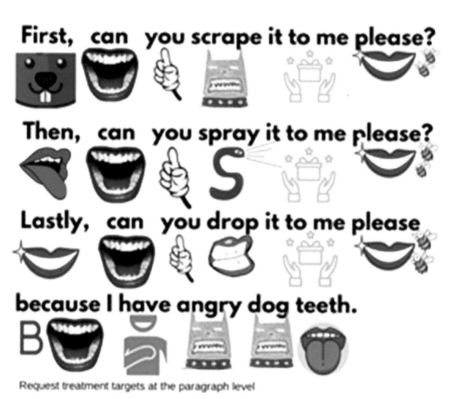

Request treatment targets at the paragraph level

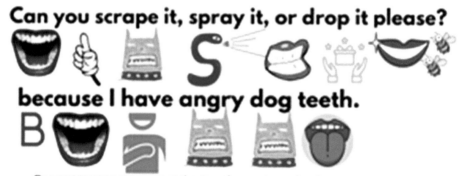

Request treatment targets at the complex sentence level

Simple 2-Element Cluster /sw/ Treatment Target

Can you sweep it to me please?

Can you sweep or squeak it to me please?

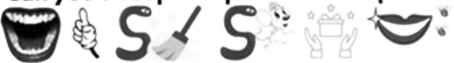

Simple treatment targets for children with difficulty with the /r/

Can you sweep or squeak it to me please?

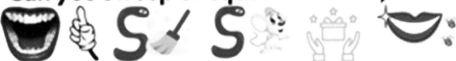

because I have angry dog teeth.

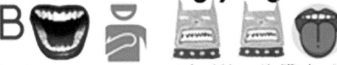

Complex sentence treatment targets for children with difficulty with the /r/

Can you scrape it, spray it, or drop it please?

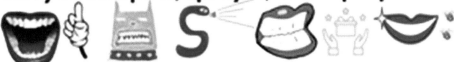

Treatment target for generalization and variation of /r/

Simple 2-Element /sw/ and 3-Element Cluster /skw/ Treatment Target

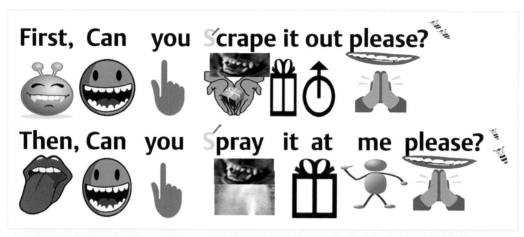

Complex Sentence Level 3-Element /skɹ/ and 3-Element /spɹ/ Cluster Treatment Target

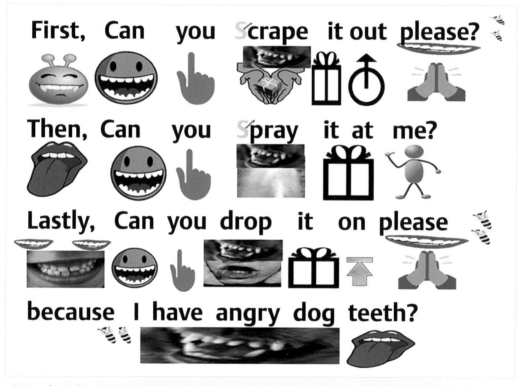

Paragraph Level Treatment Target to Ignite Maximum Gains in Speech, Language, and Sustained Attention

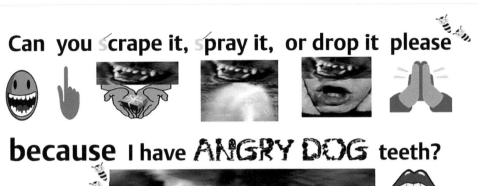

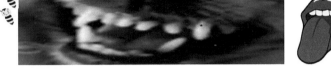

Complex Sentence Level Treatment Target for Generalization

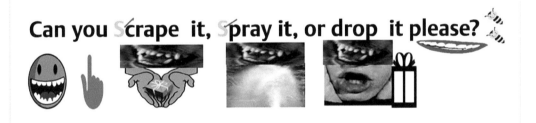

Treatment Target of Limited Syntactical Complexity for Generalization to Treat Speech Impairment Only

Can you scrape, spray, or drop it to me?

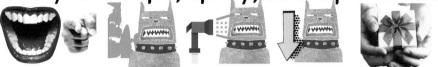

because I have angry dog teeth?

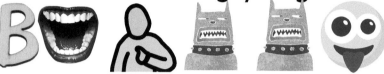

Can you scrape, splash, or drop it to me?

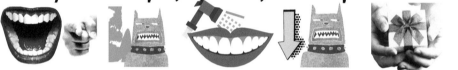

because I have angry dog teeth?

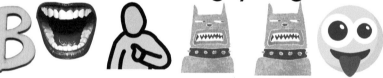

First, can you scrape it to me?

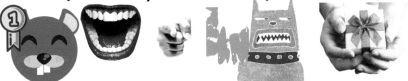

Next, can you splash it to me?

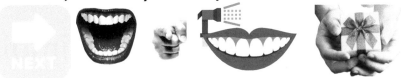

Then, can you drop it to me

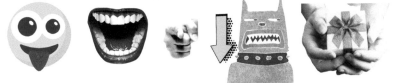

because I have angry dog teeth?

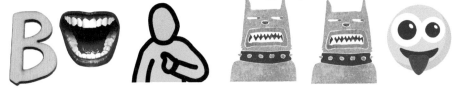

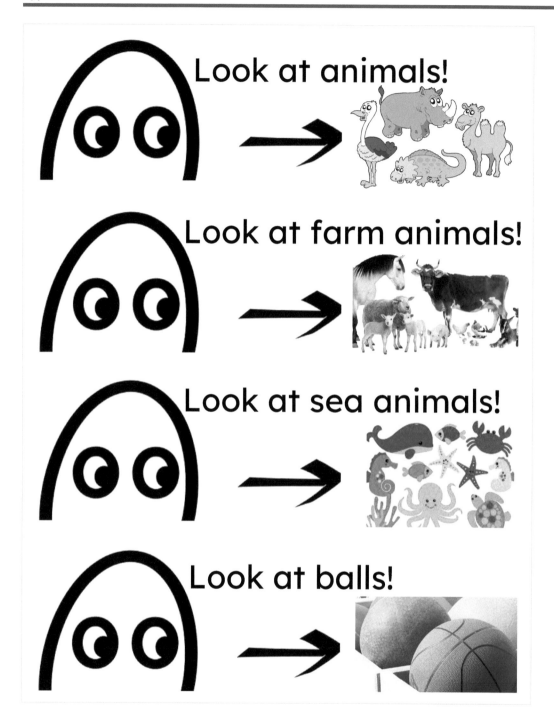

Look at animals!

Look at farm animals!

Look at sea animals!

Look at balls!

Look at blocks!

Look at body parts!

Look at books!

Look at boxes!

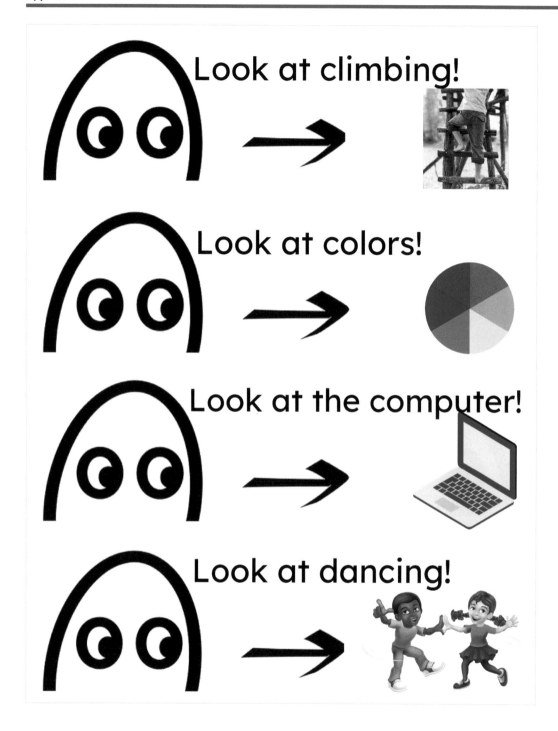

Look at climbing!

Look at colors!

Look at the computer!

Look at dancing!

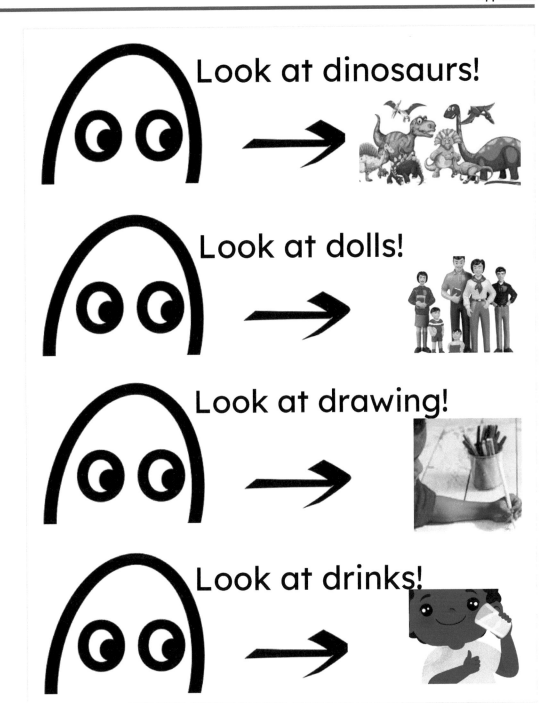

Look at dinosaurs!

Look at dolls!

Look at drawing!

Look at drinks!

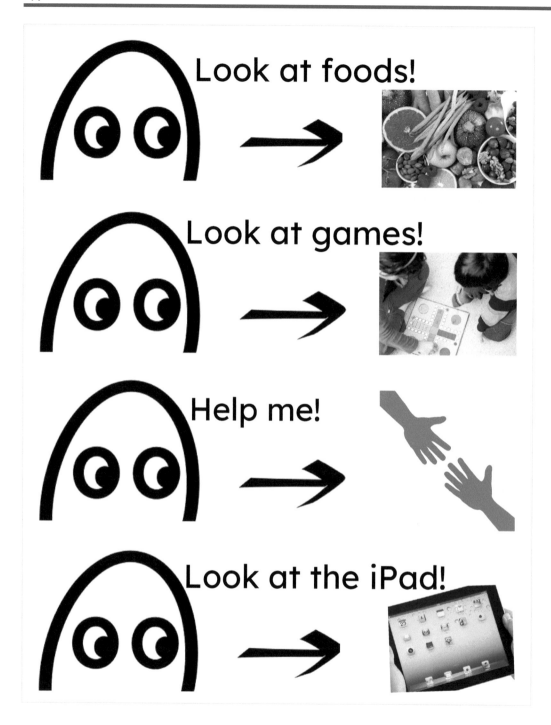

Look at foods!

Look at games!

Help me!

Look at the iPad!

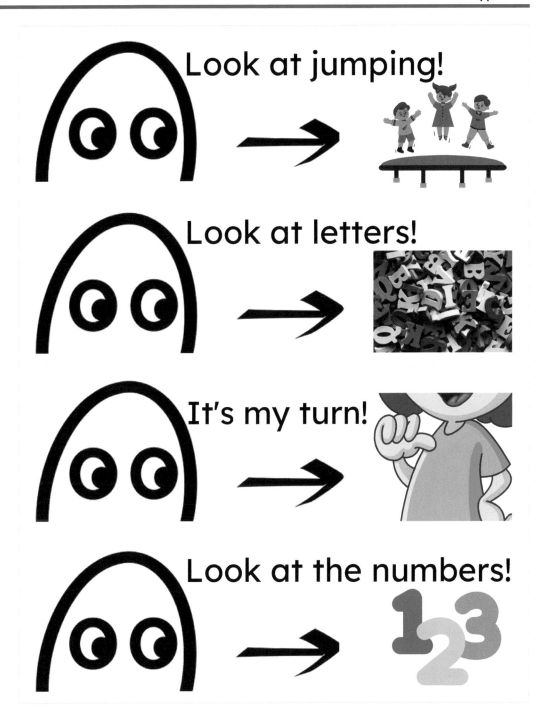

Look at jumping!

Look at letters!

It's my turn!

Look at the numbers!

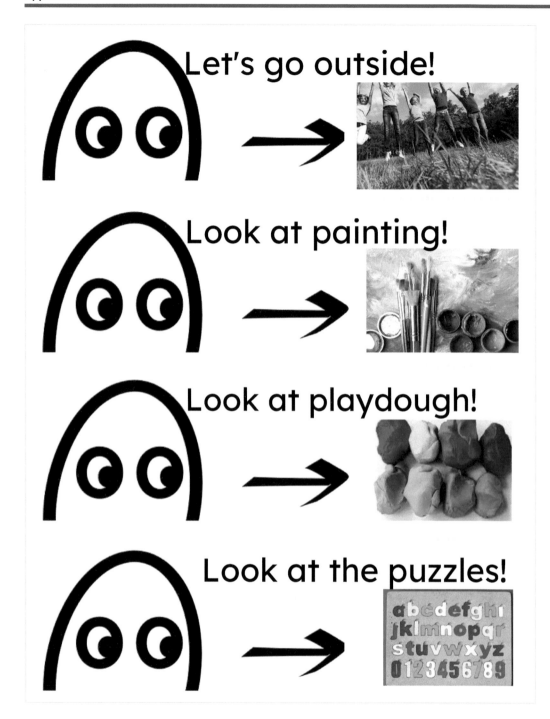

Let's go outside!

Look at painting!

Look at playdough!

Look at the puzzles!

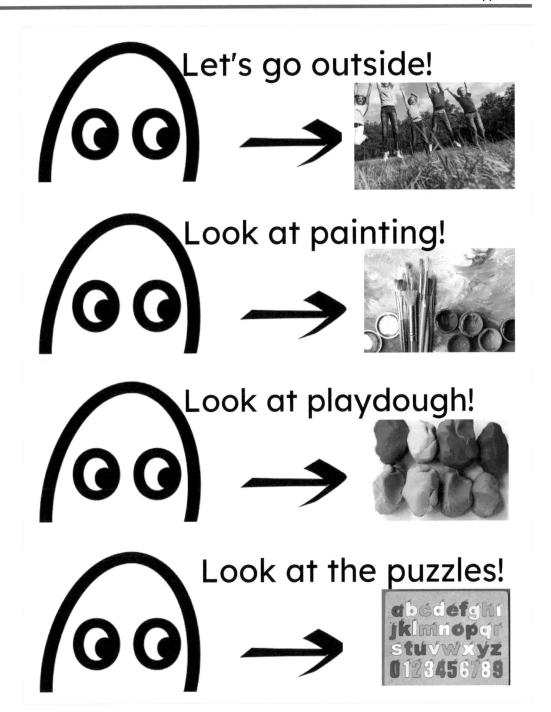

Let's go outside!

Look at painting!

Look at playdough!

Look at the puzzles!

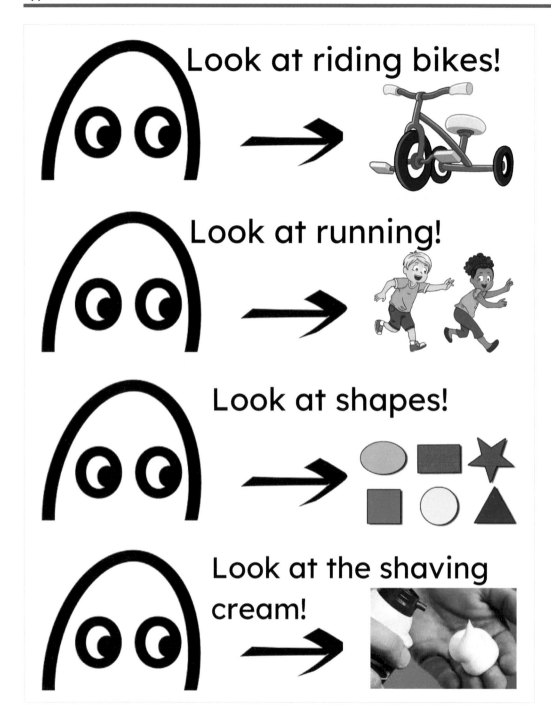

Look at riding bikes!

Look at running!

Look at shapes!

Look at the shaving cream!

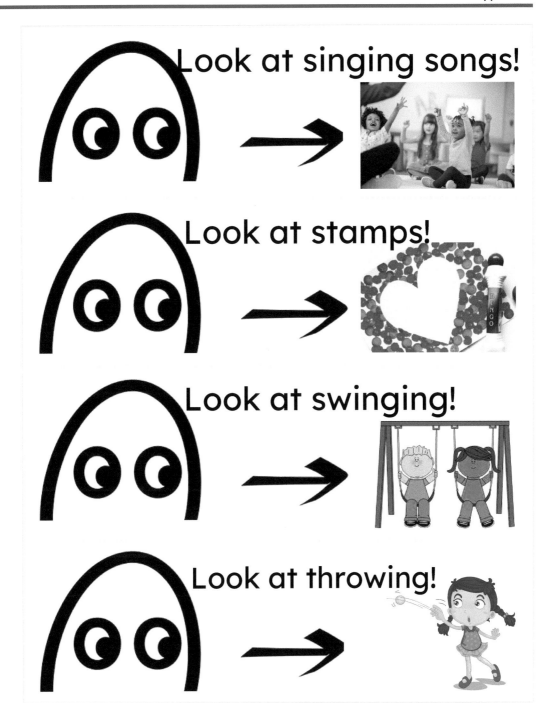

Look at singing songs!

Look at stamps!

Look at swinging!

Look at throwing!

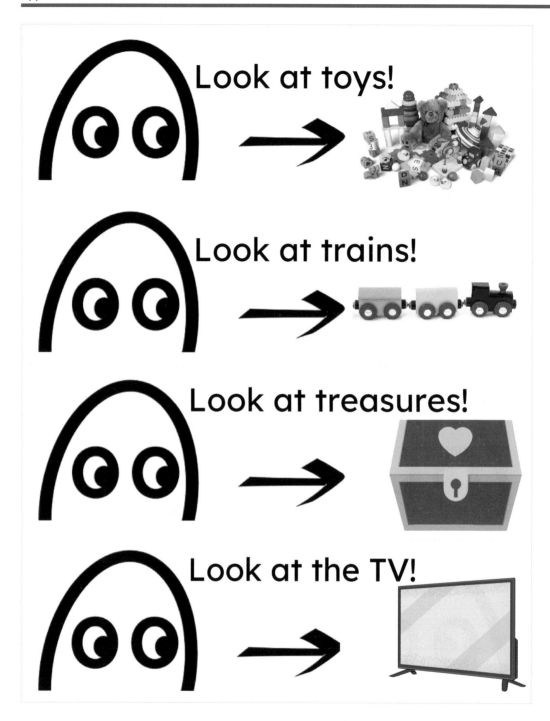

Look at toys!

Look at trains!

Look at treasures!

Look at the TV!

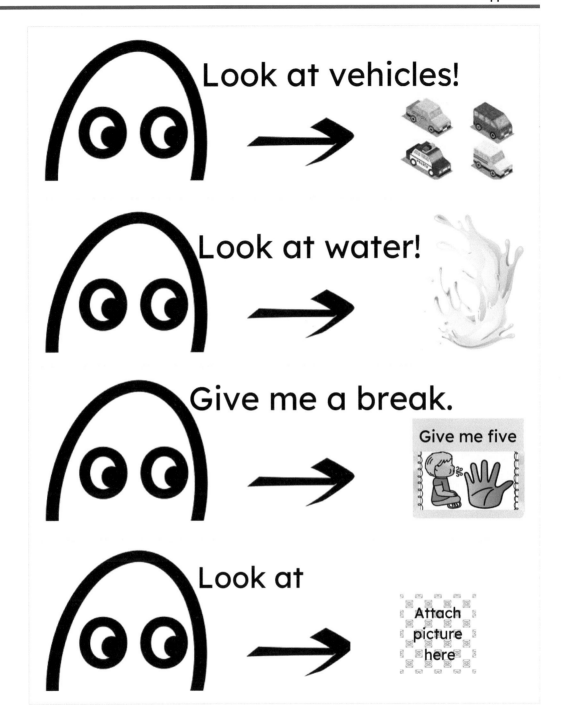

Look at vehicles!

Look at water!

Give me a break.

Give me five

Look at

Attach picture here

Index

Note: Page numbers set **bold** or *italic* indicate headings or figures, respectively.